Development of Self-Determination Through the Life-Course

Michael L. Wehmeyer • Karrie A. Shogren
Todd D. Little • Shane J. Lopez
Editors

Development of Self-Determination Through the Life-Course

Springer

Editors
Michael L. Wehmeyer
Special Education
University of Kansas
Lawrence, KS, USA

Karrie A. Shogren
Special Education
University of Kansas
Lawrence, KS, USA

Todd D. Little
Educational Psychology and Leadership
Texas Tech University
Lubbock, TX, USA

Shane J. Lopez
Gallup and The Clifton Strengths School
Omaha, NE, USA

ISBN 978-94-024-1040-2 ISBN 978-94-024-1042-6 (eBook)
DOI 10.1007/978-94-024-1042-6

Library of Congress Control Number: 2017932067

Printed on acid-free paper

This Springer imprint is published by Springer Nature
The registered company is Springer Science+Business Media B.V.
The registered company address is: Van Godewijckstraat 30, 3311 GX Dordrecht, The Netherlands

For Shane

Preface

The self-determination construct is one of the foundational constructs in the discipline of positive psychology. The millennial issue of *American Psychologist*, published in January of 2000, was dedicated to introducing the science of positive psychology and included articles on optimism, hope, creativity, and self-determination (Ryan and Deci 2000). In their landmark contribution, Ryan and Deci noted that the "fullest representation of humanity show people to be curious, vital, and self-motivated. At their best, they are agentic and inspired, striving to learn; extend themselves; master new skills; and apply their talents responsibly" (p. 68). The article's synthesis of how Self-Determination Theory (SDT) describes the impact of social contexts on self-motivation and the optimizing of a person's development, performance, and well-being firmly established the construct's importance to the new discipline of positive psychology.

As SDT grew into an important motivational metatheory, another movement embraced the self-determination construct in configuring strength-based approaches. That movement was the disability rights movement, and research and theory development in that field examined the importance of self-determination to enable people with disabilities to achieve better quality lives. The applied disciplines of special education and rehabilitation, among others, developed interventions informed by theory and research on self-determination in motivation, including research on creating autonomy-supportive classrooms, but that provided interventions that were, in essence, autonomy supportive as well and intended to promote self-determination.

This text provides a comprehensive examination of the development of self-determination in the context of two related theories of self-determination emerging from these two uses of the self-determination construct: SDT and (from the disability sphere) Causal Agency Theory. The intent is to provide a theoretical frame in which SDT and Causal Agency Theory are used to describe a lifespan approach to the development of self-determination. The text examines how organismic efforts to fulfill basic psychological needs to maintain autonomous motivation lead to causal action, which in turn leads to greater psychological need fulfillment, repeated experiences with causal action, and, ultimately, greater self-determination.

The text is structured into parts with chapters that go into depth on themes and topics pertinent to motivation, causal action, and the development of self-determination. The first part (Overview of Self-Determination and Theories of Self-Determination) provides an overview of the self-determination construct itself (Chap. 1) and of human agentic theories (Chap. 2), within which both SDT and Causal Agency Theory situate the self-determination construct. Chapter 2 culminates with the description of a theoretical model of the development of self-determination (Fig. 2.1) that forms the basis for later chapters examining such development in childhood, adolescence, and adulthood. Chapter 3 provides a look at how the development of self-determination is situated in the context of overall adolescent development and other theories pertinent to adolescent development. Chapters 4 and 5 provide detail about the two major theories covered in the text, SDT (Chap. 4) and Causal Agency Theory (Chap. 5).

The second part (Developmental Origins and Life-Course Trajectory of Self-Determination) examines issues pertaining to the development of self-determination across the lifespan utilizing the theoretical frame described in Chap. 2. Chapter 6 examines the development of self-determination during childhood, describing the development of foundational skills leading to later self-determination across childhood and, specifically, overviewing the development of foundational skills that enable children to make choices and express preferences, solve problems, engage in making decisions, set and attain goals, self-manage and self-regulate action, self-advocate, and acquire self-awareness and self-knowledge. Chapter 7 examines developmental milestones in knowledge, skills, and beliefs that emerge during adolescence and lead to enhanced self-determination, including choice making, self-initiation and planning, problem solving, decision making, goal setting and attainment, and self-regulation. The chapter concludes with a brief overview of issues in adolescent development as it pertains to motivational aspects of self-determination. In Chap. 8, attention is turned to the educational context to examine autonomy-supportive practices that lead to the development of autonomous motivation and greater self-determination. Chapter 9 examines what is known about self-determination in the disability context, while Chaps. 10 and 11 focus on self-determination in adulthood and aging life stages. This part is concluded with a chapter examining issues of culture and self-determination.

Chapters in the third part (Self-Determination Theory and Healthy Psychological and Physical Development) explore the role of self-determination in healthy psychological development, with chapters focused on the role of parenting in promoting children's psychological health (Chap. 13) and on identity development in adolescence (Chap. 14). Chapters in the final three parts address development of causal action, beginning with the fourth part (The Development of Volitional Action), which includes chapters that focus on the development of preference and choice expression (Chap. 15) and self-initiation and planning (Chap. 16). The fifth part (The Development of Agentic Action) includes chapters on the development of self-regulation (Chap. 17), goal setting and attainment (Chap. 18), problem solving (Chap. 19), decision making (Chap. 20), and pathways and agentic thinking in the development of hope (Chap. 21). The final part (Action-Control Beliefs) has a single chapter (Chap. 22) focused on the role of action-control beliefs in causal action.

Reference

Ryan, R. M., & Deci, E. L. (2000). Self-determination theory and the facilitation of intrinsic motivation, social development, and well-being. *American Psychologist, 55*, 68–78.

Contents

List of Contributors

Nicole Adams Texas Tech University, Lubbock, TX, USA

Rong Chang Texas Tech University, Lubbock, TX, USA

Edward L. Deci University of Rochester, Rochester, NY, USA

James Durham Texas Tech University, Lubbock, TX, USA

Meghann L. Fenn Oregon State University, Corvallis, OR, USA

Lisa A. Ferretti University of Albany, Albany, NY, USA

Jennifer K. Finders Oregon State University, Corvallis, OR, USA

Eriko Fukuda Texas Tech University, Lubbock, TX, USA

G. John Geldhof Oregon State University, Corvallis, OR, USA

Luther K. Griffin Texas State University, San Marcos, TX, USA

David M. Hansen University of Kansas, Lawrence, KS, USA

Nadia Jessop University of Kansas, Lawrence, KS, USA

Sheida Khamsi University of Kansas, Lawrence, KS, USA

Todd D. Little Educational Psychology and Leadership, Texas Tech University, Lubbock, TX, USA

Shane J. Lopez Gallup and The Clifton Strengths School, Omaha, NE, USA

Susana C. Marques University of Porto, Porto, Portugal

Philip McCallion University of Albany, Albany, NY, USA

Susan B. Palmer University of Kansas, Lawrence, KS, USA

Maylys Rapaport Laboratoire de Recherche sur le Comportement Social, Université du Québec à Montréal, Montréal, QC, Canada

Richard M. Ryan Australian Catholic University, Banyo, QLD, Australia

Karrie A. Shogren Special Education, University of Kansas, Lawrence, KS, USA

Bart Soenens Ghent University, Ghent, Belgium

Robert J. Vallerand Laboratoire de Recherche sur le Comportement Social, Université du Québec à Montréal, Montréal, QC, Canada

Australian Catholic University, Sydney, NSW, Australia

Maarten Vansteenkiste Ghent University, Ghent, Belgium

Michael L. Wehmeyer Special Education, University of Kansas, Lawrence, KS, USA

About the Editors

Michael L. Wehmeyer, Ph.D., is the Ross and Marianna Beach Distinguished Professor in Special Education and Associate Chairperson, Department of Special Education and Director and Senior Scientist, Beach Center on Disability and co-Director, Kansas University Center on Developmental Disabilities within the Schiefelbusch Institute for Life Span Studies, all at the University of Kansas. His research focuses on self-determination, strengths-based approaches to disability, and the application of positive psychology to the disability context. Dr. Wehmeyer has published more than 370 peer-reviewed journal articles and book chapters is an author or editor for 36 books on topics related to self-determination, positive psychology and disability, and the education of learners with intellectual and developmental disabilities and is a co-author of *Intellectual Disability: Definition, Classification, and Systems of Support*, the 11th Edition of the American Association on Intellectual and Developmental Disabilities' definition of intellectual disability as well as the Supports Intensity Scale – Children's and Adult Version.

Karrie A. Shogren, Ph.D., is a Professor in the Department of Special Education, co-Director of the Kansas University Center on Developmental Disabilities, and Associate Director of the Beach Center on Disability, all at the University of Kansas. Dr. Shogren's research focuses on self-determination and systems of support for people with disabilities as well as applications of positive psychology and strengths-based approaches to people with intellectual and developmental disabilities. Dr. Shogren has published over 100 articles in peer-reviewed journals, is the author or co-author of 10 books, and is one of the co-authors of *Intellectual Disability: Definition, Classification, and Systems of Support*, the 11th Edition of the American Association on Intellectual and Developmental Disabilities' seminal definition of intellectual disability (formerly mental retardation) as well as the Supports Intensity Scale – Children's and Adult Version.

Todd D. Little, Ph.D., is a Professor and Director of the Institute for Measurement, Methodology, Analysis and Policy at Texas Tech University. Little is widely recognized for his quantitative work on various aspects of applied SEM (e.g., modern missing data treatments, indicator selection, parceling, modeling developmental processes) as well as his substantive developmental research (e.g., action-control processes and motivation, coping, and self-regulation). In 2001, Little was elected to membership in the Society for Multivariate Experimental Psychology, and in 2009, he was elected President of APA's Division 5 (Evaluation, Measurement, and Statistics). He founded the internationally renowned "Stats Camps" (see statscamp.org). He is a fellow in APA, APS, and AAAS. In 2013, he received the Cohen award from Division 5 of APA for distinguished contributions to teaching and mentoring, and in 2015 he received the inaugural distinguished contributions award for mentoring developmental scientists from the Society for Research in Child Development.

Shane J. Lopez, Ph.D., was Gallup Senior Scientist in Residence and Research Director for the Clifton Strengths Institute. As chief architect of the Gallup Student Poll, he measured hope in over a million people. His research focused on hope, engagement, and wellbeing, particularly on links between strengths development, academic success, and overall wellbeing, and he directed the annual Gallup Wellbeing Forum. Dr. Lopez is the editor of *The Oxford Handbook of Positive Psychology* and *Positive Psychological Assessment: A Handbook of Models and Measures*, as well as more than 100 articles and chapters. He is the author of the well-regarded book, *Making Hope Happen: Create the Future You Want for Yourself and Others*. Dr. Lopez is a Fellow of the American Psychological Association.

Part I
Overview of Self-Determination and Theories of Self-Determination

Synopsis

The chapters in this part provide a comprehensive overview of the self-determination construct. Chapter 1 overviews the historical meanings and uses of the self-determination construct in philosophy, psychology, social welfare, education, and disability rights. Self-determination is framed, in this chapter, within the context of overarching theories of human agentic behavior. Human agency refers to the sense of personal empowerment involving both knowing and having what it takes to achieve goals. Human agentic theories share the meta-theoretical view that organismic aspirations drive human behaviors. An organismic perspective of self-determination portrays people as active contributors to, or "authors" of their behavior, where behavior is defined in terms of self-regulated and goal-directed actions. Chapter 2 reviews the major theories of human agentic behavior and examines the role of self-determination in each. This chapter culminates with the description of a theoretical model of the development of self-determination (Fig. 2.1) that forms the basis for later chapters examining such development in childhood, adolescence, and adulthood. Chapter 3 discusses adolescent developmental theories, first reviewing neurological growth and restructuring that occurs in the brain during adolescence. Next, cognitive and affective processes, including metacognition, self-regulation, and self-determination are described. Finally, identity development and agency and their role in adolescent development are described, followed by discussion of the role of culture and context in adolescent development. Chapters 4 and 5 provide detail about the two major theories covered in the text, SDT (Chap. 4) and Causal Agency Theory (Chap. 5).

Chapter 1
Introduction to the Self-Determination Construct

Michael L. Wehmeyer, Karrie A. Shogren, Todd D. Little, and Shane J. Lopez

Abstract Self-determination is a construct with a rich history in philosophy, social welfare, psychology, and education. This chapter overviews the origins of the self-determination construct, beginning with its application in philosophy, it's linkages to discussions of free will and volitional action, and continuing through to its implementation in motivation and personality psychology. The chapter introduces and overviews the origins of Self-Determination Theory and briefly introduces Causal Agency Theory.

This text provides a comprehensive examination of the development of self-determination in the context of two related theories of self-determination. We begin with an introduction to the self-determination construct and its historical uses in philosophy and psychology and other disciplines related to human development and behavior (education, social welfare, etc.). At the onset, it is important to understand that we position self-determination as a general psychological construct within the organizing structure of theories of human agentic behavior. Human agentic theories are discussed in Chap. 2, but at a general level, self-determination, as a psychological construct, refers to self- (vs. other-) caused action—to people acting volitionally, based on their own will. Individual chapters in this first section discuss how self-determination is defined in specific theoretical models, so the intent of this chapter is to trace the development of the construct over time, and to provide a general understanding of the construct.

M.L. Wehmeyer (✉) • K.A. Shogren
Special Education, University of Kansas, Lawrence, KS, USA
e-mail: wehmeyer@ku.edu

T.D. Little
Educational Psychology and Leadership, Texas Tech University, Lubbock, TX, USA

S.J. Lopez
Gallup and The Clifton Strengths School, Omaha, NE, USA

M.L. Wehmeyer et al. (eds.), *Development of Self-Determination Through the Life-Course*, DOI 10.1007/978-94-024-1042-6_1

Self-Determination in Philosophy

The *Oxford English Dictionary* (Simpson and Weiner 1989) identified the earliest use of the term *self-determination* as occurring in the year 1683 and defined the term as referring to the "determination of one's mind or will by itself toward an object" (p. 919). A second meaning of the term identified by the *Oxford English Dictionary* is "the action of a people in deciding its own form of government" (p. 919), with the first use of that meaning of the construct occurring in 1911. It is the first sense of the term (e.g., the personal sense) that we explore in depth in this text. As the *Oxford English Dictionary* definition shows, this personal sense of the term pertains, at its fundamental level, to issues of *human action* as a function of mind, will, and/or volition. Other definitions illustrate this basic emphasis. *Webster's Third New International Unabridged Dictionary* (Gove 1967) defined self-determination as the "determination of one's acts or states by oneself without external compulsion" (p. 2059). Similarly, the *American Heritage Dictionary of the English Language* (1992) defined self-determination as the "determination of one's own fate or course of action without compulsion; free will" (p. 814). Self-determination, in essence, refers to *acting* based on *one's own mind or free will*, without external compulsion. Finally, the *American Psychological Association Dictionary of Psychology* (VandenBos 2007) defines self-determination as "the control of one's behavior by internal convictions and decisions rather than by external demands" (p. 829).

These definitions provide an indication of the basic intent of the construct called 'self-determination' and reflect the sense of its historical antecedent, the philosophical doctrine of *determinism*. The self-determination construct emerged from centuries-old debates about free will and determinism and to understand the intent of the self-determination construct as used today one must begin with an examination of issues pertaining to determinism.

Determinism posits that events, in this context human behavior and actions, are effects of preceding causes. There are generally two forms of the philosophical doctrine, hard and soft determinism. Hard determinism is the doctrine that *every* event and *every* action is caused in accordance with causal laws that account completely for the event's or action's occurrence. Hard determinists believe that even when human actions are posited to result from mediating determinants or causes, such as wants, wishes, desires, motivations, or feelings, those same wants, wishes, desires, motivations, and feelings are, themselves, caused by specific antecedent conditions that ensure their occurrence. Alternatively, the soft determinism position argues that an act can be both *caused* and *free*. This is because, according to the soft determinist, the hard determinist mistakenly equates "caused" with "forced" or "compelled." The soft determinist believes that every action is caused somehow; but not *every* action is compelled. The indeterminist's or anti-determinist's position differs from both hard and soft deterministic positions by positing that there are *no* causes for events or actions, and that humans act completely from *free will*.

This question of *free will* verses *determinism* is generally identified by philosophers to be one of the most enduring philosophical problems of all time, bound inextricably with religious theologies about the free will of man versus the control and authority (determinism) of God. *The Catholic Encyclopedia* (Herbermann et al. 1914) stated the dichotomy as such:

> On the one hand, does man possess genuine moral freedom, power of real choice, true ability to determine the course of his thoughts and volitions, to decide which motives shall prevail within his mind, to modify and mold his own character? Or, on the other, are man's thoughts and volitions, his character and external actions, all merely the inevitable outcome of his circumstances? Are they all inexorably predetermined in every detail along rigid lines by events of the past, over which he himself has had no sort of control? This is the real import of the free-will problem.

In his important work, *An Essay Concerning Human Understanding*, published in 1690, John Locke provided a synopsis of the "free will problem." Trying to illustrate the importance of connections in human thought to understanding, Locke wrote

> this proposition "men can determine themselves" is drawn in or inferred from this, "that they shall be punished in the other world." For here the mind, seeing the connexion there is between the idea of men's punishment in the other world and the idea of God punishing; between God punishing and the justice of the punishment; between justice of punishment and guilt; between guilt and a power to do otherwise; between a power to do otherwise and freedom; and between freedom and self-determination, sees the connexion between men and self-determination (Locke 1690).

Locke is considered a soft determinist, someone who saw both causality and free will at work in human behavior. Elsewhere in the *Essay*, which was intended to establish the foundations for a new science of human understanding and knowledge, Locke hypothesized that all human thought comes from *sensation* and *reflection* and, consequently, all human action comes from human thought. Writing in an "*Abstract of the Essay*" published in 1688, he stated:

> In the thoughts I have had concerning the Understanding, I have endeavoured to prove that the mind is at first *rasa tabula*. The mind having been supposed void of all innate characters, comes to receive them by degrees as experience and observation lets them in; and we shall, upon consideration, find they all come from two originals, and are conveyed into the mind by two ways, viz. *sensation* and *reflection*. The mind, taking notice of its own operation about these ideas received by sensation, comes to have ideas of those very operations that pass within itself: this is another source of ideas, and this I call *reflection*; and from hence it is we have the ideas of *thinking*, *willing*, *reasoning*, *doubting*, *purposing*. From these two originals it is that we have all the ideas we have; and I think I may confidently say that, besides what our senses convey into the mind, or the ideas of its own operations about those received from *sensation*, we have no ideas at all (Locke 1688).

As illustrated above, Locke adamantly opposes any notion that ideas are innate as had been suggested by other philosophers, most noticeably in Descartes' declaration that we are born with the *idea* of God planted in us *by* God. All human ideas and knowledge, according to Locke, emerge from experience (sensation) and from reflection on that experience or sensation. That is, Locke's view places self-determination as a developmental phenomenon – as a guiding feature of development and as an outgrowth of developmental experiences.

Locke classified ideas as simple and complex, with complex ideas derived from relations between simple ideas, generated by reflection. Among these complex ideas were what Locke called "Modes" or ideas that combine simpler elements to form a new whole that does not exist except as a part or feature of something else. For example, we understand the 'idea' of infinity without ever having to see it exist as an actual object that can be counted. Mixed modes, which combined both sensory and reflective elements, were especially important to Locke since they encompassed the ideas of *human actions*, including the ideas of power, volition, and liberty. Locke defines power as the ability to make (active power) or receive (passive power) change (Kemerling, 2000–2001). According to Locke, the human mind has the *active* power of beginning or ceasing its own operations as activated by a preference. The exercise of that power is volition or will. Freedom or liberty (a complex mixed mode idea) is "the power to act on our volition, whatever it may be, without any external compulsion or restraint" (Locke 1690; Chapter II, XXI). Locke avoids entanglement in the free will problem by noting that the cause of the volition is irrelevant, since it is the agent, not the will, which is free. Human beings act freely just insofar as they are capable of translating their mental preferences to do or not to do into their actual performance of the action in question (Kemerling 2000–2001). Locke writes:

> Every one, I think, finds in himself a power to begin or forbear, continue or put an end to several actions in himself. From the consideration of the extent of this power of the mind over the actions of the man, which everyone finds in himself, arise the ideas of liberty and necessity. All the actions that we have any idea of reducing themselves, as has been said, to these two, viz. thinking and motion; so far as a man has power to think or not to think, to move or not to move, according to the preference or direction of his own mind, so far is a man free. Wherever any performance or forbearance are not equally in a man's power; wherever doing or not doing will not equally follow upon the preference of his mind directing it, there he is not free, though perhaps the action may be voluntary. So that the idea of liberty is, the idea of a power in any agent to do or forbear any particular action, according to the determination or thought of the mind, whereby either of them is preferred to the other: where either of them is not in the power of the agent to be produced by him according to his volition, there he is not at liberty; that agent is under necessity. So that liberty cannot be where there is no thought, no volition, no will; but there may be thought, there may be will, there may be volition, where there is no liberty (Locke 1690; Book II, Chapter XXI).

Freedom (from the Latin *libertas*), a frequent target of hard determinists like B.F. Skinner, is conceptualized as the human capacity to act (or not to act) as we choose or prefer, without any external compulsion or restraint. Freedom in this sense is usually regarded as a presupposition of moral responsibility: that is, the only actions for which I, as an autonomous person, may be praised or blamed, rewarded or punished, are just those that I perform freely (Herbermann et al. 1914). This view is the crux of the free will problem in determinism; that an omnipotent being (God) can only hold humans accountable for their behavior and actions if, indeed, those humans had the autonomy and free will to act based on their own volition as opposed to all actions being predetermined by God.

Locke's proposals about the causes of human action as both caused and volitional are important as the foundation for understanding the modern sense of the term *self-determination*. Note Locke's soft deterministic distinction that it is the *agent* (the person him or herself) who is free to act, not the action itself (since it is 'caused' by perception or sensation). From Locke and onward, determinism was gradually decoupled from the sole form of determinism considered to that point, theological determinism. Today we recognize numerous 'determinants' of human behavior, including physiological, structural, environmental, and/or organismic factors. Theories of human behavior recognize the impact on human actions and behavior of biological or genetic determinism (behavior as an effect of biological functions such as genes or neurochemicals), familial or relative determinism (human behavior as an effect of family or parental influence or treatment), environmental determinism (behavior as an effect of the environment), psychological determinism (behavior as an effect of how we perceive or understand situations), economic determinism (action as an effect of economic forces or circumstances) and so forth.

With the turn of the twentieth century and the emergence of psychology as a discipline distinct from philosophy, the philosophical discussion of determinism and self-determination as it pertains to human action and behavior becomes overshadowed by discoveries and theories in biology, psychology and anthropology. Nevertheless, even as the meaning or sense of the construct changes as it is used in other disciplines, it is important to remember that the construct's roots lie in the *free will problem* that was the basis of philosophic discussions for centuries. That is, is human behavior the effect of human thought, free will, and volition or are such actions predetermined and indeterminant? As discussed subsequently, the scope of the question altered somewhat during the twentieth century and there is currently less focus on theological determinism and more on biological, psychological, environmental or other forms of determinism. Nevertheless, self-determination still refers fundamentally to and its meanings derive directly from the philosophical debates around determinism.

Self-Determination in Psychology

In the last half of the nineteenth century the rapidly growing discipline of psychology brought its empiricism and experimentalism to bear on questions that had previously been the sole domain of introspective philosophers and, in so doing, changed the question posed by the *free will problem* slightly, from whether human behavior is the effect of free will or is predetermined to whether human behavior is caused by internal versus external forces. In essence, the anti-determinist or indeterminist view espoused in philosophy was never adopted by psychologists, leaving only the hard versus soft determinism perspectives. This separation is likely a function of several factors. The earliest psychologists were heavily influenced in the early 1900s by the perceived explanatory power of the 'new biology' which featured the merger of Darwinian evolutionary theory with the newly rediscovered mechanisms of Mendelian genetics (Cravens 1978). To the pioneers trying to establish psychology as a viable science, the new biology could, seemingly, explain the *causes* of human behavior through mechanistic and deterministic means without having to resort to the introspective techniques that dominated philosophy. Psychologists looked toward these biological models of determinism to begin to explain human behavior, focusing first on what were identified as social problems, like mental deficiency, feeblemindedness, crime, pauperism, and so forth. This focus was no more clearly in evidence then in the establishment of the field of mental measurement in the early 1900s. While Binet and Simon held what might be seen as a soft determinist position regarding intelligence, crediting both nature and nurture, the field of intelligence testing in America, led by Goddard, Terman, and Yerkes, rapidly became firmly associated with a hard determinist perspective of the hereditary nature of intelligence and, indeed, with the strong determinist position of eugenicists, which claimed social ills like crime, prostitution, and poverty were attributable almost exclusively to heritability in intelligence (or the lack thereof, feeblemindedness). Even Edward Thorndike, the founder of the mental measurement movement in education, held strongly eugenic, and thus deterministic, beliefs. The field was not exclusively hereditarian and deterministic, of course. William Bagley, in his 1925 text *Determinism in Education* rails against the assumptions of hereditarian determinists' conception of intelligence, writing:

> It is the purpose of the present paper to show that the sanction which mental measurements apparently give to this particular variety of determinism [note: referring to the hereditarian position in intelligence] is based, not upon the facts that the measurements reveal, but upon the hypotheses and assumptions that the development of the measures has involved; that these hypotheses and assumptions, while doubtless justified for certain purposes, are at basis questionable in the last degree; and that the present tendency to extend them *ad libitum* beyond a very restricted field is fraught with educational and social dangers of so serious and far-reaching a character as to cause the greatest concern (Bagley 1925, pp. 11–12).

Nevertheless, a hard deterministic view of human behavior held sway in early psychology. Skinnerian psychology rejected the claim that behavior is a function of volitional thought or ideas or, indeed, any internal mechanisms. In *Beyond Freedom and Dignity* Skinner challenged the existence of "autonomous man" and labeled as myths, illusions, or 'prescientific superstitions' all such constructs associated with 'autonomous man,' including reason, mind, values, concepts, thought, judgment, volition, purpose, memory, independence, or self-esteem. Skinner's hard deterministic position is, in essence, that all human behavior is governed (caused) by laws of operant conditioning – all functions that other psychological perspectives apply to 'autonomous man,' including volitional thought, can be explained by reinforcement contingencies. Skinner (1971) stated:

> To be for oneself is to be almost nothing. The great individualists so often cited to show the value of personal freedom have owed their successes to earlier social environments. The involuntary individualism of a Robinson Crusoe and the voluntary individualism of a Henry David Thoreau show obvious debts to society. If Crusoe had reached the island as a baby, and if Thoreau had grown up unattended on the shores of Walden Pond, their stories would have been different. We must all begin as babies, and no degree of self-determination, self-sufficiency, or self-reliance will make us individuals in any sense beyond that of single members of the human species. (pp. 123–124.)

Not surprisingly, modern behaviorists continue to hold this perspective with regard to the self-determination construct. Baer (1998) noted, in discussing "problems in imposing self-determination" (p. 50), that proposals with regard to promoting self-determination are, fundamentally, ideologies (such as personal autonomy or freedom) as opposed to behavioral science, and that if the goal of practitioners is to ensure that people with disabilities (the topic of the special issue of a journal he was commenting on) have greater choice opportunities and experience greater control, then the course of action to follow is to arrange the environments of people in ways that they want them arranged. Baer explained that this environmental control can be achieved through the use of a concurrent schedules approach, where the intervener creates two environments that differ in only one dimension, provides the person with the disability access to those environments, and measures how much time the person spends in each environment.

It was not until the establishment of the field of personality psychology as a discipline distinct from general psychology in the late 1930s that issues pertaining to self-determination were addressed with any systematic focus by psychologists. Just as the free will problem had been one of the dominant themes in philosophy in the preceding centuries, issues pertaining to causation of human behavior became central to the emerging discipline of personality psychology. In his early text titled *Foundations for a Science of Personality*, Angyal (1941) proposed that an essential feature of a living organism is its autonomy, where autonomous means self-governing or governed from inside. According to Angyal, an organism "lives in a world in which things happen according to laws which are heteronomous (e.g., governed from outside) from the point of view of the organism" (p. 33). Angyal stated that "organisms are subjected to the laws of the physical world, as is any other object of nature, with the exception that it can oppose self-determination to external determination" (p. 33). Angyal suggested that the important task for developing a *science* of personality was in identifying principle(s) of the *biological total process* – the movement of organisms from undifferentiated parts to an organized whole. He defined the "biological total process" as a trend toward autonomy and argued that the *science of personality* is, in essence, the study of two essential determinants to human behavior, autonomous-determinism (or self-determination) and heteronomous-determinism (other-determined). He noted that "in the realm of *organismic happenings* we find neither entirely autonomous nor entirely heteronomous determinants" (p. 21), and suggested a psychology of individual differences by noting that, within nature, there are marked variations in the importance and balance of autonomous and heteronomous determinants to behavior. Nonetheless, Angyal places primary importance for laying the foundation for a science of personality in the fact that a central process of an organism is the movement toward autonomous-determination. He showed this by stating:

> It would probably be generally agreed that without autonomy, without self-government, the life process could not be understood. Selection, choice, self-regulation, adaptation, regeneration are phenomena which logically imply the autonomy of the organism. Selection, that is the search for certain environmental conditions, is only possible in a being capable of self-directed activity (p. 34).

Angyal's links to issues arising from biological determinism are evident here (e.g., [natural] selection, [species] adaptation), and the central problem he poses is the degree to which human behavior is *caused* by *internal* versus *external* factors. Nonetheless, autonomous-determination, or self-determination, as described by Angyal returns the discussion to the issues characterizing the discussion of self-determination in philosophy; that of human action as both internally-determined and *volitional*. Themes of choice and autonomy that are today accepted as primary to defining the construct appear in Angyal's proposal for the new science of personality psychology, though without the baggage of philosophy's free will problem. Self-determination had moved from its philosophical alignment with the problem of free will versus *theological* determinism to one of autonomous-versus heteronomous-determination. Furthermore, Angyal's use of the term moves away from the hard determinism that dominated the psychology of previous decades toward a soft determinism that considers the importance of both nature and nurture. He noted:

> …the autonomy of the organism is not an absolute one. Self-determination is restricted by outside influences which, with respect to the organism, are heteronomous. The organism lives in a world in which processes go on independent of it. The organism asserts itself against the heteronomous surroundings (p. 38).

This use of the construct not only typifies a soft deterministic perspective, but also embodies Locke's distinction of the person being free to act, but not the action itself being free from causality.

Self-Determination in Motivational Psychology The most influential use of the self-determination construct in psychology emerged from the work of psychologists Edward Deci, Richard Ryan, and colleagues. Although Self-Determination Theory (SDT) is covered in detail in subsequent chapters, given the importance of this work in moving the application of the self-determination construct forward, it is relevant to highlight some of Deci and Ryan's early work as critical to the general or overall understanding of self-determination. Edward Deci, in an early text, *The Psychology of Self-Determination* (Deci 1980), discussed, as we have in this chapter, distinctions concerning self-determination, will, and free will. Deci argued that, despite the lack of a focus in psychology on issues of freedom and self-determination evident at that time, movement away from mechanistic theories and the recognition that "[i]nternal, mental events ... have been shown to be useful in explaining behavior, and numerous phenomena have been investigated that are relevant to the larger issue of the interplay of freedom and boundedness in human behavior" (p. 3). Such developments, suggested Deci "set the stage for an extended discussion of self-determination" (p. 3). He argued that in focusing on self-determination, "we are really raising the question, 'To what extent can people decide their own behaviors'" (p. 4). Deci (1980) answers this question as such:

> People have considerable capacity for self-determination, and the operation of will—that capacity to choose behaviors based on inner desires and perceptions—is the basis of self-determination (p. 5).

At this juncture in the development of the self-determination construct, Deci proposed that "will is the capacity of the human organism to choose how to satisfy needs" and that "self-determination is the process of utilizing will" (p. 26). Will is the "capacity for conscious choice to determine behavior" (p. 26) and is "inextricably involved with the intrinsic need for competence and self-determination" (p. 26). Further, Deci (1980) argued, "the conceptualization of intrinsic motivation as a basic human need for feeling competent and self-determining provides a framework for studying self-determination and will…" (p. 27).

In 1980, Deci and Ryan articulated a formal theory of intrinsic motivation that incorporated a central role for self-determination, and in 1985 they expanded this to be a theory of both intrinsic motivation and varied forms of extrinsic motivation. Working from White's (1959) proposal of an innate, *intrinsic* energy source, labeled by White as effectance motivation, which was theorized to motivate a wide variety of human behavior, and also building on work by cognitive theorists on personal causation and perceived locus of causality (deCharms 1968; Heider 1958), Deci and Ryan (1985) proposed that intrinsic motivation and self-determination were "necessary concepts for an organismic theory" [of motivation] (Deci and Ryan, p. 7).

In fact, Self-Determination Theory has gradually expanded over time. In 1980 Deci and Ryan presented a formal theory to explain empirical findings concerning the effects of external events on intrinsic motivation. Called *Cognitive Evaluation Theory*, it contained three primary propositions: (1) intrinsic motivation requires a sense of autonomy or self-determination; (2) intrinsic motivation also requires a sense of competence and mastery; and (3) events relevant to the initiation and regulation of intrinsically motivated behavior have three aspects (informational, controlling, and amotivating) that can be differentially salient to people, thus enhancing or undermining their motivation. Deci and Ryan (1985) later expanded SDT to include a theory of internalization and the development of autonomous forms of extrinsic motivation and self-regulation (*Organismic Integration Theory* or OIT). Still later they articulated a need based theory of well-being (BPN; *Basic Psychological Needs Theory* Deci and Ryan 2000; Ryan and Deci 2000). These formulations, along with other mini-theories are collectively described as *Self-Determination Theory* (see Chap. 4, this volume).

Importantly, Self-Determination Theory has continuously asserted the importance for modern psychology of concepts of autonomy and volition, arguing that these are not in any way problematic for a thoroughly deterministic understanding of behavior. Indeed, SDT suggests that both autonomous and controlled behaviors have distinctive neuropsychological underpinnings, and both harness both implicit and explicit mental processes (e.g., Ryan and Deci 2006).

Today *Self-Determination Theory* (SDT; Deci and Ryan 2000; Ryan and Deci 2000, 2011) represents the most extensive use of the self-determination construct in the field of psychology during the second half of the twentieth century to the present, and subsequent chapters will provide more detail on the current status of the theory. Meanwhile, other disciplines were applying the construct to their fields as well.

Self-Determination in Social Welfare

For much of the 20th Century a guiding principle of social work was the client *right* to self-determination (Biestek and Gehrig 1978; McDermott 1975). Owing much to the sense of the term as a national or political right, which emerged in the early twentieth century and which is discussed subsequently, the emphasis in social work on client self-determination became a principle that guided the way in which services should be provided by social workers. More than just a right of people in general, however, the use of the construct in social work embodies a respect and value for the rights of individuals to make choices and decisions and to, in essence, live autonomous lives.

Corporate or National Self-Determination

As mentioned previously, an alternate meaning of self-determination is as a national or political construct referring to the rights of peoples to self-governance. In his examination of national self-determination Heater (1994) attributed much of the notoriety for self-determination and its relative importance in 20th Century politics to Woodrow Wilson's famous "Fourteen Points" speech to a joint session of Congress on January 8, 1918. In this speech, Wilson outlined fourteen points for a postwar settlement that would lead to world peace. Six of the 14 referred specifically to ensuring that nations who were defeated in the war would be assured the opportunity for national self-determination. Heater noted that the twentieth century preference for national self-determination emerged from twin eighteenth century notions that the people, not monarchs, are sovereign and that the people are to be thought of as "the nation." Through the nineteenth century, the belief that a people should have the right and opportunity to determine their own government spread and gained wide acceptance, and by the twentieth century became a principal of international justice. As the twentieth century went on, this sense of the 'right of a peoples of a nation to self-governance' was adapted by other groups of people who were not identified as being the citizens of a country, but instead were self-identified by some factor (racial identity, disability status) that, in turn, was seen to result in the loss of a corporate right to self-governance. For example, one of the days of the African American holiday Kwanzaa is self-determination, referring to the rights of African Americans to shape their own corporate destinies instead of having some other group (e.g., the majority culture) shape that destiny.

Self-Determination in Disability

In the latter years of the twentieth century, the self-determination construct was applied to another civil rights cause; namely, the rights of people with disabilities for self-governance. This sense of the term is captured best by Robert Williams (1989), a national leader in the disability rights effort and a man with a disability, who stated:

> But, without being afforded the right and opportunity to make choices in our lives, we will never obtain full, first class American citizenship. So we do not have to be told what self-determination means. We already know that it is just another word for freedom. We already know that self-determination is just another word for describing a life filled with rising expectations, dignity, responsibility, and opportunity. That it is just another word for having the chance to live the American Dream (p. 16).

Not surprisingly, perhaps, the notion of a right of people with disabilities to self-determination was first raised by a philosopher, Swedish philosopher Bengt Nirje, who in 1972 authored a chapter titled *The Right to Self-Determination*, and, in the opening paragraph of that chapter, stated:

> … the choices, wishes, desires, and aspirations of a handicapped person have to be taken into consideration as much as possible in actions affecting him. To assert oneself with one's family, friends, neighbors, co-workers, other people, or vis-à-vis an agency is difficult for many persons. It is especially difficult for someone who has a disability or is otherwise perceived as devalued. But in the end, even the impaired person has to manage as a distinct individual, and thus has his identity defined to himself and to others through the circumstances and conditions of his existence. Thus, the road to self-determination is both difficult and all important for a person who is impaired. (p. 177)

Nirje's chapter appeared in the same book in which Robert Perske (1972) called for the opportunity for people with disabilities to experience the 'dignity of risk':

> The world in which we live is not always safe, secure and predictable.... Every day that we wake up and live in the hours of that day, there is a possibility of being thrown up against a situation where we may have to risk everything, even our lives. This is the way the real world is. We must work to develop every human resource within us in order to prepare for these days. To deny any person their fair share of risk experiences is to further cripple them for healthy living. (p. 199)

Self-Determination as Empowerment As illustrated by Williams, Nirje, and Perske, within the context of the disability rights and advocacy movement, the construct as a personal characteristic has been imbued with the empowerment and "rights" orientation typically associated with the sense of the term as a national or political construct. Empowerment is a term usually associated with social movements and typically is used, as Rappaport (1981) stated, in reference to actions that "enhance the possibilities for people to control their lives" (p. 15), as such, the articulation of a right to self-determination, drawing on an amalgamation of the national or corporate sense of the term and a more personal sense, has become a theme within the disability rights movement.

Self-Determination, Strengths-Based Models of Disability, and Quality of Life As the disability rights movement matured, and as civil and legislative protections (such as the Americans with Disabilities Act) began to ensure equal access to life in the community for people with disabilities, understandings of disability that focused on defects and pathology began to wane, replaced, slowly, by person-environment fit models (Wehmeyer 2013). A strengths-based approach to disability has developed roughly parallel with the growth of positive psychology as a subdiscipline, and for most of the same reasons (Shogren 2013), just as within positive psychology (Ryan and Deci 2000) self-determination took on a central role in research and practice. This central role was further enhanced by the field's shift toward models of supports delivery to people with disabilities that focused on enhancing quality of life, with enhanced self-determination conceptualized as an outcome of such a focus (Wehmeyer and Schalock 2001).

Self-Determination in Education

In the early 1990s, the growing emphasis on self-determination in the disability rights movement entered into national efforts to educate students with disabilities. Over the course of 25 years, researchers and interventionists in special education have examined the role of self-determination, and efforts to promote self-determination, on the lives of students with disabilities (see Wehmeyer et al. 2003 for overview). Many of these interventions were conceptualized more by the rights-based language used in the empowerment or disability rights movement (e.g., rights to make decisions, control one's life, live independently, etc.). Causal Agency Theory, discussed in a subsequent chapter, is one such theoretical model, conceptualizing self-determination as a dispositional characteristic (and not explicitly within a motivational framework), but drawing from and aligning with the organismic nature of SDT.

Conclusion

From its initial use in philosophy to modern usages pertaining to volitional action and autonomous motivation, the self-determination construct has proven to be a useful heuristic across multiple disciplines. The following chapters will further the examination of the construct in the larger context of human agentic theories and in adolescent development.

References

American Heritage Dictionary of the English Language, The. (1992). New York: Houghton Mifflin Company.

Angyal, A. (1941). *Foundations for a science of personality*. Cambridge, MA: Harvard University Press.

Baer, D. (1998). Problems in imposing self-determination. *Journal of the Association for Persons with Severe Handicaps, 23*, 50–52.

Bagley, W. (1925). *Determinism in education*. New York: Columbia University Press.

Biestek, F. P., & Gehrig, C. C. (1978). *Client self-determination in social work: A fifty-year history*. Chicago: Loyola University Press.
Cravens, H. (1978). *The triumph of evolution: American scientists and the heredity-environment controversy, 1900–1941*. Philadelphia: University of Pennsylvania Press.
deCharms, R. (1968). *Personal causation: The internal affective determinants of behavior*. New York: Academic Press.
Deci, E. L. (1980). *The psychology of self-determination*. Lexington: Lexington Books.
Deci, E. L., & Ryan, R. (1985). *Intrinsic motivation and self-determination in human behavior*. New York: Plenum Press.
Deci, E. L., & Ryan, R. M. (2000). The "what" and the "why" of goal pursuits: Human needs and the self-determination of behavior. *Psychological Inquiry, 11*, 227–268.
Gove, P. B. (1967). *Webster's third new international dictionary of the English language unabridged*. Springfield: Merriam-Webster.
Heater, D. (1994). *National self-determination: Woodrow Wilson and his legacy*. New York: St. Martin's Press.
Heider, F. (1958). *The psychology of interpersonal relations*. New York: Wiley.
Herbermann, C. G., Pace, E. A., Pallen, C. B., Shahan, T. J., & Wynne, J. J. (1914). *The Catholic Encyclopedia*. New York: The Encyclopedia Press. Accessed online at http://www.newadvent.org/cathen/04756c.htm on February 19, 2015.
Locke, J. (1688). *An abstract of the essay*. Accessed online at http://www.philosophypages.com/locke/k365.htm on January 2, 2016.
Locke, J. (1690). *An essay on human understanding*. Accessed online at http://www.ilt.columbia.edu/projects/digitexts/locke/understanding/title.html on February 19, 2015.
McDermott, F. E. (1975). *Self-determination in social work*. London: Routledge and Kegan Paul Ltd..
Nirje, B. (1972). The right to self-determination. In W. Wolfensberger (Ed.), *Normalization: The principle of normalization* (pp. 176–200). Toronto: National Institute on Mental Retardation.
Perske, R. (1972). The dignity of risk. In W. Wolfensberger (Ed.), *Normalization: The principle of normalization in human services* (pp. 194–200). Toronto: National institute on Mental Retardation.
Rappaport, J. (1981). In praise of a paradox: A social policy of empowerment over prevention. *American Journal of Community Psychology, 9*, 1–25.
Ryan, R. M., & Deci, E. L. (2000). Self-determination theory and the facilitation of intrinsic motivation, social development, and well-being. *American Psychologist, 55*, 68–78.
Ryan, R. M., & Deci, E. L. (2006). Self-Regulation and the problem of human autonomy: Does psychology need choice, self-determination, and will? *Journal of Personality, 74*, 1557–1585.
Ryan, R. M., & Deci, E. L. (2011). A self-determination theory perspective on social, institutional, cultural, and economic supports for autonomy and their importance for well-being. In V. I. Chirkov, R. M. Ryan, & K. M. Sheldon (Eds.), *Human autonomy in cross-cultural context: Perspectives on the psychology of agency, freedom, and well-being* (pp. 45–64). New York: Springer. doi:10.1007/978-90-481-9667-8_3.
Shogren, K. A. (2013). Positive psychology and disability: A historical analysis. In M. Wehmeyer (Ed.), *The Oxford Handbook of positive psychology and disability* (pp. 19–33). Oxford: Oxford University Press.
Simpson, G., & Weiner, W. (1989). *Oxford English dictionary*. Oxford: Oxford University Press.
Skinner, B. F. (1971). *Beyond freedom and dignity*. New York: Bantam Books.
VandenBos, G. R. (2007). *APA dictionary of psychology*. Washington, DC: American Psychological Association.
Wehmeyer, M. L. (2013). *The Oxford handbook of positive psychology and disability*. Oxford: Oxford University Press.
Wehmeyer, M. L., & Schalock, R. (2001). Self-determination and quality of life: Implications for special education services and supports. *Focus on Exceptional Children, 33*(8), 1–16.

Wehmeyer, M. L., Abery, B., Mithaug, D. E., & Stancliffe, R. J. (2003). *Theory in self-determination: Foundations for educational practice*. Springfield: Charles C Thomas Publisher, LTD..

White, R. W. (1959). Motivation reconsidered: The concept of competence. *Psychological Review, 66*, 297–333.

Williams, R. R. (1989). Creating a new world of opportunity: Expanding choice and self-determination in lives of Americans with severe disability by 1992 and beyond. In R. Perske (Ed.), *Proceedings from the national conference on self-determination* (pp. 16–17). Minneapolis: Institute on Community Integration.

Chapter 2
Human Agentic Theories and the Development of Self-Determination

Karrie A. Shogren, Todd D. Little, and Michael L. Wehmeyer

Abstract Self-determination theories are housed within theories of human agentic behavior. Human agency refers to the sense of personal empowerment involving both knowing and having what it takes to achieve goals. Human agentic theories share the meta-theoretical view that organismic aspirations drive human behaviors. An organismic perspective of self-determination portrays people as active contributors to, or "authors" of their behavior, where behavior is defined in terms of self-regulated and goal-directed actions. This chapter will review the major theories of human agentic behavior and will examine the role of self-determination in each.

Theories of human agency provide a framework for understanding human behavior. Human agentic theories, including theories of self-determination, share the meta-theoretical assumption that organismic aspirations drive human behavior (Little et al. 2006). Organismic aspirations can be understood as the drive to be active contributors to, or *agents* of, one's behavior. Thus an agentic person, driven by organismic aspirations, seeks to be the origin of his or her actions (Little et al. 2002). Human agentic theories assume that actions are volitional and that an agentic person uses self-regulated and goal-directed agentic actions to "plot and navigate a chosen course through the uncertainties and challenges of the social and ecological environments… continuously interpreting and evaluating actions and their consequences" (Little et al. 2002, p. 390). This ongoing process of navigating challenges and engaging in self-regulated, goal-directed actions gives rise to a sense of personal empowerment and action-control beliefs, or the sense that one knows and has what it takes to achieve goals, which contributes to the development of a sense of *causal agency*; that is, that the person acts with an eye toward causing an effect to accomplish a specific end or to cause or create change in his or her life. Repeated experiences of causal agency lead to enhanced self-determination.

K.A. Shogren (✉) • M.L. Wehmeyer
Special Education, University of Kansas, Lawrence, KS, USA
e-mail: shogren@ku.edu

T.D. Little
Educational Psychology and Leadership,, Texas Tech University, Lubbock, TX, USA

M.L. Wehmeyer et al. (eds.), *Development of Self-Determination Through the Life-Course*, DOI 10.1007/978-94-024-1042-6_2

In the following sections, we describe the general assumptions of human agentic theories and the features that differentiate such theories from other theories of understanding human behavior. We will also describe how human agentic theories provide a broad framework for organizing constructs related to causal agency and the development of self-determination.

Assumptions of Theories of Human Agency

Theories of human agency differ from other frameworks for understanding human behavior (e.g., theories that emphasize stimulus-response accounts of behavior) because of the assumption underlying all theories of human agency that each person is integral to his/her organismic functioning. Unlike stimulus response theories which, by and large, assume that stimuli in the environment drive behavior, agentic theories assume that the person actively shapes his or her environment and responses to that environment. Contextual factors are still highly relevant, as contexts provide supports and opportunities as well as hindrances and impediments for volitional and agentic action, but it is the individual and their drive to act as a *causal agent* (not environmental stimuli) that is the primary driver of behavior. People who consistently engage in causal action to exert causal agency are self-determined. Specifically, as individuals strive to meet basic psychological and biological needs, they engage in self-regulated, goal directed action, or *causal action*, that enables them to navigate varying environmental and contextual challenges and they become more effective in their causal action and develop a sense of *causal agenc*y and enhanced self-determination.

The process of engaging in causal action has a self-evaluative feedback process, where persons continuously interpret and evaluate their actions and the consequences of actions. This meta-cognitive monitoring shapes, on an ongoing basis, each individual's action-control beliefs about the activities that he or she is capable of in varying contexts. Specifically, people are always learning under what conditions their causal actions will have desired effects. Under optimal circumstances, this continually evolving and actively monitored self-system gives rise to a strong, integrated sense of causal agency—a self-determined person. A highly self-determined person is the primary origin of his or her actions, has high aspirations, perseveres in the face of obstacles, sees more and varied options, learns from failures, and has a strong sense of well-being. A less self-determined person is shaped by extra-personal influences, has low aspirations, struggles with problem solving and goal setting, and often feels hopeless. Thus, theories of human agency have an explicit focus on the person-environment fit. It is in the context of this interaction between personal competencies and environmental demands that people become agents of their own action or *causal agents* over their lives, and, ultimately, self-determined.

In addition to the assumptions regarding organismic aspirations and contextual influences, theories of human agency also assume that:

(a) Actions are motivated by both biological and psychological needs.
(b) When actions are directed toward self-regulated goals, this serves biological and psychological needs, both short-term and long-term.
(c) Actions are volitional and agentic and shaped by understandings about general action-control behaviors that entail self-chosen forms and functions (Deci and Ryan 2002; Little et al. 2002).

These assumptions create an organizational framework for a theoretical model of the development of self-determination (see Fig. 2.1). In the following sections, we will further describe this model, specifically discussing the various human agentic theories that contribute to an understanding of the development of self-determination.

Theoretical Model of the Development of Self-Determination

As described previously, Fig. 2.1 provides a theoretical model of the development of self-determination. At the start of this system are basic psychological needs for autonomy, competence, and relatedness proposed by Self-Determination Theory (SDT) and discussed in more detail subsequently in Chap. 4. Satisfaction of these basic needs facilitates *autonomous motivation*, defined as intrinsic motivation and well-internalized extrinsic motivation (Deci and Ryan 2012, p. 88). Consistent with assumptions of organismic theories, the interplay between the context and the individual's psychological needs satisfaction is complex and reciprocal. When a motive or motives are salient, people are in a position to select goals on the basis of their expectations about the satisfaction of these motives (Deci and Ryan 1985, p. 235). As per Fig. 2.1, these psychological needs initiate a causal action sequence that, through interaction with environmental supports and opportunities, enables the development of a "synergistic set of action-control beliefs and behaviors that provide the self-regulatory foundation that is called upon to negotiate the various tasks and challenges of the life course" (Little et al. 2002, p. 396). Action-control beliefs

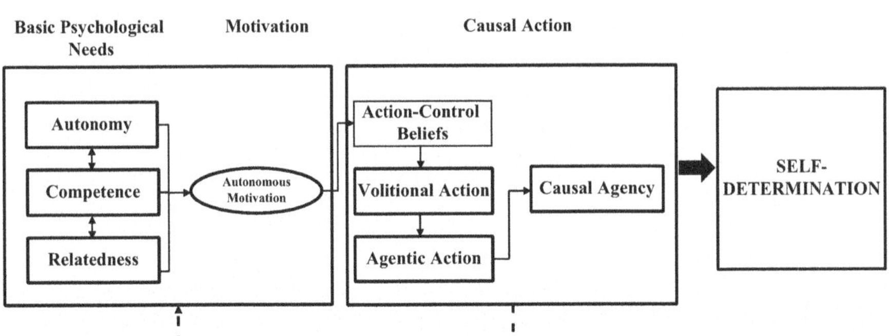

Fig. 2.1 The development of self-determination

about the link between the self and the goal (control expectancy beliefs), the links between the self and the means that are available for use to address a challenge (agency beliefs), and about which specific means are most effective for reaching one's goals (causality beliefs) (Little et al. 2002, p. 396) interact with and mediate volitional and agentic actions (employing causal and agentic capabilities), resulting in causal agency. Repeated experiences with the causal action sequence leads to multiple experiences with causal agency and, as a result, enhanced self-determination. In the following sections, we describe each of these contributors to the development of self-determination in greater depth.

Psychological and Biological Needs

As mentioned previously, a fundamental assumption of human agentic theories is that actions are motivated by both psychological and biological needs, and that if psychological and biological needs are addressed overall, well-being is supported. For purposes of this text, we are focusing on the psychological needs that motivate causal action, but, of course, biological needs also motivate action. In terms of biological needs, an assumption of human agentic theories is that all organisms require resources for physical growth and development (Hawley 1999; Little et al. 2002). These resources create an appetite for biological needs; however, to meet biological needs there is an evolutionarily duality that shapes action in pursuit of resources. On one hand, people can participate in social groups, using social connections and capital to acquire needed resources. This social group, however, can also become a source of competition as multiple people in the social group pursue resources. Within social groups, therefore, people experience both supports and threats to the attainment of resources. Ethologists describe this duality as a dominance hierarchy. Hawley (1999) further defined such hierarchies as the emergent ordering of individuals based on their relative competitive abilities. People that become highly agentic are more likely to attain needed resources, whereas those with less developed causal agency experience fewer opportunities to access resources (Hawley 1999; Little et al. 2002). Thus, contextual factors interact with the pursuit of resources to meet biological needs that shape the development of personal agency. Essentially, as people are able to meet their biological needs, they learn the types of volitional and agentic actions that enable them to access needed resources. They learn that goals can be set and met, that they can influence their environment, and that their future efforts are likely to be successful (Hawley and Little 2002). This cyclical process is why biological (and psychological needs, discussed subsequently) are foundational elements to the development of causal agency and self-determination.

Of particular focus in this text, human agentic theories also assume that there are basic psychological needs—organismic necessities for psychological growth, integrity, and wellness—that shape the development of self-determination, result in autonomous motivation, and motivate causal action (volitional action, agentic action, and action control beliefs). As mentioned previously, Self-Determination Theory (see Chap. 4 for overview) describes three fundamental psychological needs: *Competence*, *Relatedness*, and *Autonomy* (Deci and Ryan 2002). Self-Determination Theory assumes that social contexts motivate human action to meet these basic psychological needs. The need for competence is defined as the need to successfully engage, manipulate, and negotiate the environment. The need for relatedness reflects the desire for close emotional bonds and feelings of connectedness to others in the social world. The need for autonomy reflects the need to feel that one's actions are predicated on the self or volitional in nature (Vansteenkiste and Ryan 2013). These basic psychological needs serve as the "energizer of behavior" (Deci and Ryan 2012, p. 101) or, within this theoretical model of the development of self-determination, the autonomous motivation that energizes causal action.

A significant body of research has emerged documenting the efforts undertaken by individuals to address their need for autonomy (Deci et al. 1991; Vansteenkiste et al. 2012). Deci and Ryan (2012) observed that:

> To be autonomous means to behave with a sense of volition, willingness, and congruence; it means to fully endorse and concur with the behavior on is engaged in. Autonomy—this capacity for and desire to experience self-regulation and integrity—is a central force within both the life span development of individuals and in the movement of history toward greater freedom and voice for citizens within cultures and governments.
>
> In healthy individual development, people move in the direction of greater autonomy. This entails internalizing and integrating external regulations over behavior and learning to effectively manage drives and emotions. Additionally, it means maintaining intrinsic motivation and interest, which are vital to assimilating new ideas and experiences." (p. 85).

As Deci (1996) noted, "without choice, there would be no agency, and no self-regulation" (p. 222). Autonomy is therefore understood as a critical need, and actions undertaken to address this need are critical to the development of a sense of causal agency and self-determination.

As organisms take action to meet these three basic psychological needs, this energizes the development of autonomous motivation, consisting of intrinsic motivation (doing an activity because it is enjoyable) and/or internalized extrinsic motivation (doing an activity because it leads to a valued consequence separate from the activity itself) (Deci and Ryan 2012, p. 88). The interaction between the organism's efforts to meet basic psychological needs and the resultant autonomous motivation stimulates causal action, discussed in the next section.

Causal Action

While the self-system processes pertaining to psychological needs and autonomous motivation are detailed and explained by Self-Determination Theory, we turn, by and large, to Action-Control Theory (Chap. 22) and Causal Agency Theory (Chap. 5) to explain causal action and the development of causal agency leading to self-determination. As mentioned previously, human agentic theories assume that actions are volitional and that an agentic person uses causal actions to "plot and navigate a chosen course through the uncertainties and challenges of the social and ecological environments… continuously interpreting and evaluating actions and their consequences" (Little et al. 2002, p. 390). As discussed in Chap. 1 self-determined action is self-caused action. Organisms act volitionally and self-initiate action based upon conscious choices that reflect one's preferences in pursuit of goals that enhance personal well-being. The interaction between causal action and the context or environment is complex, but in essence, reflects the organism's response to opportunities or threats in the environment. As depicted in Fig. 2.2, these two classes of challenges to which the organism responds (opportunity or threat) are composed of three distinct contextual conditions. Opportunity refers to situations or circumstances that provoke the organism to engage in causal action to achieve a planned, desired outcome that is available because of the opportunity.

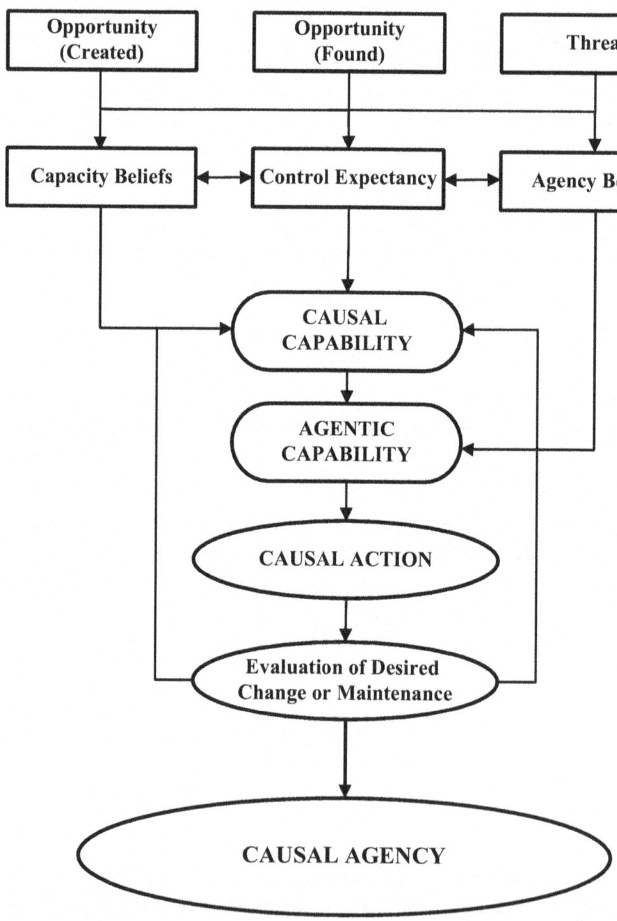

Fig. 2.2 Causal action schema

Opportunity implies that the situation or circumstance provides a chance for the person to create change or make something happen based upon his or her individual causal capability (knowledge and abilities leading to volitional action, discussed subsequently). If a person has the causal capability to act on the situation or circumstance, that situation or circumstance can be construed as an opportunity. If the person is unable to act on the situation or circumstance because of limitations to causal capability, that may be a 'missed opportunity.' However, if the person has limited causal capability, the situation or circumstance is not an opportunity. An opportunity is definitionally bound to the person's causal capability. Opportunities can be "found" (unanticipated, happened upon through no effort of one's own) or "created" (the person acts to create a favorable circumstance).

The second challenge condition, threat, involve situations or circumstances that threaten the organism's self-determination and provoke the organism to exercise causal action to maintain a preferred outcome or to create change that is consistent with one's own values, preferences, or interests, and not the values, preferences or interests of others. The interplay between autonomous motivation and these challenge conditions is, as mentioned previously, complex. In the case of created opportunities, it is the organism's autonomous motivation that directly motivates the effort to create the opportunity. In the case of found opportunities or threats, these contextual challenges emerge unsolicited by the organism, so that it is the context or the condition that triggers the autonomous motivation to take advantage of the opportunity or minimize the impact of the threat. In all cases, though, the emergence of these environmental and contextual conditions lead to the innervation of a set of action-control beliefs that mediate volitional and causal action.

Action-Control Theory The interaction between the organism's efforts to meet basic psychological needs and the resultant autonomous motivation and the environmental conditions of opportunity or threat stimulate causal action, beginning with "self-perceptions about the means and competencies one has to reach one's goals" (Little et al. 2002, p. 396). These self-perceptions are articulated through Action-Control Theory as a set of action-control beliefs:

> From this view point, the general agency system of individuals gives rise to a synergistic set of action-control beliefs and behaviors that provide the self-regulatory foundation that is called upon to negotiate the various tasks and challenges of the life course. More specifically, action-control theory focuses on the role of specific self-regulatory beliefs as mediators of motivated action (i.e., they are the proximal links to behavior). (Little, Hawley, Heinrich, & Marsland, 2002, p. 396).

These self-regulatory beliefs involve:

> *Control Expectancy Beliefs*: Control expectancy beliefs "reflect the general expectations about the link between the self and the goal" (Little et al. 2006, p. 70); they reflect "the general perception of the degree to which a person feels that he or she can attain a given goal" (Little et al. 2002, p. 396).

> *Agency Beliefs:* Agency beliefs "reflect the links between the self and the various means that they are relevant for attaining a chosen end" (Little et al. 2006; p. 71); they are "beliefs about whether these means are personally available for use" (Little et al. 2002, p. 396).

> *Causality Beliefs:* Causality beliefs "reflect general views of the utility or usefulness of a given means such as efforts, luck, or ability for attaining a particular goal" (Little et al. 2006; p. 71); they are "judgments about which specific means are most effective for reaching one's goals" (Little et al. 2002, p. 396).

Greater detail about these action-control beliefs can be found in subsequent chapters. Before moving to the operators involved in volitional and agentic action (as per Fig. 2.1), it is important to note that these interrelated action-control beliefs contribute jointly to the initiation of volitional action, but also contribute uniquely. Control expectancy beliefs are more generalized beliefs about one's ability to set and attain goals, influencing both capacity and agency beliefs as well as the initiation of volitional action. Capacity beliefs contribute more directly to the initiation of volitional action (and specific causal capabilities), while agency beliefs contribute more directly to agentic action and the agentic capabilities that energize that action. Each of these is described in greater detail in the next section.

Causal Agency Theory As will be detailed in Chap. 5 Causal Agency Theory specifies how one becomes self-determined. Within Causal Agency Theory, self-determination is defined as:

> …dispositional characteristic manifested as acting as the causal agent in one's life. Self-determined *people* (i.e., causal agents) act in service to freely chosen goals. Self-determined *actions* function to enable a person to be the causal agent is his or her life. (Shogren et al., 2015, p. 257)

Causal Agency Theory holds that self-determined action is characterized by three essential characteristics – *volitional action*, *agentic action*, and *action-control beliefs*. As has been discussed, the causal action sequence depicted in Fig. 2.2 begins with the organism's response to (or attempt to create) environmental opportunities and threats, resulting in the stimulation of action-control beliefs. In turn, these beliefs mediate causal action in the form of volitional and agentic action.

Briefly, as per Causal Agency Theory, volitional action is defined as making conscious choices based on one's preferences and engaging in self-initiated actions that promote autonomy. Agentic action refers to the process of identifying pathways that lead to specific ends and engaging in self-directing and self-regulating action to navigate environmental opportunities and threats. The primary operators in propelling volitional and agentic action involve the capability to perform causal actions or behaviors, subdivided into causal capability and agentic capability. Capability refers to the condition of being capable; that is, having *requisite mental or physical capacity to accomplish a particular task.* Two types of capabilities are important to causal agency; Causal Capability and Agentic Capability. These capabilities differentiate between the two aspects of causal action; (1) causing something to happen (e.g., Volitional Action) and (2) directing that action toward a preferred end (e.g., Agentic Action). As can be seen in Table 2.1, these capabilities provide an overarching theme for the skills and knowledge needed to develop and acquire in relation to the essential characteristics of Volitional Action and Agentic Action.

Causal capability refers to the mental or physical capacity (e.g., the ability to perform an action or behavior) that enables a person to cause or make something

Table 2.1 Component elements of Causal Agency Theory

Essential characteristics	Component constructs	Component elements
Volitional action	Autonomy	**Causal capabilities**
	Self-initiation	Choice-making skills
		Decision-making skills
		Goal setting skills
		Problem solving skills
		Planning skills
Agentic action	Self-regulation	**Agentic capabilities**
	Self-direction	Self-management skills (self-monitoring, self-evaluation, etc.)
	Pathways thinking	Goal attainment skills
		Problem solving skills
		Self-advocacy skills
Action-control beliefs	Psychological empowerment	Self-awareness
	Self-realization	Self-knowledge
	Control expectancy	
	Agency beliefs	
	Causality beliefs	

happen. Such capacities include the skills and knowledge associated with making a choice or a decision, setting a goal, solving a problem, planning a course of action; the skills and behaviors that enable self-initiation and autonomous functioning and, as such, volitional action. However, we would emphasize that limitations to the number or complexity of such capacities that might otherwise hinder causal or agentic action can, in fact, be mitigated by a wide array of supports, including technological devices, social networks and supports, and so forth, thus enabling people who might otherwise not be able to perform requisite actions to, in fact, engage in causal action and become more self-determined.

Agentic capability, in turn, involves the mental or physical capacities involved in directing behavior toward an end. Such capacities include the skills and knowledge associated with self-management, goal attainment, problem solving, and self-advocacy; the skills and behaviors that enable self-regulation, self-direction, pathways thinking and, as such, agentic action.

Conclusion

Figure 2.1 introduced a theoretical model of the development of self-determination. This process involves the stimulation of action through the organism's response to contextual and environmental challenges (opportunities, threats) that energize basic psychological needs and resultant autonomous motivation, stimulating a causal action sequence in which volitional and agentic actions are mediated by action-control beliefs, resulting in experiences of causal agency. Repeated experiences of causal agency result in enhanced self-determination. Though explained by three different theories (Self-Determination Theory, Action-Control Theory, Causal Agency Theory), all share the broad metatheoretical assumptions inherent within human agentic theories that organismic aspirations drive behavior, and that humans engage in goal-directed activity to meet basic biological and psychological needs, influenced by contextual and environmental challenges, and that, by learning to engage in volitional and agentic action and developing action-control beliefs, causal agency increases ultimately enhancing self-determination and the agentic self. The following chapters will provide more detail on specific theories and process that also influence the development of the agentic self.

References

Deci, E. L. (1996). Making room for self-regulation: Some thoughts on the link between emotion and behavior. *Psychological Inquiry, 7*, 220–223.

Deci, E. L., & Ryan, R. (1985). *Intrinsic motivation and self-determination in human behavior*. New York: Plenum Press.

Deci, E. L., & Ryan, R. M. (Eds.). (2002). *Handbook of self-determination research*. Rochester: University of Rochester Press.

Deci, E. L., & Ryan, R. M. (2012). Motivation, personality, and development within embedded social contexts: An overview of self-determination theory. In R. M. Ryan (Ed.), *The Oxford handbook of human motivation* (pp. 85–110). Oxford: Oxford University Press.

Deci, E. L., Vallerand, R. J., Pelletier, L. G., & Ryan, R. M. (1991). Motivation and education: The self-determination perspective. *Educational Psychologist, 26*(3–4), 325–346.

Hawley, P. H. (1999). The ontogenesis of social dominance: A strategy-based evolutionary perspective. *Developmental Review, 19*, 91–132.

Hawley, P. H., & Little, T. D. (2002). Evolutionary and developmental perspectives on the agentic self. In D. Cervone & W. Mishel (Eds.), *Advances in personality sciences*. New York: Guliford Press.

Little, T. D., Hawley, P. H., Henrich, C. C., & Marsland, K. (2002). Three views of the agentic self: A developmental synthesis. In E. L. Deci & R. M. Ryan (Eds.), *Handbook of self-determination research* (pp. 389–404). Rochester: University of Rochester Press.

Little, T. D., Snyder, C. R., & Wehmeyer, M. L. (2006). The agentic self: On the nature and origins of personal agency across the lifespan. In D. Mroczek & T. D. Little (Eds.), *The handbook of personality development* (pp. 61–79). Mahwah: Lawrence Erlbaum and Associates.

Shogren, K. A., Wehmeyer, M. L., Palmer, S. B., Forber-Pratt, A., Little, T. J., & Lopez, S. J. (2015). Causal agency theory: Reconceptualizing a functional model of self-determination. *Education and Training in Autism and Developmental Disabilities, 50*(3), 251–263.

Vansteenkiste, M., & Ryan, R. M. (2013). On psychological growth and vulnerability: Basic psychological need satisfaction and need frustration as a unifying principle. *Journal of Psychotherapy Integration, 23*(3), 263–280. doi:10.1037/a0032359.

Vansteenkiste, M., Sierens, E., Goossens, L., Soenens, B., Dochy, F., Mouratidis, A., … Beyers, W. (2012). Identifying configurations of perceived teacher autonomy support and structure: Associations with self-regulated learning, motivation and problem behavior. *Learning and Instruction, 22*, 431–439. doi: http://dx.doi.org/10.1016/j.learninstruc.2012.04.002

Chapter 3
A Context for Self-Determination and Agency: Adolescent Developmental Theories

David M. Hansen and Nadia Jessop

Abstract This chapter discusses adolescent developmental theories, first reviewing neurological growth and restructuring that occurs in the brain during adolescence. Next, cognitive and affective processes, including metacognition, self-regulation, and self-determination are described. Finally, identity development and agency and their role in adolescent development are described, followed by discussion of the role of culture and context in adolescent development.

The aim of this chapter is to situate the discussion of agency and self-determination within the broader context of adolescent developmental theory. There are few theories that focus solely on adolescence; most are based on lifespan models (e.g., Piaget's theory of cognitive development). There is also no shortage of theories on human development, with each theorist providing a different lens through which to view the processes of maturation, e.g., Vygotsky and Erickson. In addition to these lifespan theories, over the last twenty years there has been a flurry of neuroscience research on adolescent brain growth. At first glance, much of the neuroscience research appears void of guiding developmental theory, emphasizing instead biological or medical models of growth. However, even these biological/medical models use a default model when interpreting the findings, frequently characterizing adolescence as a "storm and stress" period of development (Hall 1904). Given the range of theories that could be included in this chapter, we narrowed the focus to those that we consider the most relevant to the processes through which adolescents' transition into adult roles in society.

To accomplish the chapter aims, we begin by first examining the foundations of adolescence—the remarkable puberty-initiated neurological growth and restructuring of adolescents' brains. Drawing on relatively recent neuroscience research, we suggest that adolescents are ontogenetically primed for developing capacities relevant for self-determination and agency. We next examine changes in fundamental cognitive and affective "processes" during adolescence: metacognition, self-regulation,

D.M. Hansen (✉) • N. Jessop
University of Kansas, Lawrence, KS, USA
e-mail: dhansen1@ku.edu

M.L. Wehmeyer et al. (eds.), *Development of Self-Determination Through the Life-Course*, DOI 10.1007/978-94-024-1042-6_3

and self-determination (i.e., basic psychological needs). Although one could argue that self-regulation is a developmental task, we chose to treat it as a cognitive-affective process that supports other developmental tasks. In the third section we focus on identity and agency development. Many consider identity the quintessential developmental task of adolescence. Identity development and agency are linked to creating purpose and meaning within society, which takes center stage as adolescents begin to assign value to their "future selves" (Markus and Nurius 1986). The fourth major section we devote to discussion of how culture and context intersect with adolescent development. The point we reach in the concluding section is that adolescence represents a unique window of opportunity for specific, accelerated development in the human lifespan.

Puberty and Adolescence

Youniss (1983) argued that "[a]dolescence is socially constructed" and, as a social construct, represents shared socio-cultural understandings and beliefs that have emerged over time as a way to 'make sense' of physical and neurological changes brought on by puberty. These shared understandings and beliefs are the basis for what we expect from and how we treat adolescents. While many of our understandings and beliefs are explicit and defined (e.g., legal culpability), just as many, if not more, are implicit and only visible in society's embedded socio-cultural norms and practices. The social construction process makes adolescence a dynamic construct, with physical and neurological changes being the only constants.

The foundation for understanding adolescence is puberty. Strictly speaking, puberty refers to three overlapping neuroendocrinological events (adrenarche, gonadarche, and growth axis activation) associated with sexual maturation, which result in reproductive capabilities characteristic of adult members of a species (Rosenblum 1990). Among humans, an early first stage of sexual maturation, andrenarche, involves an increasing production of adrenal androgens, starting between ages 6–9 in girls and 7–10 in boys, building to an apex approximately 10 years later and continuing into the 20s, although it slows considerably after this apex (Blakemore et al. 2010; Dorn et al. 2006). This increase in androgens is associated with development of pubic and axillary hair and a slightly accelerated rate of bone growth (Cutler 1991). Gonadarche is a second phase of puberty in which the hypothalamic-pituitary-gonadal (HPG) axis is "reactivated" resulting in pulsatile production of gonadotropin hormone that stimulates the release, via the follicle-stimulating and luteinizing hormones, of gonadal hormones—testosterone in males, estrogen in females (Spear 2000). Gonadarche begins around age 11 for girls, with a range of 8–14, and around age 12 for boys, with a range of 9–15 (Blakemore et al. 2010). The HPG axis is active early in life but becomes "deactivated" during childhood only to become reactivated during adolescence, which then continues to be active throughout adulthood. Coinciding with gonadarche is an increase in growth hormone (GH) production giving rise to the development of secondary sexual characteristics (e.g., breast development) and rapid growth (e.g., growth spurt) that changes body size and composition, which occurs around age 12 for girls and age 14 for boys (Blakemore et al. 2010; Spear 2000). The start of adolescence is typically associated with changes related to gonadarche and activation of the growth-axis, perhaps because these neuroendocrine events produce more visible changes in the adolescent.

The criteria for identifying the conclusion of adolescence vary greatly. We summarize this variability into two 'camps' based on operational definitions evident in the literature that can often be traced to underlying assumptions regarding adolescence as a biological and/or a social construction (e.g., nature versus nurture). The *neuro-biological* camp focuses on identifying an end of adolescence that is associated with the normalization of neuroendocrinological functions (e.g., gonadotropic functions). For the neuro-biological camp, the end of adolescence occurs approximately around age 18 (c.f. Spear 2000). The second camp focuses on *socially-constructed* definitions to identify the end of adolescence. For example, as educational requirements for gainful employment in the United States have increased, along with other macrostructural changes (Mortimer and Larson 2002), some scholars extend the upper boundaries of adolescence well into the middle 20s or even age 30 (Arnett 2000). The social-construction camp typically relies on neuroendocrinological events for the start of adolescence but then switches to social definitions to determine the endpoint.

Neurobiology of Puberty

The neuroendocrinological events of puberty result not simply in sexual maturation but they also trigger profound changes in the brain that impact "the perceptions, motivations, and behavioral repertoire of the individual" (Blakemore et al. 2010, p. 926). These changes accelerate learning for an ontogenetic purpose—to provide flexibility (neuroplasticity) to rapidly learn and adapt to environmental needs and demands, presumably to promote learning associated with functioning as a member of adult society (Bourgeois et al. 1994; Keating 2004; Spear 2000). There are two broad domains of brain changes, and each domain is associated with a specific learning potential that focuses and prioritizes the 'object' of learning. These changes support the apparent ultimate ontogenetic outcome for brain development during adolescence: the integration/coordination of affective and cognitive brain systems that make possible, but do not ensure, a more fully reflective, consciousness for self-directed thought and action (Keating 2004). We next review research findings on the two domains of brain development during adolescence in order to provide a neurobiological backdrop for understanding the normative development tasks of contemporary adolescence (e.g., identity, agency).

Neurogenesis, Pruning, and Myelination In response to hormonal events of puberty, adolescents' experience a massive overproduction and pruning of neurons (Huttenlocher 1979). The magnitude of this neuron generation (neurogenesis) and pruning is startling, with some reasonable estimates of pruning of around 30,000 synapses (connection between two neurons) *per second* in the primate brain, and a similar rate in humans during adolescence (Huttenlocher 1984; Rakic et al. 1994). Pruning is an essential process for organizing neural connections into networks that support functioning in an environment; the pattern of connections, not a greater number of neurons per se, is related to skill development and improved functioning. Only during the early years of life (e.g., ages 0–3) is the rate of neurogenesis and pruning roughly equivalent to that during adolescence. By approximately age 16, the rate of production and pruning peaks and begins to slow to adult-typical levels (He and Crews 2007; Huttenlocher 1979). One indication of this slowing of neuron production is the relative volume of grey matter (neurons). Grey matter volume is reduced and becomes roughly equivalent to adult levels around ages 18–20 (Giedd et al. 2010; Nelson et al. 2006; Sowell et al. 2001).

Myelination of the axons of neurons (white matter) is important for skill learning because it increases the efficiency and speed of neuronal firing for performing a task (e.g., cognitive, affective, or behavioral task). White matter density increases proportionally based on the degree to which specific neural pathways are repeatedly used, and thus reflects learning. The pattern of white matter development shows a linear increase throughout adolescence and it continues throughout adulthood (Paus 2010; Sala et al. 2012). The *rate* of white matter formation, however, follows a similar pattern as grey matter development, peaking and then slowing to a more adult-typical rate after age 18.

Emotional and Motivational Sensitivity Coinciding with accelerated grey and white matter changes during adolescence are alterations in incentive and emotional processing brain systems—subcortical systems. We use the term 'alteration' instead of change to indicate a more transitive or temporary state, rather than a permanent change to motivational and emotional processes systems. Overall, there is an intensification and sensitivity to affective and motivational cues and rewards, which appears tied to alterations in the number of and responsiveness to neurotransmitter receptors, such as dopamine (DA) and GABA—gamma-amino butyric acid (Somerville et al. 2010; Spear 2000). The density of dopamine receptors in the striatum, which is associated with reward motivation and movement, peaks in early adolescence and by mid-to-late adolescence the density of receptors returns to its previous levels (Casey and Jones 2010; Seeman et al. 1987). A shift in the value of incentive stimuli during adolescence appears to support greater novelty-induced reward seeking, which is frequently cited as a causal mechanism for 'characteristic'[1] adolescent sensation seeking or risk-taking behaviors that can have negative consequences (Steinberg 2008; Sturman and Moghaddam 2011). Although such implied causal relationships are commonly made, there is no compelling ontogenetic argument to support this *a priori* assumption given that such behaviors are a function of context, opportunity, and learning (Casey et al. 2006). More importantly,

[1] We avoided referring to characterizations of adolescents' behaviors as a "stereotype" but there are ample examples in the literature that fit this latter label.

raising the sensitivity of affective and motivational brains systems to coincide with the flood of new neurons and rapid pruning makes ontogenetic sense—since affect and motivation have a powerful organizing and guiding effect, serving to focus learning on relevant tasks (e.g., Rakic et al. 1994).

Puberty and Experience-Dependent Neuroplasticity

Although the rapid neuronal growth and restructuring during adolescence occurs across cortical regions, it is particularly concentrated in prefrontal cortex (PFC). PFC is implicated in numerous higher-order cognitive processes, including meta-cognition, prospective thinking, planning and organization, executive function, and response inhibition (Casey et al. 2008; Keating 2004; Luna and Sweeney 2004; Spear 2000). One of the results of changes in PFC is the "top-down" or cognitive coordination[2] of goal-directed thought and action. Luna and Sweeny (2004, p. 298) describe the coordinating function as "the ability to voluntarily/cognitively choose what stimuli or ideas will guide our behavior, and inhibit responses to competing ideas of events that could be less adaptive (Bjorklund & Harnishfeger, 1995; Dempster, 1992; Fuster, 1997)." Although children exhibit fundamental capacities for cognitive coordination, during adolescence the explosion of neurons and pruning in PFC results in the rapid expansion of existing capacities (Luna and Sweeney 2004) and the development of new ones. Cognitive coordination in PFC does not occur independent of other systems, however, rather it is subserved by "widely distributed and integrated brain systems" (Luna et al. 2010). That is, PFC co-ops existing and emerging functions of other systems to expand its own functional capacities for the voluntary/conscious *suppression* of irrelevant and off-task behaviors that could interfere with goal attainment, as well as for *advancing* salient and on-task behaviors that lead to the intended goal.

The remarkable growth in PFC, with its aim of coordinating and directing thought and behavior, often overshadows an equally important change between the top-down functions of PFC and the 'bottom-up' functions of subcortical, affective systems. During adolescence there is an increase in the number and myelination of long neuronal tracks between PFC and subcortical regions, resulting in the integration of and greater coordination between the functional capacities of affective and cognitive systems (Keating 2004; Luna and Sweeney 2004). By more fully integrating affect and cognition, there is an increase in adolescents' capacities for self-direction and regulation of effort, motivation, thought, and behavior (Casey et al. 2008).

Importantly, neurobiological changes in brain structure during adolescence only represent a *potential* for the expansion of functional capacities, rather than some ontogenetically ensured outcome of neurobiological growth. A basic function of the

[2] We avoid the term 'cognitive control' since it suggests that thinking (e.g., cold cognition) controls or supersedes affective or motivational influences instead of coordinating thought, behavior, and affect/motivation.

human brain is to learn how to successfully function within an environment by interacting with it (Amso and Casey 2006). This experience-dependent plasticity is essential for adaptive learning that is distinctive to an individual and maximizes his or her chances, not only of survival in a particular setting, but also successful functioning in it (Greenough et al. 2002a, b). Experiences in the environment influence which neurons are pruned and which ones remain; experience 'sculpts' the emergent networks of synaptic connections for functioning within an environment (Blakemore et al. 2010; Markham and Greenough 2004). Interactions with the functional demands of an environment, then, provide essential information for adaptive learning. However, different environments will vary in the types, number, and frequency of demands and experiences, e.g., their complexity (Grossman et al. 2002). Similarly, any two individuals in the same environment can perceive very different information depending on prior learning, personality, and personal interests. Thus, the experience-dependent adaptive learning hinges on experiences in an environment and on individual's past learning and propensities.

Unfortunately, neuroscience is not yet capable of examining specific neurobiological changes related to learning specific complex capacities for functioning, including capacities needed for adulthood. However, neuroscience research suggests that adolescents are developmentally primed for experience-dependent accelerated learning related to the *conscious coordination and regulation their own thoughts, affect, and behavior* (Luna and Sweeney 2004). Thus, we propose that adolescence provides a distinct neurobiological window of development that is intended to maximize chances for learning self-regulatory capacities in preparation for functioning in adult society. Furthermore, research suggests that *specific experiences within an environment play in an essential role in sculpting adolescents' brains.* Conversely, if there are not sufficient experiences during adolescence that demand learning to regulate the 'self,' there is little reason to expect such capacities to flourish.

Changes in Fundamental Cognitive and Affective "Processes"

Before examining key developmental tasks of adolescence, we examine changes during adolescence in three "processes" that operate across the different tasks: metacognition, self-regulation, and self-determination. The term 'processes' is used to indicate that we are treating them as fundamental processes of the mind (cognition, affect, and behavior) that support developmental tasks (defined below). Metacognition (c.f. Miller et al. 1970) and self-regulation (c.f. Bandura 1986) share the following conceptual core: "individuals make efforts to monitor their thoughts and actions and to act accordingly to gain some control over them" (Dinsmore et al. 2008, p. 404). The two constructs, however, have distinct research traditions, with metacognition focused on maturation of individuals' awareness of their thoughts (Moshman 1982) and self-regulation focused on development of behavioral and emotional regulation from interactions within an environment (Bandura 1982).

We also treat the basic psychological needs in Self-Determination Theory (SDT) as fundamental processes; these processes may help explain underlying intentions for metacognition and self-regulation.

Metacognition

Metacognition is essentially about individuals' monitoring of their own thinking, which includes the now classic "thinking about thinking" moniker (Miller et al. 1970). Operationally, metacognition emphasizes metacognitive knowledge and experience, goals, plans, and strategies for the intentional monitoring or regulating of one's thoughts, presumably to achieve some outcome or engage in some action. The study of metacognition has strong ties to Piagetian theory (Inhelder and Piaget 1958) with an emphasis on formal operational thinking (logical reasoning) and judgement and decision making. From a Piagetian perspective, the emergence of formal operational thinking is a hallmark of adolescence, although it is more accurate to consider it a potential development during adolescence rather than a guaranteed one (Keating 2004). Formal operation thinking can be defined as hypothetical, deductive reasoning (e.g., , hyothetico-deductive reasoning) to arrive at necessary and logical inferences, as opposed to inductive, concrete operational reasoning that begins with what is observed and then infers a hypothesis (Foltz and Overton 1995). Research indicates adolescence is associated with increased formal operational reasoning (e.g., higher-order, complex logical thinking and problem solving) but this capacity *does not* result from completion of some ontogenetic structural goal to shift thinking from concrete to formal logical processing (Klaczynski 2001a; Moshman 1998). A particular challenge in the study of metacognition as formal operations is how much this logical reasoning predominates everyday decision-making and behaviors among adolescents and adults.

Metacognition has been applied in the context of adolescent judgments and decision-making. Two fields of research, neuropsychological and cognition, indicate that everyday judgments and decision-making rarely, perhaps if ever, follow only logical-based rules (Bechara et al. 1997; Evans 1996). Instead, "heuristic" thinking is the brain's default mode for decision-making, with analytic thinking asserting itself when heuristic processing is not sufficient or does not lead to desired outcome (Klaczynski et al. 2001; Papies and Aarts 2010). In a dual processing model (heuristic and analytic thinking) *affect* directs, at least initially, attention and influences selection/application of a response that is similar or pertinent to the present context (Klaczynski 2001b). This affective processing, which is typically carried out unconsciously, provides an efficient (e.g., reduced cognitive load) and effective method for making the myriad of advantageous decisions necessary in our daily lives that would otherwise require laborious and time consuming cognitive processing (Keating 2004). In situations where previously learned responses are not sufficient to guide decisions, analytic thinking is employed to further guide the decision-making process. Research on the relative balance between heuristic and analytic thinking among adolescents indicates that analytic processing increases with age, while heuristic thinking is less age bound and more experiential and context specific (Klaczynski 2001a, b). To be clear, analytic thinking is not independent of heuristic thinking, and vice versa. Successful analytic thinking, for example, can lead to the modification of a decision-making heuristic. This line of research suggest that adolescence is associated with an increasing coordination between heuristic (e.g., affective) and analytic (e.g., cognitive) systems, which is consistent with the neurological research presented in the previous section, as well as research findings on the development of self-regulation. Finally, experiential and contextualized learning are essential to support heuristic thinking, including the heuristic thinking that has been modified through analytic processes. Thus, in order for heuristic and analytic cognition to become coordinated for (advantageous) judgment and decision-making, experiential and contextualized learning is a must.

Self-Regulation

Self-regulation focuses on decision-making and judgment aspects in the domains of behavioral and motivational regulation, as well as in more traditional cognitive domains (Zimmerman 1989, 2008; Zimmerman and Schunk 2008). At its optimum, self-regulation is the ability to "withstand temptations, persist through obstacles, and delay gratification" (Fitzsimons and Finkel 2011, p. 407). Self-regulation among adolescents (and children) has been studied primarily within the academic setting, frequently termed self-regulated learning (SRL), although it has also been applied to the sport and physical activity setting. Zimmerman (2008, pp. 166) defined SRL as "the self-directive processes and self-beliefs that enable learners to transform their mental abilities, such as verbal aptitude, into an academic performance skill, such as writing." (Academic skill in this instance refers to metacognitive processes, such as goal setting, strategy selection and monitoring.) Given the extent of research on self-regulation and SRL, we will only highlight the relevant findings for adolescents (see Boekaerts et al. 2005 for review).

Self-regulation development parallels the cognitive changes occurring during adolescence. A particularly important cognitive change associated with prefrontal cortical maturation (Paus et al. 1999; Sowell et al. 1999) is the capacity for the temporal organization of and execution of behavior, speech, and cognition (Fuster 2001). Thus, in addition to the expansion of higher-order reasoning capacities, the maturation of prefrontal cortex supports the growth of the temporal representation of goal-directed actions, including actions extending further into the future, which become integrated with inhibitory control processes (Fuster 2002). Research on self-regulation indicates that adolescents' become increasingly capable of regulating their actions through forethought, advanced planning, goal setting, and acting with intention, that is, *planfulness*, something not fully possible prior to puberty (Demetriou 2000). Thus in many respects, adolescence is the 'golden age' of regulatory development since most of the neurological growth is directed toward integration and coordination of cognition, affect/motivation, and behavior for planfulness.

An important 'outcome' of self-regulation is a growing sense that the individual has control over his or her own behavior (e.g., "self-agency"). A sense of self-agency is important because it serves to motivate and guide behaviors for goal achievement, often without much conscious deliberation (Gollwitzer and Sheeran 2006; Papies et al. 2009). However, it is only through repeatedly experiencing a sense of control over outcomes that a generalized sense of self-agency is built, and conversely, in the absence of such reinforcing experiences an individual may learn that efforts to regulate his or her actions to achieve an outcome have little benefit (Papies and Aarts 2010).

Self-Determination: Basic Psychological Needs

The exercise of volition is a basic assumption across the literature on self-regulation. The importance of volition for human development is suggested in the extensive body of research emanating from Self-Determination Theory (SDT). We acknowledge that the term 'self-determination' has been criticized, and sometime rightly so, as a Western construct that reflect an individualistic worldview. Our reading and understanding of SDT, however, suggests we take a more generic view of self-determination, and similarly of autonomy, and consider it as a motivational component of human beings that operates in distinct ways depending on the contexts (e.g., culture) in which they are learned and exercised.

Within the SDT framework, the three basic psychological needs—competence, autonomy, and relatedness—are fundamental affective processes proposed to motivate human behavior and action (Ryan and Deci 2000). Theoretically, these needs operate across the full range of cultures, domains, and social and personal contexts, although their idiosyncratic expression will also vary within these contexts. (Chaps. 2 and 4 in this book cover SDT in detail, thus we omit discussion of it here.) From a developmental perspective, the relative importance of each need could wax and wane depending on the period or age in the lifespan. Consequently, while all three needs constantly interact to affect growth across the lifespan, we suggest adolescents may particularly need to experience their 'self' as the originator of decisions and volition over actions in order to support the emergent neurological potentials (discussed in a previous section). The experience of the self being the originator of one's action becomes self-reinforcing (Deci and Ryan 2002) and an individual's environment can support or thwart this self-propagating experience of self-determination (Ryan and Deci 2000). Since volition and choice are instrumental to the experience of autonomy, an important question to address is how much choice and volition do the different environments of adolescents' daily lives permit. In schools in the United States, for example, adolescents' volitional actions can be relatively limited.

Key Developmental Tasks of Adolescence

Havighurst (1948) introduced the concept of a developmental task as a physical, cognitive, and/or emotional skill that needs to be learned during a particular period of the lifespan. Learning these specific skills (e.g., language) is integral for subsequent periods of development. The ontogeny of particular skills during a particular period results from genetically-propelled physical/neurological maturation that is affected by the environment in which it occurs. Although the concept of developmental tasks has been applied to various points in the lifespan (e.g., emerging adulthood), we prefer a narrower definition in which the emergence of new developmental tasks in the lifespan ends at a point where genetically-driven physical/neurological growth is complete, e.g., an organism has reached its mature state. We find this narrow definition helps identify a *specific learning need* that arises during a genetically-driven period physical/neurological growth, and thus also defines *specific types of experiences in an environment* that are important for supporting the development of a given task. An absence of particular experiences in an environment to support a physical/neurological learning need, then, would undermine the developmental task.

Developmental Task: Identity

Adolescence has long been associated with the search for identity or purpose—to understand one's self (e.g., "Who am I?") and role in adult society (Erikson 1968; Hill and Burrow 2012). Identity/purpose development occurs across the lifespan, but it is particularly acute during adolescence as a neurobiological push to integrate cognition and affect appear to promote questioning related to valuing and meaning. Although issues of identity/purpose extend into young adulthood and beyond in contemporary Western society, it remains a central task for adolescents (puberty through high school). Identity is important as research suggests that those with a strong sense of identity are better able to self-direct and flourish both presently and in adulthood, e.g., strive toward goals (Hill et al. 2013).

Erikson's stage of identity development has dominated Western psychology and research, although it is important to keep in mind identity was but one stage of Erikson's lifespan theory of psychosocial development (Erikson 1950, 1968). According to Erikson, individuals either successfully achieve a sense of identity during adolescence or they do not. More current thinking, however, is that achieving a sense of identity is best conceived as an ongoing process, which takes on heightened importance during adolescence. Achieving a sense of identity requires adolescents to resolve conflicts or crises regarding how they view their 'self' and their role as an adult in society. Exploring different selves and roles is an important process in Erikson's theory as exploration leads to awareness of conflicts, for example, conflict between expectations about what one should do and what one actually did. Achieving a sense of identity, then, entails progressively resolving conflicts until some stable point is reached in which conflicts become minimized, e.g., personal fidelity. Thus, identity development during adolescence is an iterative process (Crocetti et al. 2008, 2012) leading to a stable sense of self.

Theoretically, achieving a stable identity is not the only possible outcome of adolescence. Adolescents may, for example, commit to an identity without having sufficiently explored alternative options (e.g., experienced conflict from role commitment). James Marcia (1967, 1987) was instrumental in operationalizing Erikson's crisis, exploration, and commitment dimensions, leading to the differentiation of identity statuses: achieved, diffused, moratorium, and foreclosure. Within Marcia's framework (Marcia 1966, 1967), individuals with an achieved identity status have cultivated resilience since they have explored choices, made decisions on their own terms, and are not easily overwhelmed by new experiences, responsibilities, or changes in their environment. Individuals with a foreclosed status however, risk vulnerability since they tend to make a commitment before experiencing a period of intensive exploration on which to base the commitment, and their rigid adherence to the expected path precludes adaptability to ambiguous or unexpected situations (Marcia 1966, 1967; Muuss 1996). A diffused status indicates little commitment to or exploration of an identity, while a moratorium status represents active exploration without firm commitment.

Identity serves a self-regulating role by directing adolescents' attention and influencing the selection of goals and actions. Similar to Baltes (1997) self-regulation theory, Crocetti et al. (2008, 2012) suggest that the process of identity formation proceeds from the selection of identity-appropriate goals and actions, and then once enacted the goals and actions become a source of information about the value and usefulness of the identity. Over time, an adolescent may abandon, modify, or maintain her commitment to the identity. The selection and enactment of identity-relevant goals and actions is not, however, independent of socio-cultural factors. Rather the process of identity formation is embedded within the social, economic, and cultural contexts and systems in an adolescent's daily life (Cote and Levine 2014; Phinney 1989; Phinney and Chavira 1992; Phinney and Ong 2007; Schwartz et al. 2012; Sellers et al. 1998; Umaña-Taylor et al. 2014). These contexts and systems are not simply the testing grounds for adolescents' identity exploration but they also provide access to information on different identities. Not surprisingly since most of adolescents' daily lives are highly age-graded, peers are an important source of identity normative information; education is another prominent source.

A particular challenge adolescents face is learning to balance being presently guided by more immediate identity-relevant goals and actions or by more future ones (.g., possible self; Markus and Nurius 1986). The relative weighting of immediate and future identities depends on many interacting factors (e.g., personality), but we suggest support for autonomy or self-direction is essential since individuals' engage in self-directed actions that are consistent with what they value and find meaningful (Vansteenkiste et al. 2010). Encouraging adolescents' self-direction, then, would foster interest as well as the creation of purpose and meaning (Hidi and Renninger 2006; Hill et al. 2013). Thus, a greater degree of freedom to self-direct within the contexts and systems of adolescents' lives should facilitate identity development.

Developmental Task: "Real-World" Agency

The development of identity is closely linked to the development of capacities for exercising agency—a learned ability to deliberately act in order to set and achieve desired goals or outcomes (c.f. Bandura 2006; Larson 2000). Although agency can certainly be considered as a generalized pattern for engaging one's environment (Little et al. 2006), in this section we focus on a line of research by Larson and colleagues on adolescents' development of a specific set of skills for the exercise of agency within real-world, adult-typical settings (Larson and Hansen 2005; Larson and Angus 2011; Larson et al. 2005; Larson et al. 2014). In the United States, capacities for exercising agency under real-world conditions are increasingly needed across domains of adult life (Larson 2000). For example, adults need "skills to set goals, formulate plans, and work over time to achieve the goals. Most importantly, they need to do this in ways that anticipate the open-ended and not-always-logical system dynamics of real-world environments" (Larson et al. 2014, p. 3). Youth programs, such as leadership, arts, and civic action programs, are a common setting in adolescents' lives for learning skills for agency (Gootman and Eccles 2002; Mahoney et al. 2005). An important feature of youth programs is that adolescents' participation is voluntary, which should promote self-direction within this setting.

Motivationally, exercising agency under real-world conditions requires the "the ability to be motivated from within to direct attention and effort toward a challenging goal" (Larson 2000, p. 170). The key to developing this capacity is the pairing of intrinsic motivation (e.g., enjoyment) with challenge, that is, addressing the challenges and demands of a task or activity become a primary source enjoyment (Csikszentmihalyi and Rathunde 1993; Larson 2000; Moore and Hansen 2012). Intrinsic motivation (e.g., enjoyment), then, is an important, albeit not sufficient, mechanism that supports sustained engagement in an activity or task (Ryan and Deci 2000). Cognitively, exercising agency under real-world conditions requires learning "strategic thinking" skills, including planning and forethought (e.g., problem representation, tasks sequencing) that is less rigid and more adaptive, higher-order abstract reasoning for understanding and coordinating actions within complex institutional systems, and advanced perspective taking that can anticipate others' actions, intentions, and reactions (Larson and Hansen 2005; Larson and Angus 2011; Larson et al. 2014). Furthermore, these advanced motivation and cognitive capacities are predicated on the expansion of metacognition and self-regulation capacities.

Grounded theory research suggests adolescents' learn skills for the exercise of agency through three processes (Larson and Hansen 2005; Larson and Angus 2011; Larson et al. 2005; Larson et al. 2014). First, adolescents' learn agency from engaging with the *a priori* requirements (e.g., "I had to) and tactical demands (e.g., challenges of the work, such as logistics of running event) of their work on projects (Larson et al. 2005). By engaging these demands, adolescents' appear to develop strategies for self-motivation as well as creative and analytic reasoning about how to meet the demands, e.g., concrete organizing skills (Larson and Hansen 2005;

Larson et al. 2014). Second, adolescents appear to learn agency from feedback on the success and failure of their work, e.g., how effective their strategies were. Finally, adults in the youth programs can provide instrumental support as adolescents work on their projects (Larson and Angus 2011). Adults can support adolescents' learning by "keeping youth on track" (e.g., reminder of looming deadline), and by keeping control over the work with the adolescents, often resisting the urge to take over youths work to ensure intended outcomes (Larson and Walker 2010). The research of Larson and colleagues suggests adolescents are capable of learning skills to exercise "real-world" agency and that the setting and its supports can promote, or conversely thwart, their agency development.

Cultural and Agency

From a cultural psychological perspective, culture shapes the mind and the mind in turn creates culture in a cycle of mutual construction (Adams 2012). Given that adolescence is a social construct (Youniss 1983), different societies are likely to have varying constructions of what adolescence represents, how adolescents are expected to develop, and how they should behave. Moreover, because of the adolescent brain's plasticity and experience-dependent developmental systems, the cultural environment is likely to greatly affect neural reorganization during adolescence. Therefore, the ways in which adolescents' metacognition, self-regulation, and self-determination shape their expressions of identity, purpose, and agency will vary across cultures.

Cultural mandates about self-construal likely define the developmental tasks that are seen as culturally-appropriate for adolescents, which in turn are manifested in psychological tendencies (Kitayama et al. 2009; Markus and Kitayama 1991). For example, research by Higgins and colleagues has shown that while self-regulation might be a common cognitive process for all humans, there are differences in the regulatory focus of goals pursued (Higgins and Silberman 1998; Shah et al. 1998). In Western or individualistic cultures, goals that allow self-promotion tend to be favored, but in non-Western or collectivistic cultures goals that prevent social disharmony tend to be favored (Lee et al. 2000). Preferences for different types of goals may be shaped by differing parenting practices and socialization strategies that emphasize nurturance (favoring promotion goals) or security (favoring prevention goals) (Higgins and Silberman 1998). In turn, these preferences and differences in regulatory-focus may impact the types of role models that adolescents' gravitate toward (Lockwood et al. 2002) and their motivational-regulation of distal vs. proximal goal achievement (Pennington and Roese 2003). In addition, research by Kagitcibasi (2005, 2013) has shown a view of adolescent development that emphasizes individuation-separation (as opposed to a self-determination focus on autonomy and volition) may not be applicable to non-Western cultures, such as Turkey, where autonomy-relatedness in the family context is a more optimal outcome for adolescents. Similarly, in some East Asian societies, reciprocal filial piety—not emotional separation—is seen as a developmental strength or desired dispositional trait for autonomous adolescents and young adults (Pan et al. 2013).

Identity is another aspect of adolescent development that varies across cultures due to the fact that identity is shaped by the dynamic ecological systems in which the individual is embedded. For example, Côté and Levine (2014) emphasize the ecological aspects of Erikson's adolescent identity development theory in their explanation of a culture-identity framework that is influenced by macro-level structural shifts in societies over time. These authors' argue that in modern societies, adolescents' and young adults' experience an almost perpetual state of moratorium and diffusion driven by the image-oriented management of loosely structured identities in a cycle of continuous discovery. Similarly, others have theorized that globalization presents a multiplicity of pathways to adolescent identity that can complicate cultural identity formation (Arnett-Jensen 2003; Jensen et al. 2011). There is also research suggesting that hegemonic cultural globalization can lead adolescents from non-Western Caribbean cultures to incorporate aspects of Western, Americanized identities into their own local cultural identities (Ferguson and Bornstein 2012, 2015).

However, culture is not solely a deterministic force; rather, culture can be viewed as a tool for agentic identity construction. According to Holland (2001, p. 4) "identities are improvised—in the flow of activity within specific social situations—from the cultural resources at hand." In this way, tangible and intangible sociocultural/psychological affordances (such as level of education and resilience) serve as identity capital for malleable configuration of the self and strategic investment in the self and salient others or ideologies (Cote and Levine 2014). The amount of identity capital that individual adolescents are afforded in their cultural environment will vary by specific social situations, and will impact (1) the extent to which they are able to explore and master different identity roles, and (2) the level of agency that they exercise in fulfillment of valued roles (Cote and Levine 2014; Côté and Schwartz 2002). Thus, culturally-embedded learning processes shape identity and agency development (Flum and Kaplan 2012).

Conclusion

Adolescence represents a remarkable time of accelerated development, unparalleled at any other point in the lifespan after early childhood. Within the puberty-driven physical and neurological changes, societies have constructed what it means to be an adolescent, including what we think adolescents are and are not capable of. We can boil down this chapter to two major points. First, adolescents' rapidly become capable of learning skills for directing and regulating themselves, as well as making a meaningful contribution (e.g., identity) to society by learning skills for exercising agency. Second, whether or not adolescents accomplish important developmental tasks is less about their cognitive and affective capabilities than it is about how society, and the contexts within it, support these developmental tasks. Our present view is that adolescence represents a unique window of learning opportunity but this opportunity we think is being squandered, for example through overly restrictive and rigid standards-driven education that minimizes self-determination and agency, as well as pervasive age-grading across most domains of adolescents' lives that limits their access to socially relevant models of agency among adults. Without offering concrete solutions for how to support self-determination, identity, and agency, we run the risk of be a critic, but to offer 'solutions' here would far exceed the scope of the chapter. However, we suggest that asking how the settings and institutions in adolescents' life presently support or thwart these important developmental task is a needed first step in finding solutions.

References

Adams, G. (2012). Context in person, person in context: A cultural psychology approach to social-personality psychology. In *The Oxford handbook of personality and social psychology* (pp. 182–208).

Amso, D., & Casey, B. (2006). Beyond what develops when neuroimaging may inform how cognition changes with development. *Current Directions in Psychological Science, 15*(1), 24–29.

Arnett, J. J. (2000). Emerging adulthood: A theory of development from the late teens through the twenties. *American Psychologist, 55*(5), 469.

Arnett-Jensen, L. (2003). Coming of age in a multicultural world: Globalization and adolescent cultural identity formation. *Applied Developmental Science, 7*(3), 189–196.

Baltes, P. B. (1997). On the incomplete architecture of human ontogeny: Selection, optimization, and compensation as foundation of developmental theory. *American Psychologist, 52*(4), 366.

Bandura, A. (1982). Self-efficacy mechanism in human agency. *American Psychologist, 37*(2), 122.

Bandura, A. (1986). *Social foundations of thought and action: A social cognitive theory*. Englewood Cliffs: Prentice-Hall, Inc..

Bandura, A. (2006). Toward a psychology of human agency. *Perspectives on Psychological Science, 1*(2), 164–180.

Bechara, A., Damasio, H., Tranel, D., & Damasio, A. R. (1997). Deciding advantageously before knowing the advantageous strategy. *Science, 275*(5304), 1293–1295.

Blakemore, S. J., Burnett, S., & Dahl, R. E. (2010). The role of puberty in the developing adolescent brain. *Human Brain Mapping, 31*(6), 926–933.

Boekaerts, M., Pintrich, P. R., & Zeidner, M. (2005). *Handbook of self-regulation*. Burlington: Elsevier.

Bourgeois, J.-P., Goldman-Rakic, P. S., & Rakic, P. (1994). Synaptogenesis in the prefrontal cortex of rhesus monkeys. *Cerebral Cortex, 4*(1), 78–96.

Casey, B., & Jones, R. M. (2010). Neurobiology of the adolescent brain and behavior: Implications for substance use disorders. *Journal of the American Academy of Child and Adolescent Psychiatry, 49*(12), 1189–1201.

Casey, B., Amso, D., & Davidson, M. C. (2006). Learning about learning and development with neuroimaging. In *Attention and performance XXI: Processes of change in brain and cognitive development*.

Casey, B., Jones, R. M., & Hare, T. A. (2008). The adolescent brain. *Annals of the New York Academy of Sciences, 1124*(1), 111–126.

Cote, J. E., & Levine, C. G. (2014). *Identity, formation, agency, and culture: A social psychological synthesis*. New York: Psychology Press.

Côté, J. E., & Schwartz, S. J. (2002). Comparing psychological and sociological approaches to identity: Identity status, identity capital, and the individualization process. *Journal of Adolescence, 25*(6), 571–586.

Crocetti, E., Rubini, M., Luyckx, K., & Meeus, W. (2008). Identity formation in early and middle adolescents from various ethnic groups: From three dimensions to five statuses. *Journal of Youth and Adolescence, 37*(8), 983–996.

Crocetti, E., Scrignaro, M., Sica, L. S., & Magrin, M. E. (2012). Correlates of identity configurations: Three studies with adolescent and emerging adult cohorts. *Journal of Youth and Adolescence, 41*(6), 732–748.

Csikszentmihalyi, M., & Rathunde, K. (1993). The measurement of flow in everyday life: Toward a theory of emergent motivation.

Cutler, G. B., Jr. (1991). Adrenarche. In R. M. Lerner, A. C. Petersen, & J. Brooks-Gunn (Eds.), *Encyclopedia of adolescence* (Vol. I, pp. 14–7). New York: Garland Publishing.

Deci, E. L., & Ryan, R. (2002). Overview of self-determination theory: An organismic dialectical perspective. In *Handbook of self-determination research* (pp. 3–33).

Demetriou, A. (2000). Organization and development of self-understanding and self-regulation: Toward a general theory.

Dinsmore, D. L., Alexander, P. A., & Loughlin, S. M. (2008). Focusing the conceptual lens on metacognition, self-regulation, and self-regulated learning. *Educational Psychology Review, 20*(4), 391–409.

Dorn, L. D., Dahl, R. E., Woodward, H. R., & Biro, F. (2006). Defining the boundaries of early adolescence: A user's guide to assessing pubertal status and pubertal timing in research with adolescents. *Applied Developmental Science, 10*(1), 30–56.

Erikson, E. (1950). *Childhood and society: 1963*. New York: WW Norton & Co., Inc.

Erikson, E. (1968). *Youth: Identity and crisis*. New York: WW.

Evans, J. S. B. (1996). Deciding before you think: Relevance and reasoning in the selection task. *British Journal of Psychology, 87*(2), 223–240.

Ferguson, G. M., & Bornstein, M. H. (2012). Remote acculturation: The "Americanization" of Jamaican islanders. *International Journal of Behavioral Development, 36*(3), 167–177.

Ferguson, G. M., & Bornstein, M. H. (2015). Remote acculturation of early adolescents in Jamaica towards European American culture: A replication and extension. *International Journal of Intercultural Relations, 45*, 24–35.

Fitzsimons, G. M., & Finkel, E. J. (2011). The effects of self-regulation on social relationships. In *Handbook of self-regulation: Research, theory, and applications* (pp. 407–421).

Flum, H., & Kaplan, A. (2012). Identity formation in educational settings: A contextualized view of theory and research in practice. *Contemporary Educational Psychology, 37*(3), 240–245.

Foltz, C., & Overton, W. F. (1995). Proof construction: Adolescent development from inductive to deductive problem-solving strategies. *Journal of Experimental Child Psychology, 59*(2), 179–195.

Fuster, J. M. (2001). The prefrontal cortex—An update: Time is of the essence. *Neuron, 30*(2), 319–333.

Fuster, J. M. (2002). Frontal lobe and cognitive development. *Journal of Neurocytology, 31*(3–5), 373–385.

Giedd, J. N., Stockman, M., Weddle, C., Liverpool, M., Alexander-Bloch, A., Wallace, G. L., et al. (2010). Anatomic magnetic resonance imaging of the developing child and adolescent brain and effects of genetic variation. *Neuropsychology Review, 20*(4), 349–361.

Gollwitzer, P. M., & Sheeran, P. (2006). Implementation intentions and goal achievement: A meta-analysis of effects and processes. *Advances in Experimental Social Psychology, 38*, 69–119.

Gootman, J. A., & Eccles, J. (2002). *Community programs to promote youth development*. Washington, DC: National Academies Press.

Greenough, W. T., Black, J. E., & Wallace, C. S. (2002a). In Johnson, M. H., Munakata, Y., Gilmore, R. O., (Eds.), *Brain development and cognition: A reader* (2nd ed., pp. 186–216), Chapter xiv, 544 Pages. Blackwell Publishing.

Greenough, W. T., Black, J. E., & Wallace, C. S. (2002b). Experience and brain development. In M. H. Johnson, Y. Munakata & R. O. Gilmore (Eds.), ItemValueImpl (label = publication title value = brain development and cognition: A reader (2nd ed.)] blockName = text mnemonic = pub mnemonicSearchType = ExactMatch template = null) (2nd ed., pp. 186–216, Chapter xiv, 544 Pages). Malden: Blackwell Publishing. Retrieved from https://search-proquest-com.www2.lib.ku.edu/docview/620087228?accountid=14556

Grossman, A. W., Churchill, J. D., Bates, K. E., Kleim, J. A., & Greenough, W. T. (2002). A brain adaptation view of plasticity: Is synaptic plasticity an overly limited concept? *Progress in Brain Research, 138*, 91–108.

Hall, G. S. (1904). *Adolescence: Its psychology and its relations to physiology, anthropology, sociology, sex, crime, religion, and education* (Vol. II).

Havighurst, R. J. (1948). Developmental tasks and education.

He, J., & Crews, F. T. (2007). Neurogenesis decreases during brain maturation from adolescence to adulthood. *Pharmacology Biochemistry and Behavior, 86*(2), 327–333.

Hidi, S., & Renninger, K. A. (2006). The four-phase model of interest development. *Educational Psychologist, 41*(2), 111–127.

Higgins, E. T., & Silberman, I. (1998). *Development of regulatory focus: Promotion and prevention as ways of living*. New York: Springer.

Hill, P. L., & Burrow, A. L. (2012). Viewing purpose through an Eriksonian lens. *Identity, 12*(1), 74–91.

Hill, P. L., Burrow, A. L., & Sumner, R. (2013). Addressing important questions in the field of adolescent purpose. *Child Development Perspectives, 7*(4), 232–236.

Holland, D. (2001). *Identity and agency in cultural worlds*. Cambridge, MA: Harvard University Press.

Huttenlocher, P. R. (1979). Synaptic density in human frontal cortex-developmental changes and effects of aging. *Brain Research, 163*(2), 195–205.

Huttenlocher, P. R. (1984). Synapse elimination and plasticity in developing human cerebral cortex. *American Journal of Mental Deficiency, 88*(5), 488–496.

Inhelder, B. A., & Piaget, J. (1958). *The growth oflogical thinking*. New York: Basic Books.

Jensen, L. A., Arnett, J. J., & McKenzie, J. (2011). Globalization and cultural identity. In *Handbook of identity theory and research* (pp. 285–301). New York: Springer.

Kagitcibasi, C. (2005). Autonomy and relatedness in cultural context implications for self and family. *Journal of Cross-Cultural Psychology, 36*(4), 403–422.

Kagitcibasi, C. (2013). Adolescent autonomy-relatedness and the family in cultural context: What is optimal? *Journal of Research on Adolescence, 23*(2), 223–235.

Keating, D. (2004). Cognitive and brain development. In R. M. Lerner & L. Steinberg (Eds.), *Handbook of adolescent psychology* (pp. 45–84). New York: Wiley.

Kitayama, S., Park, H., Sevincer, A. T., Karasawa, M., & Uskul, A. K. (2009). A cultural task analysis of implicit independence: Comparing North America, Western Europe, and East Asia. *Journal of Personality and Social Psychology, 97*(2), 236.

Klaczynski, P. A. (2001a). Analytic and heuristic processing influences on adolescent reasoning and decision-making. *Child Development*, 844–861.

Klaczynski, P. A. (2001b). Framing effects on adolescent task representations, analytic and heuristic processing, and decision making: Implications for the normative/descriptive gap. *Journal of Applied Developmental Psychology, 22*(3), 289–309.

Klaczynski, P. A., Byrnes, J. P., & Jacobs, J. E. (2001). Introduction to the special issue: The development of decision making. *Journal of Applied Developmental Psychology, 22*(3), 225–236.

Larson, R. W. (2000). Toward a psychology of positive youth development. *American Psychologist, 55*(1), 170.

Larson, R. W., & Angus, R. M. (2011). Adolescents' development of skills for agency in youth programs: Learning to think strategically. *Child Development, 82*(1), 277–294.

Larson, R., & Hansen, D. (2005). The development of strategic thinking: Learning to impact human systems in a youth activism program. *Human Development, 48*(6), 327–349.

Larson, R. W., & Walker, K. C. (2010). Dilemmas of practice: Challenges to program quality encountered by youth program leaders. *American Journal of Community Psychology, 45*(3–4), 338–349.

Larson, R. W., Hansen, D. M., & Walker, K. (2005). Everybody's gotta give: Development of initiative and teamwork within a youth program. In *Organized activities as contexts of development: Extracurricular activities, after-school and community programs* (pp. 159–183).

Larson, R. W., Lampkins-Uthando, S., & Armstrong, J. (2014). Adolescents' development of new skills for prospective cognition: Learning to anticipate, plan, and think strategically. *Journal of Cognitive Education and Psychology, 13*(2), 232–244.

Lee, A. Y., Aaker, J. L., & Gardner, W. L. (2000). The pleasures and pains of distinct self-construals: the role of interdependence in regulatory focus. *Journal of Personality and Social Psychology, 78*(6), 1122.

Little, T. D., Snyder, C., & Wehmeyer, M. (2006). The agentic self: On the nature and origins of personal agency across the lifespan.

Lockwood, P., Jordan, C. H., & Kunda, Z. (2002). Motivation by positive or negative role models: regulatory focus determines who will best inspire us. *Journal of Personality and Social Psychology, 83*(4), 854.

Luna, B., & Sweeney, J. A. (2004). The emergence of collaborative brain function: FMRI studies of the development of response inhibition. *Annals of the New York Academy of Sciences, 1021*(1), 296–309.

Luna, B., Padmanabhan, A., & O'Hearn, K. (2010). What has fMRI told us about the development of cognitive control through adolescence? *Brain and Cognition, 72*(1), 101–113.

Mahoney, J. L., Larson, R. W., Eccles, J. S., & Lord, H. (2005). Organized activities as developmental contexts for children and adolescents. In *Organized activities as contexts of development: Extracurricular activities, after-school and community programs* (pp. 3–22).

Marcia, J. E. (1966). Development and validation of ego-identity status. *Journal of Personality and Social Psychology, 3*(5), 551.

Marcia, J. E. (1967). Ego identity status: Relationship to change in self-esteem, "general maladjustment," and authoritarianism. *Journal of Personality, 35*(1), 118–133.

Marcia, J. E. (1987). The identity status approach to the study of ego identity development.

Markham, J. A., & Greenough, W. T. (2004). Experience-driven brain plasticity: Beyond synapse. *Neuron Glia Biology, 1*(4), 351–363.

Markus, H. R., & Kitayama, S. (1991). Cultural variation in the self-concept. In *The self: Interdisciplinary approaches* (pp. 18–48). New York: Springer.

Markus, H., & Nurius, P. (1986). Possible selves. *American Psychologist, 41*(9), 954.

Miller, P. H., Kessel, F. S., & Flavell, J. H. (1970). Thinking about people thinking about people thinking about...: A study of social cognitive development. *Child Development*, 613–623.

Moore, E. W. G., & Hansen, D. (2012). Construct-validity of the engagement with challenge measure for adolescents: Structural-and criterion-validity evidence. *Psychology, 3*(10), 923.

Mortimer, J. T., & Larson, R. W. (2002). Macrostructural trends and the reshaping of adolescence. In*The changing adolescent experience: Societal trends and the transition to adulthood* (pp. 1–17). Cambridge: Cambridge University Press.

Moshman, D. (1982). Exogenous, endogenous, and dialectical constructivism. *Developmental Review, 2*(4), 371–384.

Moshman, D. (1998). Cognitive development beyond childhood. *Educational Psychology Papers and Publications*, 48.

Muuss, R. (1996). Theories of adolescents. New York: McGraw Hill.

Nelson, C. A., Thomas, K. M., & Haan, M. (2006). Neural bases of cognitive development. In*Handbook of child psychology*. New York: Wiley.

Pan, Y., Gauvain, M., & Schwartz, S. J. (2013). Do parents' collectivistic tendency and attitudes toward filial piety facilitate autonomous motivation among young Chinese adolescents? *Motivation and Emotion, 37*(4), 701–711.

Papies, E. K., & Aarts, H. (2010). Nonconscious self-regulation or the automatic pilot of human behavior. In*Handbook of self-regulation: Research, theory, and applications* (pp. 125–142). New York: Guilford Press.

Papies, E. K., Aarts, H., & De Vries, N. K. (2009). Planning is for doing: Implementation intentions go beyond the mere creation of goal-directed associations. *Journal of Experimental Social Psychology, 45*(5), 1148–1151.

Paus, T. (2010). Growth of white matter in the adolescent brain: Myelin or axon? *Brain and Cognition, 72*(1), 26–35.

Paus, T., Zijdenbos, A., Worsley, K., Collins, D. L., Blumenthal, J., Giedd, J. N., et al. (1999). Structural maturation of neural pathways in children and adolescents: In vivo study. *Science, 283*(5409), 1908–1911.

Pennington, G. L., & Roese, N. J. (2003). Regulatory focus and temporal distance. *Journal of Experimental Social Psychology, 39*(6), 563–576.

Phinney, J. S. (1989). Stages of ethnic identity development in minority group adolescents. *The Journal of Early Adolescence, 9*(1–2), 34–49.

Phinney, J. S., & Chavira, V. (1992). Ethnic identity and self-esteem: An exploratory longitudinal study. *Journal of Adolescence, 15*(3), 271–281.

Phinney, J. S., & Ong, A. D. (2007). Conceptualization and measurement of ethnic identity: Current status and future directions. *Journal of Counseling Psychology, 54*(3), 271.

Rakic, P., Bourgeois, J.-P., & Goldman-Rakic, P. S. (1994). Synaptic development of the cerebral cortex: Implications for learning, memory, and mental. *The Self-Organizing Brain: From Growth Cones to Functional Networks, 102*, 227.

Rosenblum, L. A. (1990). A comparative primate perspective on adolescence. In*Adolescence and puberty* (pp. 63–69). New York: Oxford University Press.

Ryan, R. M., & Deci, E. L. (2000). Self-determination theory and the facilitation of intrinsic motivation, social development, and well-being. *American Psychologist, 55*(1), 68.

Sala, S., Agosta, F., Pagani, E., Copetti, M., Comi, G., & Filippi, M. (2012). Microstructural changes and atrophy in brain white matter tracts with aging. *Neurobiology of Aging, 33*(3), 488–498 e482.

Schwartz, S. J., Zamboanga, B. L., Meca, A., & Ritchie, R. A. (2012). Identity around the world: An overview. *New Directions for Child and Adolescent Development, 2012*(138), 1–18.

Seeman, P., Bzowej, N. H., Guan, H. C., Bergeron, C., Becker, L. E., Reynolds, G. P., et al. (1987). Human brain dopamine receptors in children and aging adults. *Synapse, 1*(5), 399–404. doi:10.1002/syn.890010503.

Sellers, R. M., Smith, M. A., Shelton, J. N., Rowley, S. A., & Chavous, T. M. (1998). Multidimensional model of racial identity: A reconceptualization of African American racial identity. *Personality and Social Psychology Review, 2*(1), 18–39.

Shah, J., Higgins, T., & Friedman, R. S. (1998). Performance incentives and means: How regulatory focus influences goal attainment. *Journal of Personality and Social Psychology, 74*(2), 285.

Somerville, L. H., Jones, R. M., & Casey, B. (2010). A time of change: Behavioral and neural correlates of adolescent sensitivity to appetitive and aversive environmental cues. *Brain and Cognition, 72*(1), 124–133.

Sowell, E. R., Thompson, P. M., Holmes, C. J., Jernigan, T. L., & Toga, A. W. (1999). In vivo evidence for post-adolescent brain maturation in frontal and striatal regions. *Nature Neuroscience, 2*(10), 859–861.

Sowell, E. R., Thompson, P. M., Tessner, K. D., & Toga, A. W. (2001). Mapping continued brain growth and gray matter density reduction in dorsal frontal cortex: Inverse relationships during postadolescent brain maturation. *The Journal of Neuroscience, 21*(22), 8819–8829.

Spear, L. P. (2000). The adolescent brain and age-related behavioral manifestations. *Neuroscience & Biobehavioral Reviews, 24*(4), 417–463.

Steinberg, L. (2008). A social neuroscience perspective on adolescent risk-taking. *Developmental Review, 28*(1), 78–106.

Sturman, D. A., & Moghaddam, B. (2011). The neurobiology of adolescence: Changes in brain architecture, functional dynamics, and behavioral tendencies. *Neuroscience & Biobehavioral Reviews, 35*(8), 1704–1712.

Umaña-Taylor, A. J., Quintana, S. M., Lee, R. M., Cross, W. E., Rivas-Drake, D., Schwartz, S. J., et al. (2014). Ethnic and racial identity during adolescence and into young adulthood: An integrated conceptualization. *Child Development, 85*(1), 21–39.

Vansteenkiste, M., Niemiec, C., Soenens, B., Urdan, T., & Karabenick, S. (2010). Advances in motivation and achievement: The decade ahead.

Youniss, J. (1983). Social construction of adolescence by adolescents and parents. *New Directions for Child and Adolescent Development, 1983*(22), 93–109.

Zimmerman, B. J. (1989). A social cognitive view of self-regulated academic learning. *Journal of Educational Psychology, 81*(3), 329.

Zimmerman, B. J. (2008). Investigating self-regulation and motivation: Historical background, methodological developments, and future prospects. *American Educational Research Journal, 45*(1), 166–183.

Zimmerman, B. J., & Schunk, D. H. (2008). An essential dimension of self-regulated learning. In *Motivation and self-regulated learning: Theory, research, and applications*, 1.

Chapter 4
Self-Determination Theory

Nicole Adams, Todd D. Little, and Richard M. Ryan

Abstract This chapter provides an introduction to Self-Determination Theory, a macro-theory that details the origins and outcomes of human agentic action. Basic psychological needs for autonomy, competence, and relatedness in Self-Determination Theory are introduced as is the relationship of need satisfaction to intrinsic motivation and the regulation of extrinsic motivation. Mini-theories associated with self-determination are introduced, and research on self-determination summarized.

Self-Determination Theory (SDT) is one of several prominent approaches to studying human motivation (Weiner 1990). A departure from most theories that treat motivation as a unitary concept, SDT differentiates motivation into autonomous and controlled types (Deci and Ryan 2008). The initial work leading to SDT began in the 1970s and was formalized especially in the eighties by Edward L Deci and Richard M Ryan (e.g., Deci and Ryan 1980, 1985b). Since then the formal theory and applications of SDT have expanded greatly (Deci and Ryan 2000; Ryan and Deci 2000, 2011).

Today SDT represents a comprehensive macro-theory that details the origins and outcomes of human agentic action (Vansteenkiste et al. 2012). SDT is based on the *organismic paradigm* or *metatheory*; one that assumes humans are active organisms, motivated to assimilate and integrate knowledge and capacities in both their physical and social environments. (Ryan 1995). As a contrast to theories that stress the dependence of behavior on environmental or biological contingencies, SDT views human behavior as growth-oriented and proactive (Deci and Ryan 2012). According to this theory, both the bright and dark sides of human behavior—its active constructive nature and its passive and defensive manifestations are both understood as outcomes of the interaction between people's basic psychological

N. Adams (✉)
Texas Tech University, Lubbock, TX, USA
e-mail: nikadams5513@gmail.com

T.D. Little
Educational Psychology and Leadership, Texas Tech University, Lubbock, TX, USA

R.M. Ryan
Australian Catholic University, Banyo, QLD, Australia

M.L. Wehmeyer et al. (eds.), *Development of Self-Determination Through the Life-Course*, DOI 10.1007/978-94-024-1042-6_4

needs and the sources of need support or thwarting in social environments (Vansteenkiste and Ryan 2013).

SDT initially grew from a foundation of research on the effects of intrinsic and extrinsic rewards on human motivation (Deci and Ryan 1980). Early evidence suggested an external incentive such as receiving monetary reward for solving puzzles can decrease intrinsic motivation for that task (e.g., Deci 1971). Conversely, when given positive, competence relevant feedback, participants' intrinsic motivation could be enhanced. These findings prompted further study of the quality of motivation, which, before SDT, had historically been primarily studied in quantity only (Deci and Ryan 1985b, 2008).

The effects of extrinsic rewards on autonomous motivation can be understood in terms of both ones perceived locus of personal causality, or autonomy, and basic psychological needs satisfaction (Ryan and Deci 2000). deCharms (1968) originally described the concept of perceived locus of causality in terms of the "Origin-Pawn" concept, an issue he understood to be central to human motivation. To illustrate the origin-pawn concept, we describe a longitudinal study deCharms (1972) conducted to test whether treating students as origins or pawns affected their perceptions of personal causality, and indirectly, their academic achievement. Students in an experimental (trained) group were encouraged over the course of several years to determine realistic goals for themselves, know their strengths and weaknesses, determine actions they could take to reach their goals, and evaluate whether their actions were leading to the desired outcome. Compared to students in the non-trained group, students in the trained group had increased scores on measures tapping their sense of being an origin for their behaviors, and ultimately, they also showed improved academic achievement. The origin measures included categories for internal goal setting, internal determination of instrumental activity, reality perception, personal responsibility, self-confidence, and internal control. deCharms previously had referred to the underlying construct related to origin behavior as intrinsic motivation or internal causation, but emphasized the concept of origin-pawn to highlight the locus of causality associated with internal versus external motivations (1968).

Deci and Ryan (1985b) were early on influenced by both deCharms' (1968) origin-pawn distinction and by White's (1959) conceptualizations of effectance motivation as applied to intrinsic motivation. Deci and Ryan built upon these concepts in their early theorizing about the determinants of intrinsic motivation, and later expanded SDT as a full motivational theory, concerned with the energization and direction of intrinsic and extrinsic behavior (1985b).

Deci and Ryan (1985b, 2000) emphasize that SDT, as an organismic meta-theory, views humans as proactive beings with the propensity to assimilate and integrate both their internal states and their mastery and understanding of the social and environmental circumstances they encounter. Humans, that is, are viewed as striving toward growth and optimal development, not merely shaped by social learning or stimulus response pairing. Yet in order to attain optimal development and functioning, people require certain positive supports from the environment. Hence, SDT frames optimal human development as the interaction between growth-striving humans and their social environment in which *basic psychological needs* are either supported or thwarted. When needs are supported both greater growth and higher well-being result.

According to SDT, the critical social environment supports are described in terms of three specific basic psychological needs, namely the needs for competence, autonomy, and relatedness (Deci and Ryan 2000; Ryan 1995). In social environments that support the satisfaction of these needs, optimal growth and positive development are expected whereas in social environments that thwart satisfaction of any of these fundamental needs, greater passivity, alienation and ill-being are expected.

Satisfaction of the three basic psychological needs is thus a foundational concept to SDT and considered essential for maintaining intrinsic motivation and the self-regulation of extrinsic motivations (Deci and Ryan 2000). The *need for competence* reflects humans' desire to effectively master their environment and experience a sense of competence in it. An important distinction is that humans experience satisfaction of the need for competence not necessarily as an absolute level of achievement but instead as a "phenomenological" experience in which a person experiences increasing mastery and effectance (Deci et al. 2013, p. 112). The *need for autonomy* is satisfied when an individual experiences choice and volition in their action, and perceives themselves to be the origin of their actions. Autonomous actions are those that are self-endorsed, and congruent with one's values and interest (Vansteenkiste et al. 2010). Finally, the *need for relatedness* is associated with social belonging. Relatedness is a satisfaction derived from a sense of connectedness with others; to care and be cared for by others (Deci et al. 2013; Ryan and Deci 2000).

In the development of self-determination theory, Deci and Ryan incorporated the fundamental concepts of motivation and basic psychological needs into six mini-theories, each addressing different problems of motivation theory. Together, these mini-theories explain the operations of self-determination theory in a complex social world (Deci and Ryan 2012). Described below, the mini-theories are cognitive evaluative theory (CET), organismic integration theory (OIT), causality orientations theory (COT), basic psychological needs theory (BPNT), goal content theory (GCT), and relationships motivation theory (RMT). These mini-theories each explain a set of observed motivation phenomena in various domains of functioning (Ryan and Deci 2011).

Deci and Ryan (1980) first introduced *cognitive evaluation theory* (CET) to organize empirical research uncovered in experimental manipulations and field studies related to how external events could enhance or diminish intrinsic motivation. CET argues that autonomy supportive social contexts enhance intrinsic motivation, whereas controlling social contexts undermine it. In addition CET suggests that positive competence feedback enhances motivation whereas feedback suggesting incompetence diminishes it. Subsequently, Deci and Ryan introduced a new mini-theory to further explain individual differences in motivation-related behavior, proposing trait-like motivational orientations. *Causality orientations theory* (COT) proposes three different personality orientations based on people's tendencies to orient to different sources of behavioral initiation and regulation, specifying three

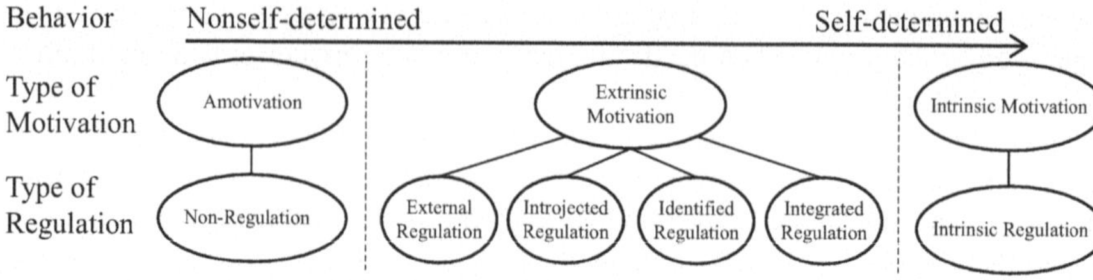

Fig. 4.1 The continuum of self-determination as described by organismic integration theory showing the variation in degree of self-determination according to the motivational and self-regulatory origins of behavior (Adapted from Ryan and Deci 2000)

types of orientation, autonomous, controlled, or impersonal (Deci and Ryan 1985a). An individual with autonomous orientation is said to orient toward internal and external cues in a way that supports their autonomy and provides information significant to their actions. An individual with controlled orientation is said to focus on external cues and contingencies in regulation actions, and thus is prone to more extrinsic and controlled types of motives. Finally, an individual with impersonal orientation is said to be especially sensitive to cues as indicators of incompetence and is linked with amotivation.

Acknowledging that most common daily activities are not intrinsically motivated, Deci and Ryan developed a third mini-theory under the SDT umbrella detailing the degree of autonomy involved in extrinsically motivated behavior. *Organismic integration theory* (OIT) explains behavior that is extrinsically motivated can be either controlled or autonomous (1985b). Thus, they recognized that motivation exists on a continuum and the quality of an individual's motivation and engagement depends on the type of extrinsic motivation they exhibited. OIT details six types of motivation existing on a continuum from extrinsic to intrinsic; amotivation, external regulation, introjected regulation, identified regulation, integrated regulation, and intrinsic motivation. Researchers have used this theory to explain how desirable behaviors that are more autonomously regulated tend to be maintained. Also, more autonomous forms of regulation have been shown to be associated with positive outcomes such as wellness, engagement, and perceived competence (Deci and Ryan 2012). Figure 4.1 illustrates the continuum of motivation from extrinsic to intrinsic and includes the source of regulation associated with each.

With mounting empirical evidence for the above mini-theories, Deci and Ryan (2000) noted continuing support for the importance of the three basic psychological needs; autonomy, competence, and relatedness (2012) for psychological well-being. They further formalized *basic psychological needs theory* (BPNT) based upon ample findings that environments and contexts where psychological needs were satisfied were associated with greater feelings of well-being, psychological health, and greater positive affect in multiple domains (Ryan et al. 2010).

Kasser and Ryan (1996) and colleagues further developed SDT by focusing research not just on *why* people were motivated to act, but also *what* they were pursuing in terms of the content focus of their goals and aspirations. The resulting theory, *goal content theory* (GCT) posits that extrinsic goals such as financial wealth, image, and fame are less likely to satisfy the three basic psychological needs compared to intrinsic goals such as personal growth, community and emotional closeness (Ryan et al. 1996, 1999). Research evidence for GCT indicates that pursuit of extrinsic goals leads to less well-being and poorer performance whereas pursuing intrinsic goals leads to greater well-being; a phenomenon best explained by increased satisfaction of the basic psychological needs (Deci and Ryan 2012).

Finally, and most recently Deci and Ryan (2014) articulated *relationships motivation theory* (RMT) to describe the need supportive elements most likely to lead to sustained and satisfying relationships. Beyond the idea that intimacy is about warmth, involvement and security, RMT argues that true relationship satisfaction depends on respect and caring for the *self* of the other. RMT helps explain variations in security of attachment as a function of autonomy support (e.g., La Guardia et al. 2000), and why parental styles such as contingent regard hamper both motivation and emotional wellness (e.g., Roth et al. 2009).

SDT's fundamental theoretical foundations; motivation , choice, and attributions, have fueled a rich empirical tradition. SDT has been applied to study a diverse array of issues such as health behavior initiation and maintenance, academics and school adjustment, psychotherapy, and sport and physical activity (Chen and Bozeman 2013; Curran et al. 2013; Gourlan et al. 2013; Vansteenkiste et al. 2013; Wang et al. 2011). Current findings in each of these domains provide additional information about the operation of the multidimensional framework of SDT as a predictor of external behavior, internal states, and other distal outcomes. For example, results of a recent meta-analysis of 184 SDT-based studies in the health domain by Ng et al. (2012) supported the interactions proposed by SDT. Overall, the findings showed that support for autonomy in the health care setting positively predicted patient competence and relatedness as well as autonomy in the health behavior domain. This analysis also showed that satisfaction of the three psychological needs was associated with moderate to strong levels of patient welfare (Ng et al. 2012). Deci et al. (1999) examined empirical evidence for another fundamental tenet of SDT; the potentially undermining effects of extrinsic rewards on intrinsic motivation. In their meta-analysis including 128 experimental studies, Deci et al. differentiated studies by the type of reward, according to cognitive evaluative theory (CET). Rewards were categorized as tangible or verbal, task-contingent or task-noncontingent, and expected or unexpected. As predicted by CET, all rewards did not affect intrinsic motivation in a uniform manner. Instead, in free-choice behavior, all tangible rewards, all expected rewards, engagement-contingent rewards, completion-contingent rewards, task-contingent rewards, and performance-contingent rewards significantly undermined intrinsic motivation. In general, positive feedback (verbal rewards) enhanced intrinsic motivation but had the opposite effect when delivered with a controlling interpersonal style. Finally a variety of randomized controlled trails have shown the efficacy of SDT as an approach to interventions (e.g., see Ryan et al. 2008).

In other recent studies researchers have applied SDT as a process model for change in physical rehabilitation for young adults with a physical disability (Saebu et al. 2013). In this study, researchers hypothesized a SDT process model for change in which perceived autonomy support during a physical activity intervention period would positively predict psychological needs satisfaction at the end of the intervention. In turn, this was expected to increase autonomous motivation and self-efficacy for physical activity which were both expected to lead to increased physical activity over the course of the intervention. Results supported the SDT process model with significant paths to each of the variables except for change in self-efficacy from autonomous motivation which was positive but non-significant (Saebu et al. 2013). SDT is also notably applied in education and academic functioning. A recent application of SDT involved examining the effects of self-talk on students' emotions and perception of their understanding new academic material. Oliver et al. (2010) assessed undergraduate students' self-talk following a lecture on research methods. According to cognitive evaluative theory, students construe their self-talk as informational or controlling, depending on the functional significance the student attaches to their inner dialogue. The perceived informational or controlling nature of this dialogue has important effects on anxiety and affect. Oliver et al. found students who evaluated their inner dialogue as informational were more likely to report positive affect following the lecture, independent of their understanding of the lecture material. Conversely, controlling self-talk was found to be associated with higher state anxiety following the lecture.

With SDT, Deci and Ryan have emphasized contextual factors and social influences play a significant role for motivation in multiple domains of human functioning. As such, an important aspect of determining sport and physical activity engagement is a coaches' role in creating an autonomy supportive atmosphere for athletes (Bartholomew et al. 2011). For example, using SDT as a framework for predicting behavioral engagement, Curran et al. (2013) found autonomy-supportive delivery of structural supports from coaches, (such as information, strategy, limits, and expectations) fostered ideal conditions for satisfaction of basic psychological needs. These contextual elements were also associated with higher levels of behavioral engagement and lower levels of behavioral disaffection.

SDT provides a comprehensive approach to the study of motivation and its associated antecedents and consequences. Deci and Ryan's multidimensional theory hinges on satisfaction of three basic psychological needs as underlying forces in motivated behavior. The six SDT mini-theories further account for behavior in multiple domains by explaining the complex interactions of environmental and contextual factors with individual traits and their learned behaviors. Viewed holistically, SDT provides a detailed framework for understanding the antecedents and consequences of intrinsic versus extrinsic motivation, and thus, human agency.

References

Bartholomew, K. J., Ntoumanis, N., Ryan, R. M., & Thogersen-Ntoumani, C. (2011). Psychological need thwarting in the sport context: Assessing the darker sides of athletic experience. *Journal of Sport and Exercise Psychology, 33*, 75–102.

Chen, C., & Bozeman, B. (2013). Understanding public and nonprofit managers' motivation through the lens of self-determination theory. *Public Management Review, 15*(4), 584–607.

Curran, T., Hill, A. P., & Niemiec, C. P. (2013). A conditional process model of children's behavioral engagement and behavioral disaffection in sport based on self-determination theory. *Journal Of Sport & Exercise Psychology, 35*(1), 30–43.

de Charms, R. (1968). *Personal causation: The internal affective determinants of behaviour.* New York: Academic Press.

de Charms, R. (1972). Personal causation training in the schools. *Journal of Applied Social Psychology, 2*, 95–113.

Deci, E. L. (1971). Effects of externally mediated rewards on intrinsic motivation. *Journal of Personality Psychology, 18*, 105–115.

Deci, E. L., & Ryan, R. M. (1980). The empirical exploration of intrinsic motivational processes. In L. Berkowitz (Ed.), *Advances in experimental social psychology* (Vol. 13, pp. 39–80). New York: Academic Press.

Deci, E. L., & Ryan, R. M. (1985a). The general causality orientations scale: Self-determination in personality. *Journal of Research in Personality, 19*, 109–134.

Deci, E. L., & Ryan, R. M. (1985b). *Intrinsic motivation and self-determination in human behavior.* New York: Plenum.

Deci, E. L., & Ryan, R. M. (2000). The 'what' and 'why' of goal pursuits: Human needs and the self-determination of behavior. *Psychological Inquiry, 11*, 227–268.

Deci, E. L., & Ryan, R. M. (2008). Facilitating optimal motivation and psychological well-being across life's domains. *Canadian Psychology, 49*, 14–23.

Deci, E. L., & Ryan, R. M. (2012). Motivation, personality, and development within embedded social contexts: An overview of self-determination theory. In R. M. Ryan (Ed.), *Oxford handbook of human motivation* (pp. 85–107). Oxford: Oxford University Press.

Deci, E. L., & Ryan, R. M. (2014). Autonomy and need satisfaction in close relationships: Relationships motivation theory. In N. Weinstein (Ed.), *Human motivation and interpersonal relationships: Theory, research and applications* (pp. 53–73). Dordrecht: Springer.

Deci, E. L., Koestner, R., & Ryan, R. M. (1999). A meta-analytic review of experiments examining the effects of extrinsic rewards on intrinsic motivation. *Psychological Bulletin, 125*, 627–668. doi:10.1037/0033-2909.125.6.627.

Deci, E. L., Ryan, R. M., & Guay, F. (2013). Self-determination theory and actualization of human potentials. In D. M. McInerney, H. W. Marsh, R. G. Craven, F. Guay, & D. M. McInerney (Eds.), *Theory driving research: New wave perspectives on self-processes and human development* (pp. 109–133). Charlotte: Information Age Publishing.

Gourlan, M., Sarrazin, P., & Trouilloud, D. (2013). Motivational interviewing as a way to promote physical activity in obese adolescents: A randomised-controlled trial using self-determination theory as an explanatory framework. *Psychology & Health, 28*(11), 1265–1286.

Kasser, T., & Ryan, R. M. (1996). Further examining the American dream: Differential correlates of intrinsic and extrinsic goals. *Personality and Social Psychology Bulletin, 22*, 280–287.

La Guardia, J. G., Ryan, R. M., Couchman, C., & Deci, E. L. (2000). Within-person variations in attachment style and their relations to psychological need satisfaction. *Journal of Personality and Social Psychology, 79*, 367–384.

Ng, J. Y., Ntoumanis, N., Thøgersen-Ntoumani, C., Deci, E. L., Ryan, R. M., Duda, J. L., & Williams, G. C. (2012). Self-determination theory applied to health contexts: A meta-analysis. *Perspectives On Psychological Science, 7*(4), 325–340. doi:10.1177/1745691612447309.

Oliver, E. J., Markland, D., & Hardy, J. (2010). Interpretation of self-talk and post-lecture affective states of higher education students: A self-determination theory perspective. *British Journal Of Educational Psychology, 80*(2), 307–323.

Roth, G., Assor, A., Niemiec, C. P., Ryan, R. M., & Deci, E. L. (2009). The emotional and academic consequences of parental conditional regard: Comparing conditional positive regard, conditional negative regard, and autonomy support as parenting practices. *Developmental Psychology, 45*, 1119–1142.

Ryan, R. M. (1995). Psychological needs and the facilitation of integrative processes. *Journal of Personality, 63*, 397–427.

Ryan, R. M., & Deci, E. L. (2000). Self-determination theory and the facilitation of intrinsic motivation, social development, and well-being. *American Psychologist, 55*, 68–78.

Ryan, R. M., & Deci, E. L. (2011). A self-determination theory perspective on social, institutional, cultural, and economic supports for autonomy and their importance for well-being. In V. I. Chirkov, R. M. Ryan, & K. M. Sheldon (Eds.), *Human autonomy in cross-cultural context* (pp. 45–64). New York: Springer. doi:10.1007/978-90-481-9667-8_3.

Ryan, R. M., Kasser, T., Sheldon, K. M., & Deci, E. L. (1996). All goals are not created equal: An organismic perspective on the nature of goals and their regulation. In P. M. Gollwitzer, J. A. Bargh, P. M. Gollwitzer, & J. A. Bargh (Eds.), *The psychology of action* (pp. 7–26). New York: Guilford Press.

Ryan, R. M., Chirkov, V. I., Little, T. D., Sheldon, K. M., Timoshina, E., & Deci, E. L. (1999). The American dream in Russian: Extrinsic aspirations and well-being in two cultures. *Personality and Social Psychology Bulletin, 25*, 1509–1524. doi:10.1177/01461672992510007.

Ryan, R. M., Patrick, H., Deci, E. L., & Williams, G. C. (2008). Facilitating health behaviour change and its maintenance: Interventions based on self-determination theory. *European Health Psychologist, 10*, 1–4.

Ryan, R. M., Bernstein, J. H., & Brown, K. W. (2010). Weekends, work, and well-being: Psychological need satisfactions and day of the week effects on mood, vitality, and physical symptoms. *Journal of Social and Clinical Psychology, 29*, 95–122.

Saebu, M., Sørensen, M., & Halvari, H. (2013). Motivation for physical activity in young adults with physical disabilities during a rehabilitation stay: A longitudinal test of self-determination theory. *Journal of Applied Social Psychology, 43*(3), 612–625. doi:10.1111/j.1559-1816.2013.01042.x.

Vansteenkiste, M., & Ryan, R. M. (2013). On psychological growth and vulnerability: Basic psychological need satisfaction and need frustration as a unifying principle. *Journal of Psychotherapy Integration, 23*(3), 263–280. doi:10.1037/a0032359.

Vansteenkiste, M., Niemiec, C., & Soenens, B. (2010). The development of the five mini-theories of self-determination theory: An historical overview, emerging trends, and future directions. In T. Urdan & S. Karabenick (Eds.), *Advances in motivation and achievement, vol. 16: The decade ahead*. Bingley: Emerald Publishing.

Vansteenkiste, M., Williams, G. C., & Resnicow, K. (2012). Toward systematic integration between self-determination theory and motivational interviewing as examples of top-down and bottom-up intervention development: Autonomy or volition as a fundamental theoretical principle. *International Journal of Behavioral Nutrition and Physical Activity, 9*, 23.

Vansteenkiste, M., Claes, L., Soenens, B., & Verstuyf, J. (2013). Motivational dynamics among eating-disordered patients with and without nonsuicidal self-injury: A self-determination theory approach. *European Eating Disorders Review, 21*(3), 209–214. doi:10.1002/erv.2215.

Wang, C. J., Koh, K. T., Biddle, S. H., Liu, W. C., & Chye, S. (2011). Physical activity patterns and psychological correlates of physical activity among Singaporean primary, secondary, and junior college students. *Journal Of Research In Health, Physical Education, Recreation, Sport & Dance, 6*(2), 3–9.

Weiner, B. (1990). History of motivational research in education. *Journal of Educational Psychology, 82*(4), 616–622.

White, R. W. (1959). Motivation reconsidered: The concept of competence. *Psychological Review, 66*, 297–331.

Chapter 5
Causal Agency Theory

Karrie A. Shogren, Michael L. Wehmeyer, and Susan B. Palmer

Abstract Causal Agency Theory is an extension of the Functional Theory of Self-Determination; both theories describe how one becomes self-determined. These theories have been widely applied in the field of special education, and conceptualize self-determination as a dispositional characteristic (enduring tendencies used to characterize and described differences between people) based on the *function* given actions serve for an individual. This chapter will introduce and overview Causal Agency Theory, tracing its evolution from the functional model of self-determined behavior and its increasing application to all people, including those with disabilities. Causal Agency Theory will provide an organizational framework for the remainder of the text.

Causal Agency Theory is a theory that explains how people become self-determined; that is, how they define the actions and beliefs necessary to engage in self-caused, autonomous action (e.g., causal action) in response to basic psychological needs and autonomous motivation as well as contextual and environmental challenges. Causal Agency Theory emerged from and is a reconceptualization of the "functional model" of self-determined behavior, first introduced in the field of special education in the early 1990s. Causal Agency Theory reflects the ongoing development, refinement, and expansion of the functional model, incorporating theoretical advances in related areas (Self-Determination Theory, Action-Control Theory) and the growth in research in positive psychology. Importantly, Causal Agency Theory aligns work conducted through the functional model of self-determined behavior with Self-Determination Theory (SDT) and Action-Control Theory to form a theoretical model of the development of self-determination (as discussed in detail in Chap. 2). The purpose of this chapter is to describe the functional model and its application to special education and related disciplines and, subsequently, to explain its evolution as Causal Agency Theory. Both the functional model and Causal Agency Theory draw on foundational understandings of self-determination as (a) self-caused action from philosophy (Chap. 1), (b) a central process of an organism in the movement

K.A. Shogren (✉) • M.L. Wehmeyer
Special Education,University of Kansas, Lawrence, KS, USA
e-mail: shogren@ku.edu

S.B. Palmer
University of Kansas, Lawrence, KS, USA

M.L. Wehmeyer et al. (eds.), *Development of Self-Determination Through the Life-Course*, DOI 10.1007/978-94-024-1042-6_5

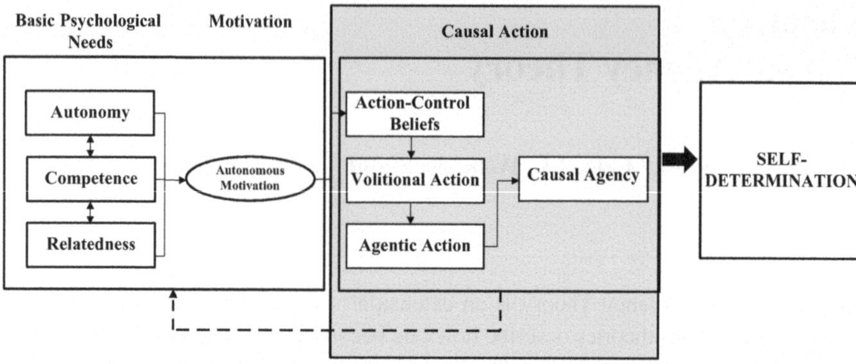

Fig. 5.1 Causal agency theory in the development of self-determination

toward autonomous determination, from personality psychology (Chap. 2), and (c) motivated by the basic psychological needs of competence, autonomy, and relatedness from SDT (Chap. 4). However, the purpose of the functional model, and now Causal Agency Theory, is to explain *how* people become self-determined; that is how they develop the actions and beliefs necessary to engage in self-caused, autonomous action that leads to causal agency. Causal Agency Theory plays a role in the development of self-determination, as introduced in Chap. 2, specifically addressing the causal action sequence leading to the experience of causal agency and, eventually, the development of self-determination. Figure 5.1 highlights the role of Causal Agency Theory in explaining the development of self-determination.

History of Causal Agency Theory: Functional Model of Self-Determined Behavior

Promoting the self-determination of adolescents with disabilities began to receive significant attention in the early 1990s in special education, as a means to enable youth and young adults with disabilities to achieve more positive outcomes pertaining to the transition from school to adulthood, such as employment, independent living, and community-inclusion. Throughout history, people with disabilities have often not been viewed as capable of being self-determined; instead the emphasis was frequently on protection, remediation, and control. However, in the last quarter of the twentieth century, changes emerged. Models of disability, referred to as social-ecological or person-environment fit models (Schalock et al. 2010; World Health Organization 2001) were introduced that conceptualized disability not as a deficit the resided within a person, but instead as a function of the interaction between personal competencies and environmental or contextual demands. Such models paved the way for a shift in emphasis in special education and related fields, from interventions that focused on fixing or curing the person, to interventions that emphasized the role of enhancing personal competency, modifying the environment or context, and providing supports that enabled people to function successfully in typical environments.

Further, professionals in the field of special education were becoming increasingly aware of and concerned about the poor transition outcomes experienced by students with disabilities (e.g., low employment rates, limited engagement in the community post-high school) (Blackorby and Wagner 1996). Relatedly, people with disabilities themselves were increasingly uniting and advocating for their right to make choices and decisions in their lives (Wehmeyer et al. 2000). As a result of this advocacy within the disability community and the concomitant focus within the field of special education on promoting positive post-school outcomes, between 1990 and 1994 the U.S. Department of Education's Office of Special Education Programs (OSEP) funded 26 model demonstration projects to develop methods, materials, and strategies to promote the self-determination of youth and young adults with disabilities during the transition from school to post-school environments (Sands and Wehmeyer 1996; Ward 1996). These projects resulted in numerous programs to promote goal-setting, problem-solving, decision-making, and self-advocacy skills and specially designed instructional methods, materials, and strategies to promote self-determination in students with disabilities (Carter-Ludi and Martin 1995; Field et al. 1998; Martin and Marshall 1996; Sands and Wehmeyer 1996; Serna and Lau-Smith 1995; Van Reusen et al. 1994; Wehmeyer et al. 1998). Several definitional frameworks for applying the self-determination construct within the special education context (Abery 1994; Field 1996; Field and Hoffman 1994; Mithaug 1996; Powers et al. 1996; Wehmeyer 1996; Wehmeyer et al. 2003, 1996) also emerged. The assumption was that by developing interventions and definitional frameworks to promote self-determination, enhanced adult outcomes related to community participation and employment would result.

Prior to this, there had been limited discussion of self-determination in the disability field. The first discussion of the importance of self-determination to people with disabilities can be traced to Bengt Nirje's (1972) chapter entitled, *The Right to Self-Determination*, in the book *Normalization: The Principle of Normalization in Human Services* (Wolfensberger 1972). Nirje applied the use of the self-determination construct within more of a rights-based framework, articulating both the right of people with disabilities to live self-determined lives and the need for environmental conditions that supported opportunities for people with disabilities to make their own decisions, and live more independently. Beyond Nirje's early 1970s call for the rights of people with disabilities to live self-determined lives, the only other application of the construct to a disability context was by Deci and Chandler (1986), who discussed the application of SDT for teachers to motivate students with learning disabilities with optimally challenging, non-repetitive, autonomy-enhancing tasks.

It was in this context that Wehmeyer (1992) proposed a 'functional' model of self-determined behavior to drive efforts to promote the self-determination of youth with disabilities. Wehmeyer defined self-determined behavior as "the attitudes and abilities required to act as the primary causal agent in one's life and to make choices regarding one's actions free from undue external influence or interference" (p. 305). Wehmeyer further elaborated, suggesting that self-determination involves "autonomy (acting according to one's own priorities or principles), self-actualization (the full development of one's unique talents and potentials) and self-regulation (cognitive or self-controlled mediation of one's behavior)" (p. 395). The notion of causal agency reflected the links of the constructs to determinism: people who are causal agents are people who make or cause things to happen in their lives, rather than others (or other things) making them act in certain ways. This early version of what has become Causal Agency Theory was developed with significant reliance on the early work of SDT theorists (Deci 1980; Deci and Ryan 1985) as discussed in Chaps. 1 and 9.

The Functional Model of Self-Determined Behavior

In 1996, Wehmeyer, Kelchner, and Richards published an empirical evaluation of the functional model of self-determined behavior, providing a refinement of the definition and the theoretical structure within which the construct was framed. It was called the 'functional' model of self-determined behavior because one could not define self-determination in a response-class manner (e.g., by a list of specific behaviors), but instead had to consider the "function" that the action served for the person. It is important to note that the functional model was intended to provide a framework to understand how children and youth became self-determined. Because of the substantial work on self-determination and motivation at that time, there was no attempt to introduce a distinct or separate motivational component.

The refined definition of self-determined behavior introduced by Wehmeyer et al. (1996) was "acting as the primary causal agent in one's life and making choices and decisions regarding one's quality of life free from undue external influence or interference" (p. 632). In a series of discriminant function analyses, the "essential characteristics" of self-determined behavior were empirically evaluated and included: autonomous functioning, self-regulation, psychological empowerment, and self-realization. These essential characteristics became the domains that were measured by *The Arc's Self-Determination Scale* (Wehmeyer and Kelchner 1995), which operationalized the functional model's structure to measure personal self-determination. The scale was validated with adolescents and adults with intellectual and developmental disabilities and shown to have strong reliability and validity (Shogren et al. 2008; Wehmeyer and Kelchner 1995).

In 2005, Wehmeyer proposed additional refinements to the functional model to address ongoing issues that were impacting the understanding (or misunderstanding) of the self-determination construct, particularly as it pertained to people with more severe intellectual disability. Many people were interpreting the construct as meaning having control over one's life, and assuming that people with the most extensive support needs were not able to be self-determined. Wehmeyer asserted that a critical element of understanding the self-determination construct was not control, but that a person acted volitionally; where volition referred to the act of making a conscious choice. Thus, he proposed a refinement to the functional model's definition, suggesting that self-determined behavior "refers to volitional actions that enable one to act as the primary causal agent in one's life and to maintain or improve one's quality of life" (p. 117). Again, this refinement emphasizes the role of acting volitionally, and, in this iteration, the fact that one acts volitionally as a causal agent.

Research with Functional Model of Self-Determination

Since the introduction of the functional model of self-determination in the 1990s, a wide range of research has established the relevance of promoting the self-determination of adolescents and young adults with disabilities (see Chap. 9 for more detailed discussion of the application of self-determination in the disability context). Promoting self-determination has been identified as a best practice in secondary education and transition services (Field et al. 1998; Shogren 2013; Wehmeyer et al. 2003, 2007). Research has consistently linked higher self-determination with the attainment of more positive academic (Fowler et al. 2007; Konrad et al. 2007; Lee et al. 2010; Shogren et al. 2012) and transition to adulthood outcomes for youth with disabilities, including more positive employment and independent living (Martorell et al. 2008; Shogren et al. 2015b; Wehmeyer and Palmer 2003; Wehmeyer and Schwartz 1997) and recreation and leisure outcomes (McGuire and McDonnell 2008), and more positive quality of life and life satisfaction (Lachapelle et al. 2005; Nota et al. 2007; Shogren et al. 2006; Wehmeyer and Schwartz 1998).

There is also a strong body of evidence that when provided instruction and supports to enhance causal action skills, students with disabilities can achieve valued life outcomes (Algozzine et al. 2001; Cobb and Alwell 2009)(discussed in greater detail in Chap. 9). Specific to the research with the functional model, a series of studies evaluated an intervention directly derived from model, the *Self-Determined Learning Model of Instruction* (SDLMI: Wehmeyer et al. 2000), Wehmeyer, Shogren et al. (2012) conducted a group-randomized, modified equivalent control group design study of 312 high school students with intellectual disability or learning disabilities using the SDLMI over a 2 year period. The SDLMI is a teaching model designed to enable teachers to teach students to self-regulate problem solving leading to educational goal attainment. The SDLMI supports students to (a) set educationally relevant and valued goals, (b) create an action plan to achieve those goals, monitor and evaluate their progress toward their goals, and (c) revise the action plan or goal as necessary based upon those evaluations that is described in detail subsequently. Students who received instruction using the SLDMI showed significant growth in their self-determination scores, compared to students who did not receive instruction, over a 2 year period. Further, students exposed to the SDLMI had significantly greater gains in their goal attainment, specifically transition goals for students with intellectual disability and academic goals for students with learning disabilities, and in their access to the general education curriculum (Shogren et al. 2012). Further, teachers perceived students who were exposed to the SDLMI as having significantly greater capacity and opportunity for self-determination (Shogren et al. 2014).

Causal Agency Theory

The functional model of self-determined behavior had utility over the past two decades to drive research and intervention pertaining to promoting the self-determination of youth with disabilities. However, with the growth of positive psychology and the growing application of universal or school-wide interventions targeting all students, including students with disabilities, an expansion of the functional model to people without disabilities, incorporating developing knowledge in the field of positive psychology became necessary. Thus, Causal Agency Theory is the most recent iteration of the theoretical framework we have used to drive our efforts to promote self-determination (Shogren et al. 2015a, b). Causal Agency Theory is derived, in part, from the functional model of self-determination and shares much with the Wehmeyer (1992, Wehmeyer 1996, 2005) definitions and conceptualizations, but has moved toward a more action-oriented focus, incorporating knowledge from the fields of motivation and positive psychology. It specifically integrates the emphasis on volitional action from the Wehmeyer (2005) definition, derived from SDT, and adds additional emphasis to agentic action and action-control beliefs. Essentially, people who act to be causal agents in their lives have the dispositional characteristic (e.g., an ongoing quality or characteristic of the person) of self-determination. This emphasis on self-determination as a dispositional characteristic defined by actions that lead to causal agency is reflected in the definition adopted by Causal Agency Theory.

Definition of Self-Determination

Within the context of Causal Agency Theory, we define self-determination as a

> …dispositional characteristic manifested as acting as the causal agent in one's life. Self-determined *people* (i.e., causal agents) act in service to freely chosen goals. Self-determined *actions* function to enable a person to be the causal agent is his or her life. (Shogren et al. 2015a, b)

Key Terms and Assumptions

Causal Agency Theory has several key terms and assumptions. First, within Causal Agency Theory, self-determination is conceptualized as a **dispositional characteristic.** A dispositional characteristic is an enduring tendency used to characterize and describe differences between people. While the assumption is that self-determined people have a tendency to act or think in a particular way, there is also a presumption of contextual variance (i.e., environmental opportunities and threats). More importantly, as a dispositional characteristic, self-determination can be measured, and variance will be observed across individuals and within individuals over time, particularly as the context changes (e.g., supports and opportunities are provided for self-determined action).

Second, is the notion of **causal agency.** As in the functional model, *causal agency* implies that it is the individual who makes or causes things to happen in his or her life. Causal agency implies more, however, than just causing action; it implies that the individual acts with an eye toward *causing* an effect to *accomplish* a *specific end* or to *cause* or *create change*. Self-determined actions enable a person to act as a causal agent. This emphasis on self-determined actions leading to causal agency is a key feature of Causal Agency Theory. Third, Causal Agency Theory is grounded in **human agentic theories** (Chap. 2) which assume that action is self-caused. Human agentic theories differentiate between self-determination as self-*caused* action and self-determination as *controlling* one's behavior. Self-determined action does not imply control over events or outcomes. Instead self-determined action refers to the degree to which action is self-caused, volitional and agentic, driven by beliefs about the relationships between actions (or means) and ends. Volitional and agentic action and action-control beliefs are central to Causal Agency Theory and reflect the essential characteristics of self-determined action under Causal Agency Theory.

Essential Characteristics of Self-Determined Actions

As shown in Fig. 5.1, these three **essential characteristics** – volitional, agentic, and action-control beliefs – are explained by Causal Agency Theory and contribute to causal agency and the development of self-determination. Thus, Causal Agency Theory builds on the basic psychological needs and autonomous motivation explained by Self-Determination Theory (Chaps. 2 and 4) and explicates the role of causal action in the development of self-determination (Chap. 2, Fig. 5.1). These essential characteristics refer not to specific actions performed or the beliefs that drive action, but to the *function* the action serves for the individual; that is, whether the action enabled the person to act as a causal agent and enhances the development of self-determination. In the following sections, each type of action is defined, and its linkages to the functional model of self-determination introduced.

Volitional Action

Self-determined people act volitionally. Volitional action is based on conscious choices that reflect one's preferences. Conscious choices are intentionally conceived, deliberate acts that occur without direct external influence. As such, volitional actions are self-initiated and function to enable a person to act autonomously (i.e., engage in self-governed action). Volitional actions involve the initiation and activation of causal capabilities—the capacity to cause something to happen—in one's life.

Agentic Action

An agent is someone who acts. Agentic action is a means by which something is done or achieved. Agentic actions are self-directed toward a goal. When acting agentically, self-determined people identify pathways that lead to a specific ends or cause or create change. The identification of pathways, or pathways thinking, is a proactive, purposive process. When acting agentically, action is self-regulated, self-directed and enables progress toward freely chosen goals. Volitional actions involve the initiation and activation of agentic capabilities—the capacity to sustain action toward a goal.

Action-Control Beliefs

In applying volitional and agentic actions, self-determined people develop a sense of personal empowerment. They believe they have what it takes to achieve freely chosen goals. They perceive a link between their action and the outcomes they experience; they develop adaptive action-control beliefs. To account for these beliefs and actions, Causal Agency Theory incorporates basic tenets of Action-Control Theory (Chaps. 2 and 22). Action-Control Theory posits three types of action-control beliefs: beliefs about the link between the self and the goal (control expectancy beliefs; "When I want to do ____, I can"); beliefs about the link between the self and the means for achieving the goal (capacity beliefs; "I have the capabilities to do _____"); and beliefs about the utility or usefulness of a given means for attaining a goal (causality beliefs; "I believe my effort will lead to goal achievement" vs. "I believe other factors – luck, access to teachers or social capital – will lead to goal achievement"). As adaptive action-control beliefs emerge, people are better able to act with self-awareness and self-knowledge in a goal-directed manner.

Environmental and Contextual Influences

As described in Chap. 2, with regard to human agentic theories generally, when acting agentically, people respond to opportunities and threats in their environment. As detailed in Chap. 2, under Causal Agency Theory, we argue that when that people respond to challenges (opportunities or threats) to their self-determination by employing volitional and agentic actions, supported and mediated by action-control beliefs. This leads to the execution of causal actions that allow people to initiate and direct their behavior to achieve a desired change or maintain a preferred circumstance or situation using their causal capabilities. Figure 2.1 provided the Causal Action schema leading to enhanced causal agency. As depicted in Fig. 5.2, the causal action sequence involving the implementation of causal and agentic

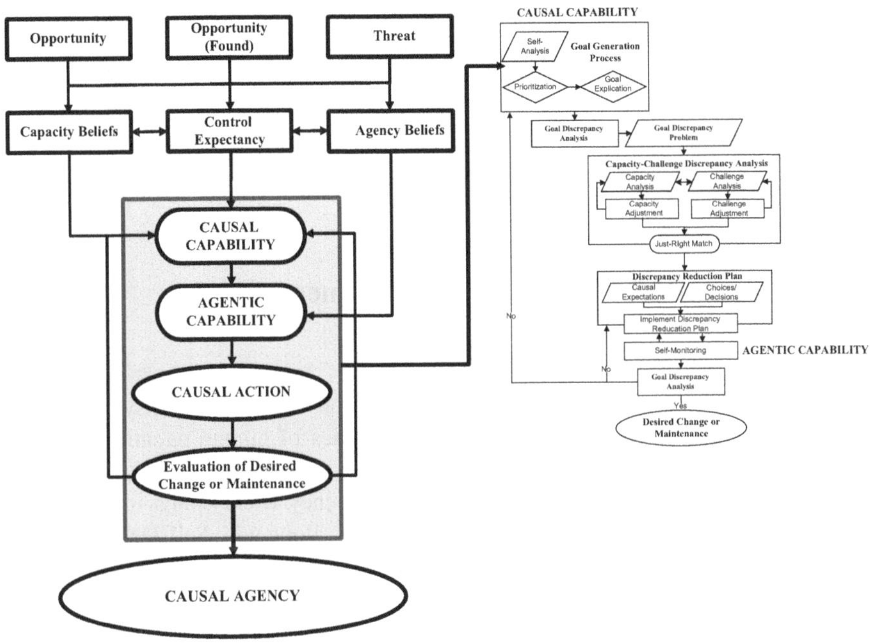

Fig. 5.2 Causal action and goal generation schemas

capabilities can be further deconstructed into a *goal generation process* leading to the identification and prioritization of needed actions. The person frames the most urgent action need in terms of a goal state, and engages in a *goal discrepancy analysis* to compare current status with goal status. The outcome of this analysis is a *goal-discrepancy problem* to be solved. The person then engages in a *capacity-challenge discrepancy analysis* in which capacity to solve the goal discrepancy problem is evaluated, and appropriate agentic actions utilizing their agentic capabilities that maximize the relationship between capacities and challenges by creating a "just-right match" between capacity and challenge to optimize the probability of solving the goal discrepancy problem.

Then, the person implements this plan and after time has passed, uses information derived from self-monitoring to self-evaluate progress toward reducing the discrepancy between current and goal status. If progress is satisfactory, the person will continue implementing the discrepancy reduction plan. If not, the person either reconsiders the discrepancy reduction plan and modifies that or returns to the goal generation process to re-examine the goal and its priority and, possibly, cycle through the process with a revised or new goal.

This process will be discussed in greater detail in Chap. 18. But, this iterative goal generation and goal discrepancy analysis using volitional and agentic actions can be taught and is increasingly internalized with repeated opportunities to engage in self-determined action, enhancing action-control beliefs. A critical part of developing causal agency is engaging in repeated opportunities to go through an iterative goal generation and discrepancy analysis process using volitional and agentic actions and developing action control beliefs. In this process a number of specific skills come into play, including expressing preferences and choice making, decision making, goal setting and attainment, self-management, and self-advocacy. These skills are called the component elements of self-determined action, and are the level at which instruction can occur and environmental supports provided.

Causal Agency Theory and the Development of Self-Determination

Causal Agency Theory defines self-determination as a general psychological construct within the organizing structure of theories of human agentic behavior. Figure 5.1 depicts the theoretical model of the development of self-determination described in Chap. 2, and depicts the role Causal Agency Theory plays in that developmental model. Causal Agency Theory contributes, along with Self-Determination Theory and Action-Control Theory, to an understanding of the development of self-determination.

References

Abery, B. H. (1994). A conceptual framework for enhancing self-determination. In M. F. Hayden & B. H. Abery (Eds.), *Challenges for a service system in transition: Ensuring quality community experiences for persons with developmental disabilities* (pp. 345–380). Baltimore: Paul H. Brookes.

Algozzine, B., Browder, D., Karvonen, M., Test, D. W., & Wood, W. M. (2001). Effects of interventions to promote self-determination for individuals with disabilities. *Review of Educational Research, 71*, 219–277. doi:10.3102/00346543071002219.

Blackorby, J., & Wagner, M. (1996). Longitudinal postschool outcomes of youth with disabilities: Findings from the National Longitudinal Transition Study. *Exceptional Children, 62*, 399–413.

Carter-Ludi, D., & Martin, L. (1995). The road to personal freedom: Self-determination. *Intervention in School and Clinic, 30*, 164–169.

Cobb, R. B., & Alwell, M. (2009). Transition planning/coordinating interventions for youth with disabilites: A systematic review. *Career Development for Exceptional Individuals, 32*(2), 70–81.

Deci, E. L. (1980). *The psychology of self-determination*. Lexington: Lexington Books.

Deci, E. L., & Chandler, C. L. (1986). The importance of motivation for the future of the LD field. *Journal of Learning Disabilities, 19*, 587–594.

Deci, E. L., & Ryan, R. M. (1985). *Intrinsic motivation and self-determination in human behavior*. New York: Plenum Press.

Field, S. (1996). Self-determination instructional strategies for youth with learning disabilities. *Journal of Learning Disabilities, 29*, 40–52.

Field, S., & Hoffman, A. (1994). Development of a model for self-determination. *Career Development for Exceptional Individuals, 17*, 159–169.

Field, S., Martin, J. E., Miller, R., Ward, M. J., & Wehmeyer, M. L. (1998). *A practical guide to teaching self-determination*. Reston: Council for Exceptional Children.

Fowler, C., Konrad, M., Walker, A. R., Test, D. W., & Wood, W. M. (2007). Self-determination interventions' effects on the academic performance of students with developmental disabilities. *Education and Training in Developmental Disabilities, 42*, 270–285.

Konrad, M., Fowler, C. H., Walker, A. R., Test, D. W., & Wood, W. M. (2007). Effects of self-determination interventions on the academic skills of students with learning disabilities. *Learning Disability Quarterly, 30*, 89–113. doi:10.2307/30035545.

Lachapelle, Y., Wehmeyer, M. L., Haelewyck, M. C., Courbois, Y., Keith, K. D., Schalock, R., … Walsh, P. N. (2005). The relationship between quality of life and self-determination: An international study. *Journal of Intellectual Disability Research, 49*(10), 740–744. doi: 10.1111/j.1365-2788.2005.00743.x.

Lee, S. H., Wehmeyer, M. L., Soukup, J., & Palmer, S. B. (2010). Impact of curriculum modifications on access to the general education curriculum for students with disabilities. *Exceptional Children, 76*, 213–233.

Martin, J. E., & Marshall, L. H. (1996). ChoiceMaker: Infusing self-determination instruction into the IEP and transition process. In D. J. Sands & M. L. Wehmeyer (Eds.), *Self-determination across the life span: Independence and choice for people with disabilities* (pp. 215–236). Baltimore: Paul H. Brookes.

Martorell, A., Gutierrez-Recacha, P., Pereda, A., & Ayuso-Mateos, J. L. (2008). Identification of personal factors that determine work outcome for adults with intellectual disability. *Journal of Intellectual Disability Research, 52*, 1091–1101. doi:10.1111/j.1365-2788.2008.01098.x.

McGuire, J., & McDonnell, J. (2008). Relationships between recreation and levels of self-determination for adolescents and young adults with disabilities. *Career Development for Exceptional Individuals, 31*(3), 154–163. doi:10.1177/0885728808315333.

Mithaug, D. E. (1996). The optimal prospects principle: A theoretical basis for rethinking instructional practices for self-determination. In D. J. Sands & M. L. Wehmeyer (Eds.), *Self-determination across the lifespan: Independence and choice for people with disabilities* (pp. 147–165). Baltimore: Paul H. Brookes.

Nirje, B. (1972). The right to self-determination. In W. Wolfensberger (Ed.), *Normalization: The principle of normalization in human services* (pp. 176–193). Toronto: National Institute on Mental Retardation.

Nota, L., Ferrari, L., Soresi, S., & Wehmeyer, M. (2007). Self-determination, social abilities and the quality of life of people with intellectual disability. *Journal of Intellectual Disability Research, 51*, 850–865. doi:10.1111/j.1365-2788.2006.00939.x.

Powers, L. E., Sowers, J., Turner, A., Nesbitt, M., Knowles, E., & Ellison, R. (1996). TAKE CHARGE! A model for promoting self-determination among adolescents with challenges. In L. E. Powers, G. H. S. Singer, & J. Sowers (Eds.), *On the road to autonomy: Promoting self-competence in children and youth with disabilities*. Baltimore: Paul H. Brookes.

Sands, D. J., & Wehmeyer, M. L. (Eds.). (1996). *Self-determination across the life span: Independence and choice for people with disabilities*. Baltimore: Paul H. Brookes.

Schalock, R. L., Borthwick-Duffy, S., Bradley, V., Buntix, W. H. E., Coulter, D. L., Craig, E. P. M., … Yeager, M. H. (2010). *Intellectual disability: Definition, classification, and systems of support* (11th ed.). Washington, DC: American Association on Intellectual and Developmental Disabilities.

Serna, L. A., & Lau-Smith, J. (1995). Learning with a PURPOSE: Self-determination skills for students who are at risk for school and community failure. *Intervention in School and Clinic, 30*, 142–146.

Shogren, K. A. (2013). *Self-determination and transition planning*. Baltimore: Brookes.

Shogren, K. A., Lopez, S. J., Wehmeyer, M. L., Little, T. D., & Pressgrove, C. L. (2006). The role of positive psychology constructs in predicting life satisfaction in adolescents with and without cognitive disabilities: An exploratory study. *The Journal of Positive Psychology, 1*, 37–52.

Shogren, K. A., Wehmeyer, M. L., Palmer, S. B., Soukup, J. H., Little, T. D., Garner, N., & Lawrence, M. (2008). Measuring self-determination: Examining the relationship between The Arc's Self-Determination Scale and the AIR Self-Determination Scale. *Assessment for Effective Intervention, 33*, 94–107.

Shogren, K. A., Palmer, S. B., Wehmeyer, M. L., Williams-Diehm, K., & Little, T. D. (2012). Effect of intervention with the Self-Determined Learning Model of Instruction on access and goal attainment. *Remedial and Special Education, 33*, 320–330. doi:10.1177/0741932511410072.

Shogren, K. A., Plotner, A. J., Palmer, S. B., Wehmeyer, M. L., & Paek, Y. (2014). Impact of the Self-Determined Learning Model of Instruction on teacher perceptions of student capacity and opportunity for self-determination. *Education and Training in Autism and Developmental Disabilities, 49*, 440–448.

Shogren, K. A., Wehmeyer, M. L., Palmer, S. B., Forber-Pratt, A., Little, T. J., & Lopez, S. J. (2015a). Causal agency theory: Reconceptualizing a functional model of self-determination. *Education and Training in Autism and Developmental Disabilities, 50*(3), 251–263.

Shogren, K. A., Wehmeyer, M. L., Palmer, S. B., Rifenbark, G. G., & Little, T. D. (2015b). Relationships between self-determination and postschool outcomes for youth with disabilities. *Journal of Special Education, 53*, 30–41. doi:10.1177/0022466913489733.

Van Reusen, A. K., Bos, C. S., Schumaker, J. B., & Deshler, D. D. (1994). *The self-advocacy strategy for education and transition planning*. Lawrence: Edge Enterprises, Inc..

Ward, M. J. (1996). Coming of age in the age of self-determination: A historical and personal perspective. In D. J. Sands & M. L. Wehmeyer (Eds.), *Self-determination across the life span: Independence and choice for people with disabilities*. Baltimore: Paul H. Brookes.

Wehmeyer, M. L. (1992). Self-determination and the education of students with mental retardation. *Education and Training in Mental Retardation, 27*(4), 302–314.

Wehmeyer, M. L. (1996). Self-determination as an educational outcome: Why is it important to children, youth and adults with disabilities? In D. J. Sands & M. L. Wehmeyer (Eds.), *Self-determination across the life span: Independence and choice for people with disabilities* (pp. 15–34). Baltimore: Paul H. Brookes.

Wehmeyer, M. L. (2005). Self-determination and individuals with severe disabilities: Re-examining meanings and misinterpretations. *Research and Practice for Persons with Severe Disabilities, 30*, 113–120. doi:10.2511/rpsd.30.3.113.

Wehmeyer, M. L., & Kelchner, K. (1995). *The Arc's Self-Determination Scale*. Arlington: The Arc National Headquarters.

Wehmeyer, M. L., & Palmer, S. B. (2003). Adult outcomes for students with cognitive disabilities three-years after high school: The impact of self-determination. *Education and Training in Developmental Disabilities, 38*, 131–144.

Wehmeyer, M. L., & Schwartz, M. (1997). Self-determination and positive adult outcomes: A follow-up study of youth with mental retardation or learning disabilities. *Exceptional Children, 63*, 245–255.

Wehmeyer, M. L., & Schwartz, M. (1998). The relationship between self-determination and quality of life for adults with mental retardation. *Education and Training in Mental Retardation and Developmental Disabilities, 33*, 3–12.

Wehmeyer, M. L., Kelchner, K., & Richards, S. (1996). Essential characteristics of self-determined behavior of individuals with mental retardation. *American Journal on Mental Retardation, 100*, 632–642.

Wehmeyer, M. L., Agran, M., & Hughes, C. (1998). *Teaching self-determination to students with disabilities: Basic skills for successful transition*. Baltimore: Paul H. Brookes Publishing Co..

Wehmeyer, M. L., Palmer, S. B., Agran, M., Mithaug, D. E., & Martin, J. E. (2000a). Promoting causal agency: The Self-Determined Learning Model of Instruction. *Exceptional Children, 66*, 439–453.

Wehmeyer, M. L., Bersani Jr., H., & Gagne, R. (2000b). Riding the third wave: Self-determination and self-advocacy in the 21st century. *Focus on Autism and Other Developmental Disabilities, 15*(2), 106–115.

Wehmeyer, M. L., Abery, B., Mithaug, D. E., & Stancliffe, R. (2003). *Theory in self-determination: Foundations for educational practice*. Springfield: Charles C. Thomas Publishing Company.
Wehmeyer, M. L., Agran, M., Hughes, C., Martin, J. E., Mithaug, D., & Palmer, S. (2007). *Promoting self-determination in students with developmental disabilities*. New York: Guilford.
Wolfensberger, W. (1972). *Normalization: The principle of normalization in human services*. Toronto: National Institute on Mental Retardation.
World Health Organization. (2001). *International classification of functioning, disability, and health*. Geneva: Author.

Part II
Developmental Origins and Life-Course Trajectory of Self-Determination

Synopsis

The second part (Developmental Origins and Life-Course Trajectory of Self-Determination) examines issues pertaining to the development of self-determination across the lifespan utilizing the theoretical frame described in Chap. 2. Chapter 6 explores the early development of foundational skills that enable children to make choices and express preferences, solve problems, engage in making decisions, set and attain goals, self-manage and self-regulate action, self-advocate, and acquire self-awareness and self-knowledge. Chapter 7 provides an examination of the foundational skills, knowledge, and beliefs leading to the development of causal and agentic capabilities and action control beliefs during the adolescent years. The chapter overviews developmental milestones in knowledge, skills, and beliefs that emerge during adolescence and lead to enhanced self-determination, including choice making, self-initiation and planning, problem solving, decision making, goal setting and attainment, and self-regulation. The chapter concludes with a brief overview of issues in adolescent development as it pertains to motivational aspects of self-determination. Chapter 8 introduces the importance of autonomy-supportive classrooms, and why it is important to promote students' autonomy in learning, including providing guidelines on how to promote student-centered teaching practices that support student's autonomy. Chapter 9 turns the focus to the disability context, and provides an overview of research in special education and related disciplines, as driven by Causal Agency Theory. We then discuss the knowledge and information from this literature base that can inform knowledge pertaining to self-determination, in general. The next two chapters focus on self-determination in adulthood. Self-determination is about volitional action and, in large measures, pursuing one's passions. Chapter 10 introduces the concept of passion, and describes its relationship to self-growth and development. The Dualistic Model of Passion is highlighted, and two types of passion, harmonious and obsessive, defined. Research on passion is described, including work to identify the prevalence of passion, to develop a measure of passion, the Passion Scale, and to test the validity of passion constructs. Chapter 11 looks at aging and considers theoretical perspectives on independence and self-determination as people age by examining the positive support of aging in place and the challenges experienced when dementia, self-neglect or abuse, and the approaching of end of life become part of older age. A particular consideration is given to both the compromises and the opportunities presented by being the recipient of caregiving. The final chapter in this part explores the impact of context, namely cultural factors, on the development of self-determination. The influence of one's personal culture and cultural norms and beliefs on the development of self-determination are reviewed. The role of Causal Agency Theory in understanding influence of culture on the development of self-determination, and research on the operationalization of self-determined action in diverse cultures is presented.

Chapter 6
The Development of Self-Determination During Childhood

Susan B. Palmer, Michael L. Wehmeyer, and Karrie A. Shogren

Abstract Although self-determination is associated with adolescent development, the antecedents and precursors of its development lie within the development of foundational skills during the early childhood years. Adolescents become self-determined as they learn, refine, and practice knowledge, skills, beliefs and actions that enable them to respond to contextual and environmental challenges (opportunities, threats) that energize basic psychological needs and resultant autonomous motivation, stimulating a causal action sequence in which volitional and agentic actions are mediated by action-control beliefs, resulting in experiences of causal agency. This chapter explores the early development of foundational skills that enable children to make choices and express preferences, solve problems, engage in making decisions, set and attain goals, self-manage and self-regulate action, self-advocate, and acquire self-awareness and self-knowledge.

Although self-determination is associated with adolescent development, the antecedents and precursors of its development lie within the development of foundational skills during the early childhood years (Doll et al. 1996; Palmer 2010; Wehmeyer and Palmer 2000; Wehmeyer et al. 1997). Adolescents become self-determined—that is, having the dispositional characteristic of self-determination—as they learn, refine, and practice knowledge, skills, beliefs and actions that enable them to respond to contextual and environmental challenges (opportunities, threats) that energize basic psychological needs and resultant autonomous motivation, stimulating a causal action sequence in which volitional and agentic actions are mediated by action-control beliefs, resulting in experiences of causal agency. The specific knowledge, skills, beliefs, and actions are identified as component elements within Causal Agency Theory (Table 6.1) and include learning to make choices and express preferences, solve problems, engage in making decisions, set and attain goals,

S.B. Palmer (✉)
University of Kansas, Lawrence, KS, USA
e-mail: spalmer@ku.edu

M.L. Wehmeyer • K.A. Shogren
Special Education, University of Kansas, Lawrence, KS, USA

M.L. Wehmeyer et al. (eds.), *Development of Self-Determination Through the Life-Course*, DOI 10.1007/978-94-024-1042-6_6

Table 6.1 Component elements of self-determination under Causal Agency Theory

Essential characteristics	Component constructs	Component elements
Volitional action	Autonomy	**Causal capabilities**
	Self-initiation	Choice-making skills
		Decision-making skills
		Goal setting skills
		Problem solving skills
		Planning skills
Agentic action	Self-regulation	**Agentic capabilities**
	Self-direction	Self-management skills (self-monitoring, self-evaluation, etc.)
	Pathways thinking	Goal attainment skills
		Problem solving skills
		Self-advocacy skills
Action-control beliefs	Psychological empowerment	Self-awareness
	Self-realization	Self-knowledge
	Control expectancy	
	Agency beliefs	
	Causality beliefs	

self-manage and self-regulate action, self-advocate, and acquire self-awareness and self-knowledge.

The lives of young children are, necessarily, still mediated primarily by adults, who care for their physical, social, and psychological needs; nurture and support their growth, development, and education; and ensure their safety and protection. As Summers et al. (2014) noted, "since young children remain dependent upon others for caregiving and support, they are not developmentally ready to act in a self-determined manner, fundamentally due to a lack of maturity, experience, and overall capabilities" (p. 175). However, although young children are not causal agents in their own lives, the acquisition of skills, knowledge, and abilities and the experiences that lead to self-determination in adolescence have their developmental roots in early childhood development. As such, we refer to *building the foundations for self-determination* in early and middle childhood when discussing the development of these component elements (Palmer et al. 2012).

This chapter provides a broad look at the development of foundational knowledge, skills, and beliefs leading to the development, use, and refinement of causal and agentic capabilities (which enable one to engage in volitional and agentic action) and action-control beliefs that, in turn, enable experiences of causal agency, repeated experiences of which lead to enhanced self-determination. The actual developmental aspects of most of these foundational skills are discussed in subsequent chapters, so this chapter provides a broad look at these foundational skills, or component elements, as identified in Table 6.1.

Environment and the Development of Self-Determination

Human agentic theories "share the meta-theoretical view that organismic aspirations drive human behaviors" (Little et al. 2006, p. 61), and that people are active contributors to their behavior. Such organismic approaches "acknowledge the complex interplay between a person and their environment" (Shogren 2013a, p. 496). Further, "contexts reflect specific constellations of features at both the molar and micro levels that both constrain and afford behavior" (Little et al. 2002, p. 390) and an individual "both influences and is influenced by the contexts in which she or he acts and develops" (p. 390). For example, the very nature of self-regulation, discussed in detail in Chap. 17, involves one's interaction with the 'molar and micro levels' of the environment. An agentic person engages in self-regulated and goal-directed action, they "plot and navigate a chosen course through the uncertainties and challenges of the social and ecological environments… continuously interpreting and evaluating actions and their consequences" (Little et al. 2002, p. 390). As noted in Chap. 2, in fact, causal action (which leads to the development of self-determination) is action in response to opportunities or threats in one's environment that provoke organisms to engage in volitional and causal action and employ action-control beliefs to act as a causal agent in one's life.

Abery and colleagues (Wehmeyer et al. 2003) have written extensively about ecological processes at work in issues pertaining to self-determination, noting that "viewed from an ecological perspective, the exercise of self-determination can be conceived as a by-product of an ongoing interaction, across the life span, between individuals and the environments in which they function" (p. 65). Abery and Stancliffe (2003) used Bronfenbrenner's (1979) ecological systems theory to identify the wide array of environmental influences—at the microsystem, mesosystem, exosystem and macrosystem levels—that influence the expression and development of self-determination.

According to Causal Agency Theory, opportunities or threats that require causal action can be generated by the child him or herself (e.g., created opportunities), or emerge from any level of the ecological system (found opportunities, threats). As Fig. 6.1 illustrates, a myriad of environmental factors alone and in combination and at various levels of the ecosystems require causal action. Changes in family status or school variables, either at the district level or the teacher level, may directly impact the development of a child's self-determination, as can interactions among systems at the mesosystem level (for example, family-school conflict), changes or issues at the exosystem level (school board policy or decisions, access to health care) or at the macrosystem level (new legal protections).

Little et al. (2006) note that action-control beliefs differentiate over a child's elementary years, and become *domain* as well as *means* specific. Children begin to understand that different domains of functioning "have different challenges and require different skills" (Little et al. 2006, p. 397). Further, children develop means-specific beliefs as they begin to differentiate between outcomes associated with luck versus effort or ability or, importantly to the development of causal agency, between

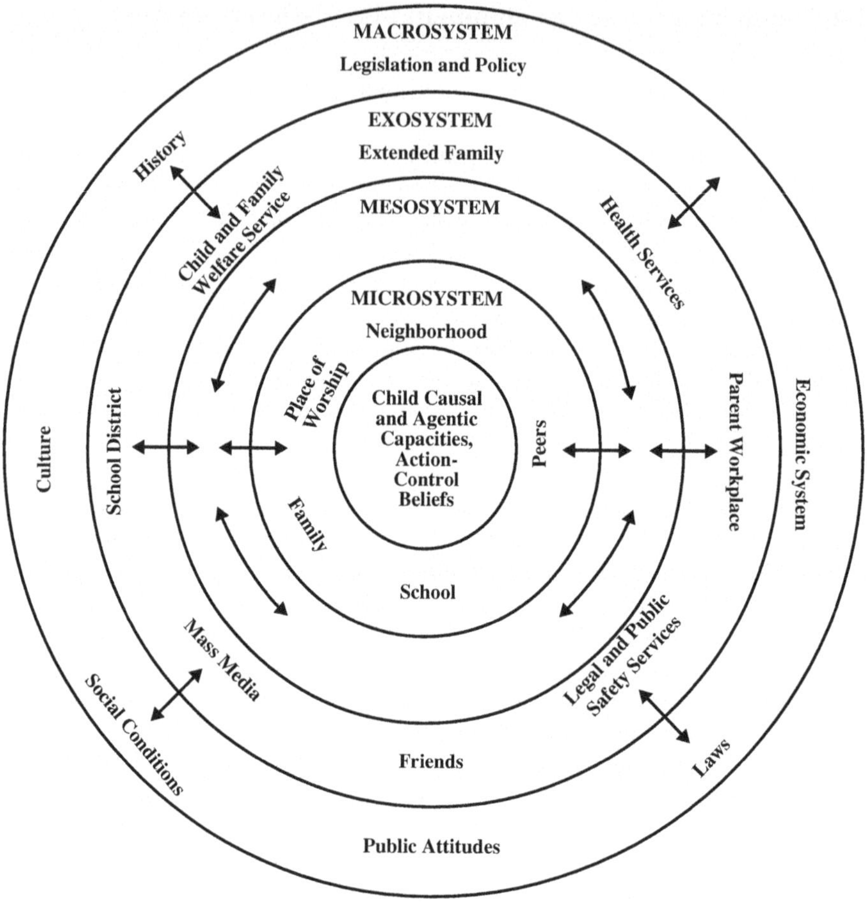

Fig. 6.1 Ecologocial system impacting child causal action and self-determination based upon Bronfenbrenner

outcomes associate with others or powerful others and self. Such differentiation occurs as a function of caregiver-child interactions, the exercise of autonomy and competence, opportunities associated with an expanding social context (Little et al. 2006).

Deci and Ryan (2012) noted that "contexts vary in the degree to which they support the individuals' autonomy versus control their behaviors, thoughts, and feelings" (p. 86). As has been noted in reference to Bronfenbrenner's ecological system theory, SDT posits that "both proximal interpersonal contexts (e.g., the behavior of people's parents or managers) and distal contexts (e.g., the cultural norms and economic structures of their society) can variously support or undermine intrinsic motivation…" (p. 86). Most of the research within SDT has addressed the former (proximal interpersonal contexts), though Deci and Ryan observe that, even then, distal contexts influence those proximal contexts (e.g., teachers work within the context of school districts).

Foundational Skills to the Development of Self-Determination

So, acknowledging the critical role in environment and context in the experience of causal action and the development of self-determination, we now turn to look at the development of specific skills—skills related to causal and agentic capacity, or the capabilities to initiate, regulate, and sustain causal action—across childhood, and we begin by noting that broad developmental tasks of children often involve component elements of self-determination. For example, in infancy to preschool, developmental tasks include attachment to caregiver (Ainsworth and Bell 1974), language development (Dale 1976), differentiation of self from the environment (Damon 1983), and self-control and compliance (Macoby and Martin 1983). For middle childhood, tasks are school adjustment, academic achievement, getting along with peers, and rule-governed conduct (Masten and Coatsworth 1998). However, although these broad developmental milestones are important to the development of skills leading to later self-determination, there are specific skills that warrant particular attention that enable children to exercise causal and agentic capabilities.

Choice-Making Skills

Chapter 15 discusses the development of Preference and Choice Expression, so a detailed discussion on developmental issues will be held until that chapter. Choice making is fundamental to dignity, responsibility, and opportunity and is a basic human right that is important for the development of self-determination (Shogren 2013b). Volition is, of course, the expression of conscious choice, and the expression of preferences is central to autonomous motivation, causal action, and self-determination. Essentially, there are two components to the act of making a choice. First, an individual identifies a preference and then, the act of choosing completes this skill (Reid et al. 2001). Thus, someone engaged in choice-making must have at least two options from which to choose, then determine a preference for one of the options, and finally, indicate their selection. Wehmeyer et al. (2007), suggest a person should be familiar with the options, be able to choose without coercion, and clearly be able to express a preference in some modality, not necessarily vocally or through pointing (Wehmeyer 2003).

Choice supports autonomy, increases motivation to learn, and may prevent problem behaviors (Bambara and Kroger 2005). Deci and Ryan (1985) observed that "[w]hen autonomy-oriented, people use available information to make choices and to regulate themselves in pursuit of self-selected goals" (p. 154). Young children engage in rudimentary choice-making very early in life. Infants and young children often choose through eye gaze or pointing at one option instead of another (Stern 1985). Between 15 and 18 months, young children can choose two familiar objects upon request; by 2-years-of age, a child can choose one object from a group of five upon request (Rossetti 1990). Strategies for preference and choice making are often used as language acquisition techniques with young children or children who experience language delays (McCormick et al. 2003). Being able to point to a preferred object or activity precedes making a verbal choice and encourages engagement with the function of language. Practitioners can decide whether to use exact objects, visual representations of objects, or verbal cues to represent an array of choices, depending on the child's understanding of abstract representation.

Adults can ensure choices are valid and reasonable, that there is enough information to make wise choices, and immediately and consistently respond to a child's choices. Older children and youth must connect choice making and consequences of a choice, to consider the outcomes of choice and make responsible choices with regard to what will occur next.

Problem-Solving Skills

Problem-solving skills are those skills which enable a person to identify one or more solutions to a problem. Chapter 19 covers the development of problem solving in greater detail. Problem solving is "what children do when they have a goal in mind but are encountering an obstacle to reaching the goal and do not know how to achieve it" (Landy 2002. p. 474). The challenge for problem solvers, according to Landy, is determining causation, believing in a good outcome, and choosing a solution related to the problem. First one must understand what the problem is and then be able to generate at least one solution to the problem. With more possible solutions, decision-making comes into play, so the problem solver must then assess the value of each of the possible solutions, choose a solution, implement the solution, and decide whether or not the problem is solved.

Social problem solving for young children often involves a need to work through problems in social interaction such as sharing a valued possession with others, getting along with peers, or resolving disagreement between children (Ramani and Brownell 2014). Addressing social linkages, children who are judged to be securely attached appear to be better problem solvers, concentrate better, plan, and use strategies in efficient ways (Landy 2002). Cognitive problem solving emphasizes critical thinking skills related to outcomes more academic in nature, such as solving a problem about how to accomplish school work. But, these strategies for social and cognitive problem solving overlap and are less unique, beyond the emphasis of purpose for social or cognitive purposes (Wehmeyer et al. 2007).

The child development literature includes a number of theories on children's mental processing and problem solving. Perspective taking evolves at around 4 years of age when children begin to understand that the thoughts, motivations, and desires of others are different from their own, which helps the ability to consider all perspectives regarding problem solving (Selman 1980). Others see executive function (developing between 12 months and 5 years of age) supporting problem solving. Executive function is a general term with "widespread influences on the organization of behavior and behavioral control" (Buss and Spencer 2014, p. 1). Planning, forming mental representations, and the ability to attend to relevant stimuli are part of executive functioning that support problem solving (Best and Miller 2010; Garon et al. 2008). Executive functioning can be understood in age-related increases in complexity of rules children can formulate and use when solving problems, and is closely associated with development of self-regulation (Zelazo et al. 2003).

Another dominant cognitive theory, that of Piaget (1963), described the adaptation to invariant schemas or plans children make to understand their world. But some authors believe Piagetian theory may have constrained our understanding of problem solving (Sigler 1996; Willatts 1990). Although Piagetian theory suggests children begin to problem solve around the age of 4 years, Sigler (1996) looked at within-child variability to conceptualize changes in children's strategies. Sigler (1996) views thinking processes within an overlapping waves metaphor, which purports children have access to a number of strategies for problem solving and can choose adaptively among the strategies depending on the situation and application. Instead of a stair-step, normative description, Siegler theorizes that children use multiple ways of thinking about problems with continuously changing frequency, rather than simple replacement of old strategies to become more efficient strategy users. Farrington-Flint et al. (2009) investigated the variability of children's problem solving in math and reading in an applied study of 50 children between ages 5 and 7 years. In general, children moved over time from less sophisticated procedural strategies for problem solving to much more efficient methods, and those who successfully used strategies in math also used more advanced strategies in reading tasks.

Concentrating on more than one idea, manipulating solutions, making decisions about what is important or not, and evaluating solutions makes problem solving a task for children often activated and achieved through scaffolding by adults. Scaffolding provides support to operate within a zone of proximal development - where one is now and somewhat beyond, to learn and grow in abilities (Vygotsky 1962).

Young children use social problem solving on shared goals within cooperative play in preschool settings (Ramani and Brownell 2014). Through social play, children can begin to practice problem solving in a controlled context within everyday routines. Shared goals require the mutual understanding of the task, the final product or goal outcomes, and the process needed to fulfill the outcome – problem solving (Tomasello 2009). Although children beginning at 18 months occasionally solved a cooperative task problem (Brownell and Carriger 1990, 1991), by 24-months-of age, this activity was more consistent. In a series of studies, children at ages 2 and 3 years were able to attend to the task, monitor the actions of their cooperative partner, and accommodate their actions together to solve the problem (Brownell and Carriger 1991). Although problem solving and goal setting are interdependent, we address each as a single component.

Decision-Making Skills

As noted, problem-solving skills are those skills which enable a person to identify one or more solutions to a problem. Alternatively, decision-making skills refer to a broader set of skills that incorporate problem-solving and choice-making skills in a process to select one of several already identified solutions. Decision making involves considering alternate courses of action, thinking about the consequences of each action, whether each consequence is possible, choosing the best alternative, and taking action on the choice/decision that is made (Furby and Beyth Marom 1992). Although seemingly a simple action, decision making is a "complex mental function influenced by the multiple interactive processes of cognition, motivation, and emotion" (Hickson and Khemka 2013, p.211).

Young children can begin to make decisions earlier in life with support, but more independent decision making improves with the development of perspective taking. Selman (1980) conducted a series of cross-sectional interview studies to identify stages within the ongoing process of children beginning to understand the point of view of another person over time. At 3 years extending to 6 years of age, children take more egocentric, undifferentiated roles, but notice people are different from them and have different thoughts and feelings. Between 6 and 8 years of age, children can detect that two different people have different perspectives or opinions on things that can lead decisions in two different directions in a more unilateral style. Then between 8 and 10 years, children grasp a somewhat more reciprocal, self-reflective type of role taking in understanding other people can evaluate their own actions. By 10–12 years, according to Selman, children use mutual role taking and often take two points of view simultaneously as a perspective in the decision making process. Finally, between 12 and 15 years of age, youth can assume a more interdependent role within perspective taking by viewing decisions from the perspective of others as well as their own views.

Decision making is an aspect of adaptive social functioning – reflecting on past events, considering the present environment, and making decisions and future predictions. Garon and Moore (2004) studied the development of decision making in 69 children ages three, four, and six using a child-adapted version of an adult gaming task. As expected, the 6-year-olds were better able to understand the task and performed significantly better than the younger children. Later in childhood, children and then adolescents showed even higher performance levels on the decision making task (Blair et al. 2001). Although young children often use some of the same decision rules as adults do, children in elementary grades can begin to use statistical information to make social judgments. Craig and Myers (1963) found similar results with two-choice, sequential decision making with children in Kindergarten not implementing consistent, logical patterns of selection, but fourth- and eighth- graders making decisions similar to those of adults, identifying patterns and repeating these selections in relevant conditions. This ability to use decision rules increases with age in parallel with biases in decision making such as stereotypical thinking or social beliefs about groups of people (Jacobs and Klacqynski 2002). But there is little research to document relationships among age, emotions, and decision making processes.

Individuals use decision making skills to initiate volitional action in response to environmental demands and to maintain agentic action. However, as with problem solving, there is no single developmental path regarding decision making. Although we realize problem solving, use of memory strategies, and other cognitive skills increase with age, even young children are capable of making decisions about known activities and options, especially with adult guidance (Jacobs and Klacqynski 2002). The more children know about a particular instance or set of options, the better their ability to make decisions (Sigler 1996). Decision making is part of problem solving, described subsequently, wherein a problem is identified and various solutions are posed with a decision about a course of action needed to complete the problem solving process (Agran and Wehmeyer 2005).

Goal Setting and Attainment

A goal is a plan, a target for what one wants to accomplish: goals can be simple or complex and inherently encourage individuals to be more involved in focused actions (Doll and Wehmeyer 2005). Steps in formal goal setting begin with goal identification, looking at options, choosing and acting, and evaluating to either finalize completion or revise goals. Chapter 18 provides a detailed description of goal setting and attainment. Obviously, goal-related actions are at the heart of causal action, causal agency, and self-determination. Bullock and Lutkenhaus (1988) stated that "much of human activity is volitional: one acts in order to achieve a particular outcome or goal" (p. 664). Bullock and Lutkenhaus described the development of volitional action over time in the context of outcome completion. Even though infants display intentional action, a child is more likely to attain outcomes when they develop skills to regulate behavior for goal attainment. Infants begin to recognize intentional relations between actors and goals as precursors to intentional actions of goal setting (Gerson 2014). For instance, at 6 months of age, habituation studies show that infants are able to grasp the relation between actor and object (Gerson and Woodward 2013) and at 7 months, infants imitate other's behavior by reaching for the same toy as experimenters (Hamlin et al. 2008). By 11 months, infants are able to anticipate the expected goal prior to any action, and even anticipate goals with multistep sequences (Cannon and Woodward 2012). These underlying abilities for goal direction precede later volitional action to accomplish formalized goals. Although young children can detect goal-directed activity, depending upon their familiarity with the context, Trabasso et al. (1992) found at age four, children are able to identify a goal in a series of pictured events, and at age five, can link goals and actions.

For young children, formal goals are generally set by adults, with minimal child involvement. However, a series of studies involving goal-directed planning and shopping for a specific event at a pretend grocery store conducted by Hudson and

Fivush (1991) showed children's planning becoming more complex and flexible with age. For example, 3-year-olds could carry out simple planning and execution of a plan or goal with support. Four-year-olds showed transitional abilities, which become more solid at 5-years-of age, when children show flexible planning and execution of more complex ideas. Children can be involved in some aspect of goal completion, including self-monitoring of goal attainment behaviors (King-Sears and Carpenter 2005). But, with age, it is important to involve children in the act of setting and attaining self-selected goals, to encourage the development of volitional action (Wehmeyer and Palmer 2000).

Domain and Means Specific Beliefs

Means-end or causal beliefs "represent behavior-event contingencies internalized partly through repeated person/environment interactions" (Geldhof and Little 2011, p. 49) and contribute to causal action (Little and Lopez 1996). Means-end beliefs can be classified into three categories: a) interagentic mean-end beliefs for personal effort and personal attributes (ability), b) beliefs about powerful others and luck, and c) unknown or unknowable causes (Skinner 1990). Younger children tend to overestimate their role as a causal agent, but between ages 7 and 10 years, there is a reduction in this thought pattern, and belief in causal agency diminishes. Then, between 10 and 12 years of age, children are able to increase their differentiation of means-end beliefs. Throughout this process the individual is becoming more of becoming an active agent in their own development (Hawley and Little 2002).

An added consideration for development of means-end beliefs is whether one can distinguish between effort and ability. Nicholls (1978) identified four levels of reasoning about ability and effort: at first, efforts and outcome are not distinguished as cause and effect (5–9 years), between 7 and 9 years children attribute outcome solely to effort, between 10 and 11 years, an inconsistent ability/effort connect is present, until by age 12 years ability is correctly inferred from effort and outcome. Folmer et al. (2008) confirmed these levels in a study of 166 children, ages five to fifteen. Children and youth who believed "effort and ability are important causes of actual school performance also performed better than those who believed less in the causal relevance of these dimensions" (Little et al. 1999, p. 816). In other words, believing in a positive outcome of effort and ability was beneficial.

Beyond volitional action, one must enact agentic action, which involves the ability to self-regulate, keep goals in mind to work toward completion, and monitor progress toward goal attainment. By the end of the second year of life, children firmly self-recognize and become more involved in problem-solving tasks that are part of goal setting and attainment. In one study, intentional tasks of block building and clean-up were presented to 82 children in the following age groupings: 15–18 months, 19–22 months, 23–28 months, and 29–35 months (Bullock and Lutkenhaus 1988). Each task had a standard, with examples and specific directions. Results showed the frequency of outcome-oriented behavior increased with age, with the children 23 through 35 months showing outcome-directed behavior in all tasks. These children were able to understand the standard for each task and accomplish the tasks in an acceptable manner, often by making adjustments, as needed (Bullock & Lutkenhaus). Children increasingly learn to understand how to self-regulate and self-correct during tasks to bring about goal attainment, generating multiple pathways to achieve their goal, using agentic action.

Self-Regulation

Self-regulation skills are critical to the development of self-determination, as discussed in greater detail in Chap. 17. Self-regulation is a response system to help individuals regulate coping responses to aspects within their environment, making decisions about how to act, to act, to evaluate outcomes of their action, and to revise the plan, if needed, according to Whitman (1990). Karoly (1993) viewed self-regulation as an internal process directing goal-guided activities over time and across contexts, describing agentic action. These definitions are examples of many that exist, depending on the theory posed or the aspects of thought or behavior considered. Self-regulation and mechanisms related to this construct are integrated into broader theories of development (Denissen et al. 2013) and have been mentioned already in regard to problem solving and goal setting. In infancy, self-regulation may be associated with eating, sleeping, and adjusting to the environment. But as a child grows and develops, self-regulation becomes more complex, involving "patterns of physical, psychological, educational, and social need" (Mithaug 2003, p. 137).

Early self-regulation is influenced by physical environments and caregiver interactions with infants, beyond the basic psychological makeup of an individual. Adults can learn to read each child's signals and provide consistent caregiving to provide reasonable order, predictable routines, and periods of quiet and activity. Bronson (2000) stated that "from the earliest months of life, the environment can support a child's intrinsic capacity to be rewarded by prediction, effectance, and control" (p.180). Shonkoff and Phillips, (Shonkoff and Phillips 2000) typify the development of self-regulation as "a cornerstone of early childhood development that cuts across all domains of behavior" (p.3). Thus, self-regulation is viewed broadly, encompassing complex behaviors and emotional control in a number of activities under regulatory control of an organism. Although there are a number of individual differences within developing children, as children become more autonomous, they need to become more self-regulating to be able to function in personal and social settings (Bronson 2000; Shonkoff and Phillips 2000). Being self-regulated earlier in life predicts later self-regulated behavior (Mischel et al. 1989; Moffitt et al. 2011).

The capacity to develop self-regulation is present at birth (Barkley 1997; Kopp 1982) and by 3 months of age, many infants can calm or self-quiet for brief periods, sleep regularly, have a predictable eating schedule, quiet when picked up, and have cycles of other predictable states (Landy 2002). As infants become children, self-regulation may involve different behaviors or previous behaviors may have different functions (i.e. crying in infancy is a form of signaling to caregivers, but later it is perceived as a sign of social immaturity) (Shonkoff and Phillips 2000). Cultural implications and expectations of families, individually or driven by ethnic affiliation, interfere with a clear and concise picture of the development of self-regulation (Rogoff 2003), but overall the business of infancy is about sleeping, eating, and growing with the help of adult caregivers (Landy 2002).

Self-regulation is often associated with behavior regulation as a type of self-control or "ability to contain and manage his own behavior without relying on caregivers to guide him", (Landy 2002, p. 369). In this manner, self-regulation is paired with the child internalizing expectations for behavior, including expectations for what is acceptable and not acceptable in different contexts. Indeed, self-regulation is an important topic during early childhood and school readiness for formal education beginning at age 5 or 6 years of age (Shonkoff and Phillips 2000).

Regarding early school success, McClelland and Cameron (2011) define self-regulation as "the capacity of controlling or directing one's attention, thoughts, emotions, and actions", (p.136). The increasing demands for self-regulation challenge children, parents, and teachers when children begin to attend school. In this context, McClelland and Cameron suggest the multiple demands of school imply self-regulation has nuances related to executive function, including attentional or cognitive flexibility, voluntarily focusing and sustaining attention to task, working memory, and inhibitory control (Shonkoff and Phillips 2000).

During the school years, self-regulation is often applied to the context of learning. Zimmerman (2008) connects self-regulation to learning as "the self-directive processes and self-beliefs that enable learners to transform their mental abilities, such as verbal aptitude into an academic performance skill", (p.166). Within self-regulated learning, including activities of children in elementary grades and beyond, one must consider whether or not a learner displays personal initiative, perseverance, and adaptive skills as part of motivational feelings and beliefs and metacognitive strategies (Zimmerman and Schunk 2007).

Other researchers typify self-regulation within an action-control model (Skinner et al. 1988), or as bidirectional person-environment interactions leading individuals "to develop beliefs about actors, means, outcomes, and their interrelationships" (p. 47, Geldhof and Little 2011). The action-control model places the agentic self within goal setting and accomplishment that applies at later ages in childhood. This model of *selection, optimization*, and *compensation* (SOC; Baltes and Baltes 1990) describes a fully self-regulated person interacting with the environment, especially during adolescence and later. But first, one must grasp means-end beliefs, previously described within problem solving, to understand causality of actions. Within means-end beliefs, as discussed earlier in the chapter, one can develop a personal strategy specific to oneself in determining effective outcomes within goal setting developing action-control beliefs.

Conclusions

This chapter has provided a broad look at the development of skills that are foundational to the development of self-determination in adolescence. Table 6.2 provides a snapshot of the development of these component elements as described in this chapter.

Returning, though, to the discussion early in the chapter with regard to the role of environment in the development of self-determination, it is important to consider the progression described in Table 6.2 and in narrative in this chapter in the context of not only proximal, but also distal environmental and contextual factors. To assist in the development of self-regulation over the age span, Bronson (2000) stresses the importance of family environments for self-control and self-regulation, and this is obviously equally true for the development of self-determination. Effective child-rearing practices - having a set of expectations, challenges, a range of options, and support systems within the environment, and promoting children's individual perception of their own competence and abilities are critical. It is important for families (and other adults) to be emotionally supportive, responsive to children, be consistent in responses and expectations, encourage responsibility, and teach problem solving strategies to support growth to meet the needs of the culture. Problem solving is "enhanced by interactions with parents and caregivers that encourage a sense of competence, self-efficacy, and problem solving that show warmth, acceptance, responsiveness, and delight in achievement (Landy 2002, p. 485).

Table 6.2 Developmental progression of foundational skills for later self-determination

Early childhood (2–5 years)	Early elementary (6–8 years)	Late elementary (9–11 years)
Self-awareness and self-knowledge		
Have a sense of self as being separate from caregivers.	Accurately label the feelings of happy, sad, afraid, and angry.	Actively seek information about task performance in order to fine-tune approach.
Understand their own feeling states and recognize them in a pictured person.	Understand how different dispositional characteristics might be expressed in different situations	
Understand that people have characteristic features (dispositional characteristics).	Selected approaches to tasks reflect accurate understanding of personal competencies.	
Tend not to self-reflect on their own thinking.		

(continued)

Table 6.2 (continued)

Early childhood (2–5 years)	Early elementary (6–8 years)	Late elementary (9–11 years)
Domain and means specific beliefs		
Self-descriptions of abilities are strikingly inaccurate and capricious.	Self-estimates of ability become stable and global across tasks.	More adept at comparing performance to a peer group and less likely to inflate achievement.
Typically overestimate the quality of their performance relative to others.	Begin to understand that task abilities can be compared among children.	Use self-evaluations as the basis for appropriate decisions to request help.
Can accurately judge the quality of their work compared to models or templates.	Understand ability as a place on a peer continuum of task performance.	Distinguish between luck and effort and understand that games of chance cannot be improved with effort or ability.
Attribute success or failure to effort rather than ability or luck.	Believe that practice can improve their performance on games of chance.	
Choice-making, Problem-solving and decision-making skills		
Routinely express preferences, verbally or non-verbally.	Can decide what kind of instructional support is required.	Understand what is required to state a preference regarding medical treatment.
Can think of solutions to social problems similar to those of older children, although fewer pathways identified and less detailed.	Able to describe 50% more solutions to social problems than younger children.	Monitor problem solving and systematically modify their approach in the face of evidence that isn't working.
Language comes to replace nonverbal gestures as the primary mode of expressing preferences.	Can use language-based rules to mediate problem solving	Capable of identifying the risks and benefits of therapy.
Choices tend to reflect instantaneous whims.		
Goal setting and attainment skills		
Play reflects children's preconceptions about their future lives.	Set goals that get them to learn information.	Can set goals to increase skills and abilities, will set moderately difficult goals, take reasonable risks, and can cope with failure.
	With teacher praise for incremental increases, can gradually increase a personal work goal.	Differentiate between goals related to ability, effort, and performance.

References

Abery, B. H., & Stancliffe, R. J. (2003). An ecological theory of self-determination: Theoretical foundations. In M. L. Wehmeyer, B. H. Abery, D. E. Mithaug, & R. J. Stancliffe (Eds.), Theory in self-determination: Foundations for educational practice (pp. 25–42). Springfield: Thomas.

Agran, M., & Wehmeyer, M. L. (2005). Teaching problem solving to students with mental retardation. In M. L. Wehmeyer & M. Agran (Eds.), *Mental retardation and intellectual disabilities: Teaching students using innovative and research-based strategies* (pp. 255–271). Washington, DC: AAMR.

Ainsworth, M. D., & Bell, S. M. (1974). Mother-infant interaction and the development of competence. In K. Connolly & J. Bruner (Eds.), *The growth of competence* (pp. 97–118). New York: Academic Press.

Baltes, P. B., & Baltes, M. M. (1990). Psychological perspectives on successful aging: The model of selective optimization with compensation. In P. B. Baltes & M. M. Galtes (Eds.), *Successful aging: Perspectives from the behavioral sciences* (pp. 1–34). New York: Cambridge University Press.

Bambara, L. M., & Kroger, F. (2005). Opportunities for daily choice making. In M. L. Wehmeyer & M. Agran (Eds.), *Mental retardation and intellectual disabilities: Teaching students using innovative and research-based strategies* (pp. 213–233). Washington, DC: AAMR.

Barkley, R. A. (1997). *ADHD and the nature of self-control*. New York: Guailford Press.

Best, J. R., & Miller, P. H. (2010). A developmental perspective on executive function. *Child Development, 81*, 1641–7660. doi:10.1111/j.1467-8624.2010.01499.x.

Blair, R., College, E., & Mitchell, D. (2001). Somatic markers and response reversal: Is there orbitofrontal cortex dysfunction in boys with psychopathic tendencies? *Journal of Abnormal Child Psychology, 29*, 499–511.

Bronfenbrenner, U. (1979). *The ecology of human development: Experiments by nature and design*. Cambridge, MA: Harvard University Press.

Bronson, M. B. (2000). *Self-regulation in early childhood: Nature and nurture*. New York: Guildford.

Brownell, C. A., & Carriger, M. (1990). Changes in cooperation and self-other differentiation during the second year of life. *Child Development, 61*, 1164–1174.

Brownell, C. A., & Carriger, M (1991). Collaboration among toddler peers: Individual contributions to social contexts. In L. Resnick & J. Leivine (Eds.), Perspectives on socially shared cognitions (pp365–383, Washington, DC: APA.

Bullock, M., & Lutkenhaus, P. (1988). The development of volitional behavior in the toddler years. *Child Development, 59*, 664–674.

Buss, A. T., & Spencer, J. P. (2014). *The emergent executive: A dynamic field theory of the development of executive function, Monographs of child development* (Vol. 79). Ann Arbor: Society for Research in Child Development.

Cannon, E. N., & Woodward, A. L. (2012). Infants generate goal-based action predictions. *Developmental Science, 15*, 292–298.

Craig, G. J., & Myers, J. L. (1963). A developmental study of sequential two-choice decision making. *Child Development, 34*, 483–493.

Dale, P. S. (1976). *Language development: Structure and function*. New York: Holt Rinehart and Winston.

Damon, W. (1983). *Social and personality development*. New York: Norton.

Deci, E. L., & Ryan, R. M. (1985). *Intrinsic motivation and self-determination in human behavior*. New York: Plenum.

Deci, E. L., & Ryan, R. M. (2012). Motivation, personality, and development within embedded social contexts: An overview of self-determination theory. In R. M. Ryan (Ed.), *The Oxford handbook of human motivation* (pp. 85–110). Oxford: Oxford University Press.

Denissen, J. J. A., van Aken, M. A. G., Penke, L., & Wood, D. (2013). Self-regulation underlies temperament and personality: An integrative developmental framework. *Child Development Perspectives, 7*, 255–260.

Doll, B., & Wehmeyer, M. L. (2005). Teaching goal setting and decision making to students with developmental disabilities. In M. L. Wehmeyer & M. Agran (Eds.), *Mental retardation and intellectual disabilities: Teaching students using innovative and research-based strategies* (pp. 273–296). Washington, DC: AAMR.

Doll, B., Sands, D. J., Wehmeyer, M. L., & Palmer, S. B. (1996). Promoting the development of self-determined behavior. In D. J. Sands & M. L. Wehmeyer (Eds.), *Self-determination across the life-span* (pp. 65–90). Baltimore: Paul H. Brookes Publishing.

Farrington-Flint, L., Vanuxem-Cotterill, S., & Stiller, J. (2009). Patterns of problem-solving in children's literacy and arithmetic. *British Journal of Developmental Psychology, 27*, 815–834.

Folmer, A. S., Cole, D. A., Sigal, A. B., Benbow, L. D., Satterwhile, L. F., Swygert, K. E., & Ciesla, J. A. (2008). Age-related changes in children's understanding of effort and ability: Implications for attribution theory and motivation. *Journal of Experimental Child Psychology, 99*, 114–134.

Furby, L., & Beyth Marom, R. (1992). Risk taking in adolescence: A decision-making perspective. *Developmental Review, 12*, 1–44.

Garon, N., & Moore, C. (2004). Complex decision making in early childhood. *Brain and Cognition, 55*, 158–170.

Garon, N., Bryson, S. E., and Smith, I. M. (2008). Executive function in preschoolers: A review using an integrative framework. *Psychological Bulletin, 134*, 31–60. doi: 10-1037/0033-2909.134.1.31.

Geldhof, G. J., & Little, T. D. (2011). Influences of children's and adolescents' action-control processes on school achievement, peer relationships, and coping with challenging life events. In R. M. Lerner, J. V. Lerner, E. P. Bowers, S. Lewin-Bizan, S. Gestsdottir, & J. B. Urban (Eds.), *Thriving in childhood and adolescence: The role of self-regulation processes, New directions for child and adolescent development* (Vol. 133, pp. 45–59). San Francisco: Jossey-Bass.

Gerson, S. A. (2014). Sharing and comparing: How comparing shared goals broadens goal understanding in development. *Child Development Perspectives, 8*, 24–29.

Gerson, S. A., & Woodward, A. L. (2013). The goal trumps the means: Alignment of goals is more beneficial than alignment of means in means-end training. *Infancy, 18*, 289–302. doi:10.1111/j.1532-7078.2012.0012.x.

Hamlin, J. K., Hallinan, E. V., & Woodward, A. L. (2008). Do as I do: 7-month-old infants selectively reproduce others' goals. *Developmental Science, 11*, 487–494. doi:10.1111/j.1467-7687.2008.00694.x.

Hawley, P. H., & Little, T. D. (2002). Evolutionary and developmental perspectives on the agentic self. In D. Cervone & W. Mischel (Eds.), *Advances in personality science* (pp. 177–195). New York: Guilford.

Hickson, L., & Khemka, I. (2013). Problem solving and decision making. In M. L. Wehmeyer (Ed.), *The Oxford handbook of positive psychology and disability* (pp. 198–225). New York: Oxford University Press.

Hudson, J. A., & Fivush, R. (1991). Planning in the preschool years: The emergence of plans from general event knowledge. *Cognitive Development, 6*, 393–415.

Jacobs, J. E., & Klacqynski, P. A. (2002). The development of judgment and decision-making during childhood and adolescence. *Current Directions in Psychological Science, 11*, 145–149.

Karoly, P. (1993). Mechanisms of self-regulation: A systems view. *Annual Review of Psychology, 44*, 23–52. doi: 0066-4308/93/0201-0023.

King-Sears, M. E., & Carpenter, S. L. (2005). Teaching self-management to elementary students with developmental disabilities. In M. L. Wehmeyer & M. Agran (Eds.), *Mental retardation and intellectual disabilities: Teaching students using innovative and research-based strategies* (pp. 235–253). Washington, DC: AAMR.

Kopp, C. (1982). Antecedents of self-regulation: A development perspective. *Developmental Psychology, 25*, 343–354.
Landy, S. (2002). *Pathways to competence: Encouraging healthy social and emotional development in young children*. Baltimore: Paul H. Brookes Publishing.
Little, T. D., & Lopez, D. F. (1996). Children's action-control beliefs and emotional regulation in the social domain. *Developmental Psychology, 32*, 299–312.
Little, T. D., Stetsenko, A., & Maier, H. (1999). Action-control beliefs and school performance: A longitudinal study of Moscow children and adolescents. *International Journal of Behavioral Development, 23*, 799–823.
Little, T., Hawley, P., Henrich, C., & Marsland, K. (2002). Three views of the agentic self: A developmental synthesis. In E. L. Deci & R. M. Ryan (Eds.), *Handbook of self-determination research* (pp. 389–404). Rochester: University of Rochester Press.
Little, T. D., Snyder, C. R., & Wehmeyer, M. (2006). The agentic self: On the nature and origins of personal agency across the lifespan. In D. K. Mroczek & T. D. Little (Eds.), *Handbook of personality development* (pp. 61–80). Mahwah: LEA.
Macoby, E. E., & Martin, J. (1983). Socialization in the context of the family: Parent-child interaction. In E. M. Hetherington (Ed.), *Handbook of child psychology, Socialization, personality, and social development* (Vol. 4, pp. 1–101). New York: Wiley.
Masten, A. S., & Coatsworth, J. D. (1998). The development of competence in favorable and unfavorable environments: Lessons from research on successful children. *American Psychologist, 53*, 205–220.
McClelland, M. M., & Cameron, C. E. (2011). Self-regulation and academic achievement in elementary school children. *New Directions for Child and Adolescent Development, 133*, 29–44.
McCormick, K. M., Jolivette, K., & Ridgley, R. (2003). Choice making as an intervention strategy for young children. *Young Exceptional Children, 6*, 3–10. doi:10.1177/109625060300600202.
Mischel, W., Shoda, Y., & Rodriguez, M. L. (1989). Delay of gratification in children. *Science, 244*, 933–338.
Mithaug, D. E. (2003). Explaining what we don't know about self-determination. In M. L. Wehmeyer, B. H. Abery, D. E. Mithaug, & R. J. Stancliffe (Eds.), *Theory in self-determination: Foundations for educational practice* (pp. 134–154). Springfield: Thomas.
Moffitt, T. E., Arseneault, L., Belsky, D., Dickson, N., Handox, R. J., Harrington, H., … Caspi, A. (2011). A gradient of childhood self-control predicts health, wealth, and public safety. *Proceedings of the National Academy of Sciences, 108*, 2393–2698.
Nicholls, J. G. (1978). The development of the concepts of effort and ability, perception of academic attainment, and the understanding that difficult tasks require more ability. *Child Development, 49*, 800–814.
Palmer, S. B. (2010). Self-determination – A life-span perspective. *Focus on Exceptional Children, 42*, 1–16.
Palmer, S., Summers, J. A., Brotherson, M. J. Erwin, E., Maude, S., Stroup-Rentier, V. …Haines, S. (2012). Building a foundation for self-determination in early childhood: An inclusive model for children with disabilities. Topics in Early Childhood Special Education, 33, 38–47. doi:10.1177/0271121412445288
Piaget, J. (1963). *The origins of intelligence in children*. New York: Norton.
Ramani, G. B., & Brownell, C. A. (2014). Preschoolers' cooperative problem solving: Integrating play and problem solving. *Journal of Early Childhood Research, 12*, 92–108.
Reid, D. H., Parsons, M. B., & Green, C. W. (2001). Evaluating the functional utility of congregate day treatment activities for adults with severe disabilities. *American Journal on Mental Retardation, 106*, 460–469.
Rogoff, B. (2003). *The cultural nature of human development*. Oxford: Oxford University Press.
Rossetti, L. (1990). *The Rossetti infant-toddler language scale*. East Moline: LinguiSystems, Inc..
Selman. (1980). *The growth of interpersonal understanding: Developmental and clinical analyzes*. New York: Academic Press.

Shogren, K. A. (2013a). A social-ecological analysis of the self-determination literature. *Intellectual and Developmental Disabilities, 51*, 496–511.
Shogren, K. A. (2013b). *Self-determination and transition planning*. Baltimore: Paul H. Brookes.
Shonkoff, J. P., & Phillips, D. A. (2000). *From neurons to neighborhoods: The science of early childhood development*. Washington, DC: National Academy Press.
Sigler, R. S. (1996). *Emerging minds: The process of change in children's thinking*. Oxford: Oxford University Press.
Skinner, E. A. (1990). Age differences in the dimensions of perceived control during middle childhood: Implications for developmental conceptualizations and research. *Child Development, 61*, 1882–1890.
Skinner, E. A., Chapman, M., & Baltes, P. B. (1988). Beliefs about control, means-ends, and agency: A new conceptualization and its measurement during childhood. *Journal of Personality and Social Psychology, 54*, 117–133.
Stern, D. (1985). *The interpersonal world of the infant*. New York: Basic Books.
Summers, J. A., Brotherson, M. J., Erwin,E. J., Maude,S. P., Palmer, S. B., Haines, S. J., … Zheng, Y. Z. (2014). Family reflections on the foundations of self-determination in early childhood. *Inclusion, 2*, 175–194. doi: 10.1352/2326-6988-2.03.175.
Tomasello, M. (2009). *Why we cooperate*. Cambringe, MA: MIT Press.
Trabasso, T., Stein, N., Rodkin, P., Park, M., & Baughan, C. (1992). Knowledge of goals and plans in the on-line narration of events. *Cognitive Development, 7*, 133–170.
Vygotsky, L. S. (1962). *Thought and language*. Cambridge, MA: MIT Press.
Wehmeyer, M. L. (2003). Self-determination: A review of the construct. In M. L. Wehmeyer, B. H. Abery, D. E. Mithaug, & R. J. Stancliffe (Eds.), *Theory in self-determination: Foundations for educational practice* (pp. 5–24). Springfield: Thomas.
Wehmeyer, M. L., & Palmer, S. B. (2000). Promoting the acquisition and development of self-determination in young children with disabilities. *Early Education & Development, 11*, 465–481.
Wehmeyer, M. L., Sands, D. J., Doll, B., & Palmer, S. B. (1997). The development of self-determination and implications for educational interventions with students with disabilities. *International Journal of Disability, Development and Education, 44*, 305–328.
Wehmeyer, M. L., Abery, B. H., Mathaug, D. E., & Stancliffe, R. M. (2003). *Theory in self-determination: Foundations for educational practice*. Springfield: Charles C. Thomas.
Wehmeyer, M. L., Agran, M., Hughes, C., Martin, J. E., Mithaug, D. E., & Palmer, S. B. (2007). *Promoting self-determination in students with developmental disabilities*. New York: Guilford Press.
Whitman, T. L. (1990). Self-regulation and mental retardation. *American Journal on Mental Retardation., 94*, 373–376.
Willatts, P. (1990). Development of problem-solving strategies in infancy. In D. F. Bjorklund (Ed.), *Children's strategies: Contemporary views of cognitive development* (pp. 23–56). Hillsdale: Erlbaum.
Zelazo, P. D., Muller, U., Frye, D., & Marcovitch, S. (2003). *The development of executive function in early childhood, Monographs of the society for research in child development, 68, Serial no.27*. Boston: Blackwell Pub.
Zimmerman, B. J. (2008). Investigating self-regulation and motivation: Historical background, methodological developments, and future prospects. *American Educational Research Journal, 45*, 166–183. doi:10.31032/0002831207312909.
Zimmerman, B. J., & Schunk, D. H. (2007). Motivation: An essential dimension of self-regulated learning. In D. H. Schunk & B. J. Zimmerman (Eds.), *Motivation and self-regulated learning: Theory, research, and applications* (pp. 1–30). Mahwah: Lawrence Erlbaum.

Chapter 7
The Development of Self-Determination During Adolescence

Michael L. Wehmeyer and Karrie A. Shogren

Abstract The intent of this chapter is to provide an examination of the foundational skills, knowledge, and beliefs leading to the development of causal and agentic capabilities and action control beliefs during the adolescent years. The chapter overviews developmental milestones in knowledge, skills, and beliefs that emerge during adolescence and lead to enhanced self-determination, including choice making, self-initiation and planning, problem solving, decision making, goal setting and attainment, and self-regulation. The chapter concludes with a brief overview of issues in adolescent development as it pertains to motivational aspects of self-determination.

Chapter 3 situated the development of self-determination within the broader context of adolescent development and the development of self-identity and agency. Chapter 6 examined the development, during childhood years, of foundational knowledge, skills, and beliefs leading to the development, use, and refinement of causal and agentic capabilities and action-control beliefs that enable experiences of causal agency and lead to enhanced self-determination. The intent of this chapter is to book-end Chap. 6 by providing an examination of the foundational skills, knowledge, and beliefs leading to the development of causal and agentic capabilities and action control beliefs during the adolescent years. Instead of situating self-determination in the context of adolescent development, which was accomplished in Chap. 3, this chapter overviews developmental milestones in knowledge, skills, and beliefs that emerge during adolescence and lead to enhanced self-determination.

As we have noted, adolescents become self-determined—that is, manifest the dispositional characteristic of self-determination—as they learn, refine, and practice knowledge, skills, beliefs and actions that enable them to respond to contextual and environmental challenges (opportunities, threats) that energize basic psychological needs and resultant autonomous motivation, stimulating a causal action sequence in which volitional and agentic actions are mediated by action-control beliefs, resulting

M.L. Wehmeyer (✉) • K.A. Shogren
Special Education,University of Kansas, Lawrence, KS, USA
e-mail: wehmeyer@ku.edu

M.L. Wehmeyer et al. (eds.), *Development of Self-Determination Through the Life-Course*, DOI 10.1007/978-94-024-1042-6_7

Table 7.1 Component elements of self-determination under Causal Agency Theory

Essential characteristics	Component constructs	Component elements
Volitional action	Autonomy	**Causal capabilities**
	Self-initiation	Choice-making skills
		Decision-making skills
		Goal-setting skills
		Problem-solving skills
		Planning skills
Agentic action	Self-regulation	**Agentic capabilities**
	Self-direction	Self-management skills (self-monitoring, self-evaluation, etc.)
	Pathways thinking	Goal-attainment skills
		Problem-solving skills
		Self-advocacy skills
Action-control beliefs	Psychological empowerment	Self-awareness
	Self-realization	Self-knowledge
	Control expectancy	
	Agency beliefs	
	Causality beliefs	

in experiences of causal agency. The specific knowledge, skills, beliefs, and actions are identified as component elements within Causal Agency Theory (Table 7.1), and it is to these component elements that we turn to describe the development of self-determination during adolescence.

The following discussion of the development of causal action (and, consequently, self-determination) is structured according to Causal Agency Theory's essential characteristics—Volitional Action, Agentic Action, Action-Control Beliefs—and their respective component constructs and component elements.

Development of Component Elements of Volitional Action

Choice-Making Skills

Volitional action involves making conscious choices that reflect one's preferences, interests, values, and goals. Conscious choices are intentionally conceived, deliberate acts that occur without undue external influence. As such, volitional actions are self-initiated and function to enable a person to act autonomously (i.e., engage in self-governed action). The major developmental milestones associated with the expression of preferences and making choices are, essentially, achieved during early childhood and elementary years, as detailed in Chaps. 6 and 15. Where issues pertaining to choice making emerge during adolescence involve the role of choice making (willingness to choose) in decision making—involving the tendency of younger adolescents to seek conformity and to be more influenced by peers in making a decision than are older adolescents--and issues of choosing and preference pertaining to weighing risks and benefits of actions. These issues, in turn, relate to the broader issue of the development of autonomy and volitional functioning. As per SDT, autonomy refers to the development of enhanced volitional functioning (rather than strictly the development of independence), and the major developmental task associated with choice making or the expression of preferences in adolescence (and the major task of parents who are trying to provide autonomy supports) involves youth increasing their volitional functioning through repeated and supported expressions of preferences (Soenens et al. 2007).

Self-Initiation and Planning

Chapter 16 details developmental aspects of self-initiation and planning skills. To act volitionally, actions must not only involve conscious choices that reflect one's preferences, but must also be intentionally conceived (planned) and self-initiated. As Nurmi (1991) noted, "adolescents are faced with a number of normative age-specific tasks … set by their parents, peers, and teachers, most of which concern expected life-span development and which, therefore, emphasize the importance of thinking about the future" (p. 1). Adolescence is, obviously, a period of intense interest in future plans, from career to education to personal life experiences. Nurmi situates future-oriented thinking in terms of three processes: motivation, planning, and evaluation. In the context of our proposed framework pertaining to the development of self-determination (see Figure 5.1), the basic need for autonomy, competence, and relatedness lead to autonomous motivation, which in response to opportunities and threats in the environment, trigger the causal action sequence. An autonomous motivation results in goals, which trigger planning activities, which when implemented, are evaluated.

The development of future orientation and planning involve the acquisition of skill sets that include anticipatory knowledge, problem definition, and strategy selection and improved metacognition and metarepresentation skills. These later emerge in early adolescence. As discussed in detail in Chap. 19, by late elementary ages, children have acquired the basic skills they need for planning, but during adolescence these skills become increasingly sophisticated as young people acquire better understandings of causal attributions and linkages between current action and future outcomes.

Development of Component Elements of Agentic Action

Problem-Solving Skills

Choice-making skills are critical to volitional action, but once one has acted based upon preferences, one must sustain that through agentic action. Agentic action is a means by which something is done or achieved. Such action is self-directed and goal oriented, and requires the implementation of a number of skills, including problem-solving skills. As covered in detail in Chap. 19, a problem involves "existing or anticipated life situations or tasks that require responses for adaptive functioning, but for which no effective coping responses are immediately identifiable or available to the individual" (Nezu 2004, p. 3). As discussed in Chap. 6, during early years, the development of problem-solving skills focuses on the development of perspective taking, planning, forming mental representations, and the ability to attend to relevant stimuli (Best and Miller 2010). Because so many problems involve social interactions or social situations, early development also focuses on learning social norms and activities, like cooperation and mutual understandings of social actions (Ramani and Brownell 2014).

By late elementary school, children begin to be able to identify problem situations and more systematically modify their approach in the face of evidence that what they are doing is not working. As such, the early adolescent years are crucial in the development of problem solving. During this time span, beginning around age 12, the ability of young adolescents to cognitively understand and process information from complex situations matures. As adolescents become increasingly independent, the opportunities for encountering (and learning to solve) social, academic, and other types of problems increase. Over time, adolescents are able to improve both the quality of the solutions they come to when faced with a problem, but also to increase the number of possible solutions they can generate.

Of particular importance for the development of self-determination is the development of social problem-solving skills. Rubin and Krasnor (1986) identified a number of skills that develop through adolescence that impact the development of problem solving:

- Recognition of interpersonal problems.
- Ability to generate alternative solutions to problems.
- Means-end thinking (ability to generate step-by-step means).
- Ability to identify consequences of social acts.
- Ability to identify and understand motives and behaviors of others (Rubin and Krasnor 1986).

Decision-Making Skills

The decision-making process incorporates both problem-solving and choice-making skills, and thus, developmentally, is situated primarily in adolescence. Chapter 20 details the development of decision making, but in essence, the development of many of the skills associated with, particularly, problem-solving (though also planning and future orientation) are incorporated into the emergence of decision-making capacity. As adolescents age, they gain more experience solving problems, develop the capacity to weigh pros and cons, and mature in the decision-making process. Much of the development during adolescence involves maturation, experience, and opportunity.

An area of particular focus in adolescence is the development of consequential thinking. As adolescents develop inductive and deductive reasoning skills they develop the capacity to consider consequences of action, but issues of maturity, peer networks and desires for conformity, and emotionality may come to play in whether adolescents apply that knowledge to the decision to engage in risky behavior. Modecki (2016) found that adolescents generally under-appreciate risks. Modecki identified several risk cognitions that come into play in judging risk: risk probability (estimations of the probability or likelihood of risk), risk identification, risk tolerance, risk salience (level of care about negative outcomes should they occur), and risk preference (relative importance of possible risk in relations to possible benefits of behavior) and found that adolescents scored less adaptively in all of these risk cognition areas except for risk probability. Efforts to focus on these various cognitions are likely important in development. Finally, recent research (Jackman and MacPhee 2015) has suggested that self-esteem and future orientation are strong predictors of risk engagement.

Self-Advocacy Skills

The development of self-advocacy skills—those skills involved in the action of representing oneself or one's views or interests—are, by necessity, linked to the development of self-identity, as discussed in Chap. 3. Young adolescents begin to "develop more abstract characterizations of themselves, and self-concepts become more differentiated and better organized" (Steinberg and Morris 2001, p. 91). This identity begins to be shaped by issues such as personal beliefs, cultural customs, and personal capacities. With regard to the latter, adolescents evaluate themselves both globally but across various dimensions as well (e.g., academics, athletics, appearances, social networks, etc.). Early on, social comparisons are important, but become less so over time. Younger adolescents may describe themselves in "ways that are occasionally discrepant (e.g., shy with friends, outgoing at home)"(Steinberg and Morris 2001, p. 91), but these discrepancies decline in later adolescence.

Among the skills that become important to self-advocacy are compromise, negotiation, persuasion, and effective communication, as well as self-awareness. Self-advocacy is inherently goal oriented, so the developmental issues associated with goal setting and attainment (next section) are important here. In general, these skills emerge in late adolescence, as youth have a stronger and more stable self-identity, can delay gratification by looking at future benefits, can engage more systematically in decision making and problem solving, and can self-regulate emotions and have more mature conflict resolution skills.

Goal Setting and Attainment Skills

As noted in Chap. 18, autonomy-focused goal-oriented action is, in many ways, at the heart of causal agency and the development of self-determination; goals energize action to satisfy psychological needs, motivate organisms to use resources and energy in one direction rather than another direction, and, in essence, enable someone to act as a causal agent in one's life. Successful goal pursuit is associated with positive affect and higher well-being (Brunstein 1993). Goals are guided by previous learning experiences, individual characteristics, social and cultural norms, and opportunities afforded by one's context (Nurmi 1991). Goal setting and attainment is the fulcrum of causal action.

The early development of goal setting and attainment revolves around children's understanding of causality and, later, differentiating between aspects such as effort and luck, contingency and uncontrollability, and practice and ability. As such, part of the developmental trajectory of goal-directed behavior lies in the development of instrumental and communicative agency; the understanding of intent and intentionality, causality, and means-end action (Gergely 2011). In adolescence, developmental issues in goal setting and attainment mirror many of those discussed for other areas in this chapter, particularly problem solving and the issues of future orientation and planning.

Researchers consistently note that goal content usually reflects the important issues of a person's life period (age) (though influenced by cultural and gendered norms), and one developmental change in goal orientation from childhood to adolescence is that the nature of goals set change… in early adolescence, goals tend to focus on leisure activities, with school/education goals increasing from middle to late adolescence, and occupation, family, and property goals increasing in late adolescence and early adulthood (Brunstein 1993). In the nature of these goals, once can see developmental changes in self-identity, future orientation, and maturity, as well as the capacity to deal with more cognitively complex goals. Consistent with emerging planning abilities, planning for goal attainment increases during early to mid-adolescence. Expectations of goal realization between early to mid-adolescence remains stable, but in late adolescence, confidence in goal attainment increases (Brunstein 1993). Factors related to the family, such as parental support, involvement, nurturance, and aspirations, are related to maturity in adolescents' beliefs of goal attainability, while the influence of peers on goal setting is mixed; goals focused on such social outcomes as being popular or accepted have been show to have some linkages with risk factors for engagement in higher risk behaviors (Brunstein 1993).

Self-Regulation

In Chap. 17, self-regulation is viewed in the context of development as the bidirectional causal interactions between individuals and their contexts (developmental regulations); self-regulation is the person's impact on developmental regulations. As discussed in Chap. 6, self-regulation involves goal-directed action, and like other areas of skill development discussed in this chapter, shares a developmental trajectory incorporating issues of goal setting, future orientation, and metacognition. Successful self-regulation during adolescence involves increased awareness of one's future self, an orientation toward distal (future) goals, and the skills to be an active actor in one's own actions.

Early developmental components leading to self-regulation involve learning to control emotions, attention to detail, self-monitoring and evaluation, and, to a large measure, the neural development that allows for the development of mental representations necessary for goal setting and attainment, problem solving, and, ultimately, self-regulation (Gestsdottir and Lerner (2008). As described in Chap. 5, Causal Agency Theory defines causal agency in terms of volitional, and thus intentional action and self-regulation requires the development of intentionality; comprised, in large measure, of skills related to goal setting, problem solving, planning and so forth. These developmental advances are augmented by development in cognitive and self-control areas that facilitate delayed gratification, better planning skills, and more accurate self-evaluations. Gestsdottir and Lerner (2008) also pointed out that, as is the case with all of the domains discussed here, self-regulation "functions within a social context that is defined by parents, peers, and the larger society" (p. 213). Identity formation is also critical in the development of self-regulation, as young people understand themselves and others, and particularly the way others think, she or he can form representations of herself or himself in contexts that involve the need for self-regulation (Gestsdottir and Lerner 2008). Within SDT, the reciprocity "among a person's identity, his or her identity, his or her goals and goal-directed actions, and self-evaluations creates a dynamic system between identity and self-regulatory actions" (Gestsdottir and Lerner 2008, p. 214).

We have referred several times to the fact that the developmental sequence for skills leading to volitional and causal action are influenced by contexts, cultures, and familial factors. An organismic approach to understanding the developing person explicitly focuses on the interface between the self and surrounding environmental context. In fact, within Causal Agency Theory, contexts provide challenges (e.g. opportunities or threats) that are catalysts for actions. As noted in Chap. 5, a challenge is any circumstance that engages a person's abilities or resources to resolve a problem or threat as well as to achieve a goal. Human actions reflect responses to socio-contextual challenges. Challenging circumstances elicit volitional actions aimed at maintaining or enhancing a person's sense of personal agency. Given that self-regulation is a person's impact on developmental regulations, obviously, one needs to consider the development of self-regulation and contexts in multiple ways.

Development of Component Elements of Action-Control Beliefs

Another operant in causal action involves the emotions, feelings, and other affective components that influence human behavior. For example, emotions (a response involving physiological changes as a preparation for action) often are evoked in response to challenges, be they opportunities (joy, excitement) or threats (anger, anxiety) that heighten or limit the organism's capacity to respond. Similarly, feelings are cognitively-mediated emotions with long lasting impacts on both causal and agentic capability, thereby influencing the ways that the person will respond to future challenges.

Action-Control Theory posits that during the life course, individuals develop key beliefs that mediate autonomously-motivated causal actions (e.g., volitional, agentic) in response to environmental challenges: control expectancy beliefs (beliefs about the link between the self and the goal); capacity beliefs (beliefs about link between the self and the means for achieving the end); and causality beliefs (beliefs about the utility or usefulness of a given means for attaining a goal). Chapter 22 discusses these Action-Control Beliefs in greater detail. But, the obvious developmental milestones pertaining to the development of these action-control beliefs are those discussed previously related to self-identity, attributions of causality, means-end deductions, goal setting and attainment, and problem solving.

Unlike other dimensions of causal action discussed in this chapter, the development of action-control beliefs differentiates over time such that by adolescence, such beliefs become domain specific and means specific. That is, adolescents gradually understand that "different domains of functioning have different challenges and require different skills" (Little et al. 2002).

SDT and Adolescent Development

The prior sections examined the development of skills pertaining to causal action. This section provides a brief overview of issues in adolescent development as it pertains to motivational aspects (that is, with regard to SDT). This issue is discussed in detail in Chap. 14.

Of course, the most important factor in healthy development and motivation is the relationship between the adolescent and his or her parents or caregivers (La Guardia and Ryan 2002). The development of autonomy and relatedness, particularly, require a shift in parent/caregiver-adolescent interactions, from more direct parental structuring of environments in childhood to maintaining reasonable limits but also providing optimal challenges during adolescence. As per La Guardia and Ryan (2002):

> The SDT view of adolescent development is quite different from [the] traditional formulation. According to SDT, the process of individuation indeed concerns internalization of values, identity development, and extrafamilial relatedness. However, none of these developmental tasks is seen as necessitating separateness, independence, or "breaking away" from parents. In fact, such detachment is viewed as neither "natural" nor particularly healthy. Instead, separateness, rebelling, or breaking away are seen as reactions to familial and cultural conditions that frustrate psychological needs (p. 197).

So, consistent with SDTs view of autonomy as referring to the development of enhanced volitional functioning (rather than strictly the development of independence), developmental issues are focused on supporting volitional functioning through repeated and supported expressions of preferences and not simply *independence*.

Much of the work on development in adolescence pertaining to SDT has focused on identity development. La Guardia (2009) noted that according to SDT, "identities are adopted in the service of … basic psychological needs (p. 92). In essence, people are drawn to "activities, roles, and relationships that promote basic psychological needs" and "will avoid or engage only with significant costs to their well-being those domains or activities that threaten basic needs" (La Guardia 2009, p. 93). Such action in the service of basic psychological needs shapes and forms an adolescent's identity. Chapter 14 discusses these issues of identity development in much more detail.

In addition, as detailed in Chap. 14, adolescence is an important time for the internalization of behavioral regulation, during which extrinsically-motivated actions become self-endorsed and internally regulated. La Guardia and Ryan (2002) pointed out that opportunities to express competence impact intrinsic motivation in adolescence.

Conclusions

As was noted in Chap. 6, adolescents become self-determined—that is, having the dispositional characteristic of self-determination—as they learn, refine, and practice knowledge, skills, beliefs and actions that enable them to respond to contextual and environmental challenges (opportunities, threats) that energize basic psychological needs and resultant autonomous motivation, stimulating a causal action sequence in which volitional and agentic actions are mediated by action-control beliefs, resulting in experiences of causal agency. The specific knowledge, skills, beliefs, and actions are identified as component elements within Causal Agency Theory (Table 7.1) and include learning to make choices and express preferences, solve problems, engage in making decisions, set and attain goals, self-manage and self-regulate action, self-advocate, and acquire self-awareness and self-knowledge. It is the development of these component elements, across childhood and adolescence, that enable young people to act as causal agents in their lives, and, eventually, become more self-determined.

References

Best, J. R., & Miller, P. H. (2010). A developmental perspective on executive function. *Child Development, 81*, 1641–7660.

Brunstein, J. C. (1993). Personal goals and subjective well-being: A longitudinal study. *Journal of Personality and Social Psychology, 65*, 1061–1070.

Gergely, G. (2011). Kinds of agents: The origins of understanding instrumental and communicative agency. In U. Guswami (Ed.), *The Wiley-Blackwell handbook of childhood cognitive development* (2nd ed., pp. 76–105). London: Wiley-Blackwell.

Gestsdottir, S., & Lerner, R. M. (2008). Positive development in adolescence. The development and role of intentional self-regulation. *Human Development, 51*(3), 202–224.

Jackman, D. M., & MacPhee, D. (2015). Self-esteem and future orientation predict adolescents' risk engagement. *The Journal of Early Adolescence*. doi:10.1177/0272431615602756.

La Guardia, J. G. (2009). Developing who I am: A self-determinatoin theory approach to the establishment of healthy identies. *Educational Psychologist, 44*(2), 90–104.

La Guardia, J. G., & Ryan, R. M. (2002). What adolescents need: A self-determination theory perspective on development within families, school and society. In F. Pajares & T. Urdan (Eds.), *Academic motivation of adolescents*. IAP: Greenwich.

Little, T. D., Hawley, P. H., Henrich, C. C., & Marsland, K. W. (2002). Three views of the agentic self: A developmental synthesis. In E. L. Deci & R. M. Ryan (Eds.), *Handbook of self-determination research*. Rochester: University of Rochester Press.

Modecki, K. L. (2016). Do risks matter? Variable and person-centered approaches to adolescents problem behavior. *Journal of Applied Developmental Psychology, 42*, 8–20.

Nezu, A. M. (2004). Problem solving and behavior therpay revisited. *Behavior Therapy, 35*, 1–33.

Nurmi, J.-E. (1991). How do adolescents see their future? A review of the development of future orientation and planning. *Developmental Review, 11*, 1–59.

Ramani, G. B., & Brownell, C. A. (2014). Preschoolers' cooperative problem solving: Integrating play and problem solving. *Journal of Early Childhood Research, 12*, 92–108.

Rubin, K. H., & Krasnor, L. R. (1986). Social-cognitive and social behavioral perspectives on problem solving. In M. Perlumutter (Ed.), *Cognitive perspectives on children's social and behavioral development: The Minnesota symposia on child psychology* (Vol. Vol. 18, pp. 1–68). Hillsdale: Erlbaum.

Soenens, B., Vansteenkiste, M., Lens, W., Luyckx, K., Goossens, L., Beyers, W., et al. (2007). Conceptualizing parental autonomy support: Adolescent perceptions of promotion of independence versus promotion of volitional functioning. *Developmental Psychology, 43*(3), 633–646.

Steinberg, L., & Morris, A. S. (2001). Adolescent development. *Annual Review of Psychology, 52*, 83–110.

Chapter 8
Enhancing Students' Motivation with Autonomy-Supportive Classrooms

Rong Chang, Eriko Fukuda, James Durham, and Todd D. Little

Abstract Motivation is one of the most important factors that influences how students will approach learning. This chapter introduces the importance of autonomy-supportive classrooms, and why it is important to promote students' autonomy in learning. First, we describe how students can be motivated to learn from the viewpoint of Self-Determination Theory (SDT) and the factors that may support students' motivation in learning. Second, we present five practical guidelines on how to promote student-centered teaching practices that support student's autonomy: (a) communication of teacher's expectations and acknowledgement of student's feelings; (b) provision of more choices and removal of controlling events for learning; (c) student's active participation; (d) positive and informational feedback, and (e) structured guidance. Finally, the factors negatively contribute to insufficiency of teacher's autonomy are also examined.

People are motivated to regulate their behavior (Niemiec and Ryan 2009; Ryan and Deci 2000a). In the sphere of education, motivation is one of the most important factors that determines the approach students will take to learning and how they pursue developing their knowledge. A core question that remains for educators and researchers to understand is why some students exhibit a higher motivation profile for learning compared to their peers. In addition to evaluating the type and directions of classroom behaviors students partake in, Self-Determination Theory (SDT) seeks to address the issues related to the promotion of students' interests in learning, confidence in performance, and value of learning outcomes (Deci et al. 1991). From this perspective, students' active participation in learning is contingent on their fulfillment of basic psychological needs (Deci and Ryan 2000; Ryan and Deci 2000a). Research (Dignath et al. 2008; Kistner et al. 2010; Niemiec and Ryan 2009; Sierens et al. 2009) suggests that social support in the classrooms is an important facilitator of self-regulated learning because it promotes need satisfaction.

R. Chang (✉) • E. Fukuda • J. Durham
Texas Tech University, Lubbock, TX, USA
e-mail: rong.chang@ttu.edu

T.D. Little
Educational Psychology and Leadership, Texas Tech University, Lubbock, TX, USA

M.L. Wehmeyer et al. (eds.), *Development of Self-Determination Through the Life-Course*, DOI 10.1007/978-94-024-1042-6_8

Self-Determination Theory of Motivation

Intrinsic and Extrinsic Motivation for Learning

Self-Determination Theory (SDT) of motivation posits that the difference of people's behaviors not only exist in the amounts of motivation individuals exhibit, but in the types of motivations individuals have (Ryan and Deci 2000a). Thus, SDT distinguishes a continuum along intrinsic to extrinsic motivation as regulatory processes in learning (Deci and Ryan 2000; Ryan and Deci 2000a, b). Intrinsic motivation is inherent in individuals' own interests and satisfaction that the behaviors are enacted not from any external impetus (Deci and Ryan 2000; Ryan and Deci 2000a). When intrinsically motivated, a person will behave in a manner that is motivated by their own pursuits and their actions are fully self-determined. Students may enjoy math class because math itself is interesting and attractive to them. Their engagement in math is "curiosity-driven" even in the absence of any external rewards or controls such as grades or parental pressure (Deci and Ryan 1985; White 1959). There is evidence showing that students with innate curiosity and interests are more involved and satisfied with the learning tasks presented to them (Deci et al. 1981b, 1991). This involvement leads to satisfaction of the needs for autonomy and competence within the individual, which in turn leads to better academic outcomes. Therefore, a student's inherent tendency to learn is a valuable resource educators and researchers should tap into in order to develop methods that cultivate student motivation in the classroom (Flavell 1999; Ryan and Deci 2000a, b).

On the other hand, it is also understandable that the materials students are required to learn may not always be attractive to them at the immediate sense, and the learning tasks students are required to participate in may not reflect their personal utility (Ryan and Deci 2000a). At such moments, it is the environmental and interpersonal factors that compel students to learn. When students' behaviors are controlled by the presentation of external incentives, they are thereby extrinsically motivated. Extrinsic motivation refers to the behaviors which are performed in order to attain a separate outcome that is beyond the presented activity (Deci and Ryan 2000; Ryan and Deci 2000a). It is notable that extrinsically motivated behavior does not mean that engagement in the activity is not emanated from the sense of self. According to the levels of autonomy, external motivations are classified into four forms that fall along the fully extrinsic to intrinsic motivation continuum – external regulation, introjected regulation, identified regulation and integrated regulation (Deci and Ryan 1985).

External regulation is the least autonomous type of extrinsic motivation, and refers to behaviors that are maintained or performed by way of external rewards and punishments; that is, behaviors will not be sustained once the external controls are removed. For example some students might listen in the classroom because they notice the teacher is staring at them. The behaviors are maintained only to avoid the punishment from the teacher, thus these students are likely to be inattentive as soon as the teacher stops looking. Introjected regulation refers to behaviors that are performed to satisfy contingent self-esteem. For example, a student might study hard for an exam in order to avoid anxiety and to preserve the self-pride related to academic performance. Although this regulation contains some internal feeling, it is still quite controlling because learning behaviors are enacted to avoid the internal pressure. Conversely, identified regulation is more autonomous and self-determined, these behaviors are enacted because the person has identified the values of the outcomes. A student might exert a good deal of effort into studying the writing and literature classes very hard because of his or her desire to be a journalist in the future. In this way, the student has identified the importance of these classes.

Integrated regulation is the most self-determined form of externally regulated behavior; here, an individual has integrated the values of the learning activity into his or her sense of self–this process that transfers the external values of task into internal regulation is viewed as the internalization process. Studies have found that when perceived value of the task and sense of self are higher, students are more willing to engage in the learning activities and they exhibit greater persistence (Grolnick et al. 1991; Niemiec et al. 2006; Black and Deci 2000). Therefore, optimal internalization of external motivation "is essential for students' self-initiation and maintained volition for educational activities that are not inherently interesting or enjoyable" (Niemiec and Ryan 2009).

In sum, both intrinsic motivation and the different flavors of extrinsically motivated behaviors are intentional but vary in their degree of autonomy. The different types of motivation reflect how a person perceives the locus of causality. In the classroom settings, regardless if the motivation is intrinsic or extrinsic, with more autonomy and the higher the self-regulation for learning, then students are more likely to enjoy the class (Ryan and Connell 1989), gain deeper conceptual understanding (Benware and Deci 1984; Grolnick and Ryan 1987; Ying Hwa et al. 2012), and show less depression and anxiety (Black and Deci 2000; Niemiec et al. 2006; Ryan and Connell 1989). Notably, Ryan and Connell (1989) compared two types of extrinsically motivated students – introjected and identified regulation. They found no difference in the degree persistence and effort toward learning that the late elementary school students displayed. Students who were more introjected, however, reported more depression and remorse; whereas students who were more identified expressed higher interests and enjoyment for the class.

Nurture Intrinsic Motivation and Promote Internalization

Both intrinsic and extrinsic motivation are not permanent personal characteristics. They can change depending on the relation between the person and the activity itself (Kusurkar et al. 2011; Ryan and Deci 2000a). A student's motivation in learning may move from highly controlled regulation to self-determined, and vice versa (Deci 1975). Therefore, elements that sustain intrinsic motivation and promote internalization of extrinsic motivation are perhaps the greatest factors needed to be present in the classroom to promote student learning.

As mentioned, SDT posits that well-being and motivation are dependent on the satisfaction of the three basic psychological needs for competence, relatedness, and autonomy (Deci and Ryan 2000; Jang et al. 2009; Niemiec and Ryan 2009; Ryan and Deci 2000a). The need for competence refers to the need to feel capable of mastering the tasks, performing the effective actions, and reaching the expected outcomes (Deci and Ryan 1985; Ryan and Deci 2000a; White 1959). In the classroom, students' competence can be supported by veridical and supportive feedback from teachers, and by providing tasks that are challenging but within the ability of a given student to reach. Multiple studies (Blanck et al. 1984; Vallerand and Reid 1984; Harackiewicz and Larson 1986) have demonstrated that positive feedback, including good grades and appropriate praise can enhance motivation for learning by increasing perceived competence. If the positive feedback is not administrated in an autonomy supportive way, however, intrinsic motivation cannot be sustained (Fisher 1978; Deci et al. 1991; Ryan 1982). In particular, if the praise students receive is contingent on what they are told or forced to do, the feeling of being controlled undermines students' autonomy and feelings of self-determination. The more external controlled behaviors would strengthen the external regulation in students.

Another need SDT posits is relatedness, which refers to the need for secure and satisfying interpersonal relations (Deci and Ryan 1985; Ryan and Deci 2000a). Anderson et al. (1976) found that children lost their intrinsic motivation when they were denied by the social context they desired to join. In the classroom, students' relatedness can be strengthened by the teachers showing interpersonal respect and communicating frequently with students. Importantly, autonomy supportive environments promote feelings of being valued and the process of learning becomes more enjoyable and less anxiety provoking (Deci et al. 1991; Ryan 1991). In other words, satisfying the need for autonomy is essential to have students more involved and self-determined in the class.

Support for competence and relatedness will enhance intrinsic motivation and internalization only if they are administrated in an autonomy supportive environment (Ryan 1982; Grolnick and Ryan 1989). Autonomy refers to being able to have free choices on the tasks and goals, and self-initiating of one's own actions (Ryan and Deci 2000a; Ryan 1991). In other words, promoting a student-centered classroom environment. Intrinsically motivated people need to make choices based on their own needs and decide the ways they would like to attain these needs. In this regard, support for autonomy allows individuals to strive for self-realization and self-determination (Little et al. 2002, 2006). Both Swann and Pittman (1977) and Zuckerman et al. (1978) found that when students were allowed to make choice themselves, they tend to be more engaged, spend more time on the activities, and were more intrinsically motivated than those who were directly assigned the tasks. Benware and Deci (1984) found that college students who learned material with an active purpose to teach another student reported higher intrinsic motivation and presented better conceptual learning than those who learned in order to be tested.

In fact, numerous studies (Ryan 1982; Grolnick and Ryan 1989) supported this postulation that students' motivation, performance, and development are maximized in the classroom if the support of autonomy is provided.

Importance of Autonomy Supportive Teaching

Optimal support of autonomy in the classroom should be provided from the teachers, given that teachers, by definition, play the leading role in the teaching and learning process (Kusurkar et al. 2011; Reeve et al. 2004; Patrick and Williams 2009; Williams and Deci 1999; Young 2005). Many studies have examined the different consequences produced by either autonomy supportive or controlling teaching behaviors. Deci et al. (1981b), for example, found that those elementary students assigned to autonomy supportive teachers displayed higher intrinsic motivation and perceived competence compared to those assigned to controlling teachers. Similar results were found by Ryan and Grolnick (1986). In another study by Tsai et al. (2008), results showed that students' interests were enhanced in the classes when teachers were autonomy supportive, and reduced in the classes that teachers were controlling. Even for those uninteresting learning activities, the perceived autonomy support can promote the internalization of extrinsic regulation and facilitate them understand the personal value in those activities. Williams and Deci (1996) found that medical students who perceived higher support for autonomy from their instructors reported higher autonomous self-regulation and competence for the tasks. Vallerand et al. (1997) assessed different types of motivated students and showed that the autonomy supports from teachers were positively related to the self-determined process such as intrinsic motivation and identified self-regulation; whereas controlling teaching behaviors led to external regulation. Ying Hwa et al. (2012) studied adaptive-profile students (i.e., high self-efficacy, metacognition, & task values) versus maladaptive-profile students. Results showed that the adaptive profile was highly correlated with the perceptions of the autonomy supportiveness.

Implications of Providing Autonomy-Supportive Classroom

Autonomy-Supportive Teaching Practices

A large body of research (e.g., Grolnick and Ryan 1989; Ryan 1982; Vallerand et al. 1997) supports the postulation that students' motivation, performance, and development are maximized under autonomy supportive teaching behaviors. Thus, we presented four practical suggestions for teachers on how to support students' autonomy in the classroom based on the research evidences.

Communicate Frequently to Present the Expectations and Acknowledge Students' Feelings

There is plenty of information teachers can communicate with their students about such as the content and structure of the class and expected outcomes. With the clear knowledge of the class design, students are able to make study plans and accommodate their needs with the class (Koh et al. 2009). On the contrary, students that are unsure about what they are supposed to learn have to be dependent on immediate teachers' behaviors. Such dependency can easily lead a student to feel less respected and strongly controlled by the teacher, which will diminish the student's feeling of relatedness and autonomy.

More importantly, communication can also promote the internalization of extrinsic motivation. Because not all the learning materials and tasks are inherently interesting to all students, communication allows students to explore their interests with a minimum of pressure. Students are also able to receive emotional support and acknowledgment from their teachers. This form of communication enhances students' feelings of relatedness and autonomy for engaging the learning tasks. Additionally, teachers are able to identify students' needs and acknowledge their feelings through good communication (Kusurkar et al. 2011). Student feedback allows teachers to modify the class well. The modification of learning materials and activities can better facilitate the development of perceived competence and relatedness in students. Meanwhile, teachers can help students understand the value of the learning materials or their personal utility to perform the learning activities, which gradually guide students to realize an optimal internalization of uninteresting activities.

Offer More Choices and Remove Controlling Events in Learning

External limits such as deadlines of assignments, competitions, and tests have been found to decrease self-determination (Amabile et al. 1976; Deci et al. 1981a). Achieving an autonomy supportive classroom requires teachers to provide more options to their students when it is possible. For example, allowing students choices on a particular topic supports autonomy because students search for and find materials in which they are most interested. With more choices, students are allowed to make plans to direct their own learning behaviors. It helps them feel closely related to the learning materials (Katz and Assor 2007). Thus, students' internal guidance and perceived competence result sin higher intrinsic motivation. The choices also represent teachers' respect and trust on students' competence. Multiple studies have found that students become more intrinsically motivated when they are offered the opportunities to make choice on their own (Deci et al. 1994; Swann and Pittman 1977; Zuckerman et al. 1978).

Allow Students to Participate Actively

Learners should not be subjected to classrooms that make them passive observers. In a passive learning environment, students have little responsibility for the information and therefore is dependent on the teacher for everything. Teachers who continuously lecture stiffil student engagement; instead, frequently pausing to allow students to discuss what they know, and determine what they still want to know engages students in the learning process. In this way, students are able to share their ideas and opinions, and feel related to the learning activities.

Mere exposure to information does very little to help students learn the information. Offering some challenging tasks during the learning process is identified as the effective way to foster students' involvement (Dev 1997). The learning tasks should be challenging but within students' ability reach (Black 1996; Dev 1997). Such problem solving situations can make students feel autonomous and competence, and become active participants in their own learning.

Provide Positive and Informational Feedback

Students' motivation can be dramatically enhanced by appropriate feedback about what they have done. Veridical positive feedback increases students' perceived competence, and thus increases their self-efficacy in performing the similar activities (Blanck et al. 1984; Vallerand 1983). However, not all the positive feedback can increase self-determination. The feedback should be informative and constructive enough to present the support for autonomy (Ryan 1982). False praise begets false beliefs about one's self and one's capabilities. If students are praised for what they are self-initiated to act upon, tend to show higher perceived competence and autonomy, and thus become more intrinsic motivated. Conversely, if students receive positive praise for what they are told to do, they may feel more controlled and lose their intrinsic motivation for the task.

Provide Structured Guidance

Structured teaching practice is another instructional style which promotes students' autonomy in the classroom. Structure is defined as the extent and clarity of expectations that teachers provide to students as well as the methods to achieve desired educational outcomes (Jang et al. 2010). Structured teacher's instructional behaviors are characterized by (a) explicit, detailed, and easily understandable directions; (b) action plans to guide students' ongoing activity; and (c) constructive feedback on how students can control outcomes (Jang et al. 2010; Skinner and Belmont 1993). Structure can be implemented in either controlling or autonomy-supportive manners. When it is provided in the autonomy-supportive manner, learning outcomes are enhanced while these outcomes decrease when provided in a controlling manner. Empirical evidence was provided by Furtak and Kunter (2012). They found that German 7th grade students in a structured classroom learned science lessons significantly better, perceived more choices, and rated instructions more positively than those in a simply autonomy supporting environment. Jang et al. (2010) also reported that students' behavioral engagement was predicted by autonomy support and structure when trained observers rated high school classrooms. Consequently, autonomy-supportive classrooms incorporating structured teaching practices maximize the learning outcomes.

Although students in Western cultures benefit from structure (Jang et al. 2010; Sierens et al. 2009), it may be more beneficial to students in cultures where the socialization process is formed thorough regularity and respect for authority figures' directions (Wang et al. 2007). In such cultures, autonomy-supportive teaching practices can be highly ambiguous as students need to make more individual decisions. These students, for example learners in East Asian cultures (e.g., China, Japan, and Korea), may thrive in more certain learning environments (i.e., structured environments; Szeto et al. 2011). Oga-Boldwin and Nakata (2015) reported that Japanese elementary school students experience autonomy-support when an autonomy-supportive environment is combined with structure, which they defined as supportive-structure. Supportive structure was found to strongly influence students' class engagement and autonomy satisfaction. Thus, structure is an essential component to support students' autonomy.

Insufficiency in Teachers' Autonomy

With all the benefits of an autonomy supportive classroom, learning is still, unfortunately, driven by external controls and evaluation is typically offered with rewards or punishments (Niemiec and Ryan 2009). In order to promote an autonomy supportive classroom, we need to understand why teachers in the classroom often refuse to be autonomous.

First, controlling teaching behaviors reflect the external pressures that are placed on teachers (Deci et al. 1991; Ryan and Brown 2005). With more teaching pressures received from those above in the hierarchy, teachers' willingness to try different teaching activities is undermined (Deci et al. 1982; Pelletier et al. 2002; Roth et al. 2007). In such situations, teachers devote their time to presenting the required information to students in order to reach the academic demands asked by the school. In addition, teachers' controlling practices can also be due to the teaching beliefs which are shaped by educational experiences the teachers have received during their student time. Another contributing factor to controlling teaching behaviors comes from students' behaviors. Students' maladaptive behaviors of learning can easily reduce teachers' enthusiasm to apply autonomy supportive teaching ways (Jelsma 1982). That is, teachers tend to be more controlling to students if they believe those students are less interested in the learning materials or not involved in the activities. On the other hand, teachers are more willing to try autonomous teaching practices if students are highly motivated and regulated.

Conclusion

Teachers' autonomous behaviors are essential to create autonomy supportive classrooms. According to the research, it is important for educational administrators and policy makers to consider how to motivate teachers' autonomy supportive behaviors in the class room (Deci and Ryan 2002; Deci et al. 1991; Niemiec and Ryan 2009). Instead of putting unrealistic academic demands on educators, we should encourage an autonomous environment that allows more freedom for teachers to determine teaching content and structures for themselves which in turn enhances the autonomy supportive experiences of the students.

Authors' Note This work was partially supported by grant NSF 1053160 (Wei Wu & Todd D. Little, co-PIs) and by the Institute for Measurement, Methodology, Analysis, and Policy (Todd D. Little, Director) at Texas Tech University. Correspondence should be directed to Rong Chang (Rong.Chang@ttu.edu) or Todd D. Little (yhat@ttu.edu or yhat@statscamp.org).

Todd D. Little is founder and director of the annual Stats Camp (statscamp.org) and the director of the Institute for Measurement, Methodology, Analysis, and Policy (IMMAP) at Texas Tech University. He is a professor in the Research, Evaluation, Measurement, and Statistic Program of the Educational Psychology Department at TTU. He owns and receives remuneration from Yhat Enterprises, LLC, which runs educational workshops such as Stats Camp (statscamp.org), and processes his royalties and his fees for consulting on statistics and methods with life-science science researchers.

References

Amabile, T. M., DeJong, W., & Lepper, M. R. (1976). Effects of externally imposed deadlines on subsequent intrinsic motivation. *Journal of Personality and Social Psychology, 34*, 92–98.

Anderson, R., Manoogian, S. T., & Reznick, J. S. (1976). The undermining and enhancing of intrinsic motivation preschool children. *Journal of Personality & Social Psychology, 34*(5), 915–922.

Benware, C., & Deci, E. L. (1984). Quality of learning with an active versus passive motivational set. *American Educational Research Journal, 21*, 755–765.

Black, S. (1996). The truth about homework. *American School Board Journal, 183*(10), 48–51.

Black, A. E., & Deci, E. L. (2000). The effects of instructors' autonomy support and students' autonomous motivation on learning organic chemistry: A self- determination theory perspective. *Science Education, 84*, 740–756.

Blanck, P. D., Reis, H. T., & Jackson, L. (1984). The effects of verbal reinforcement of intrinsic motivation for sex-linked tasks. *Sex Roles, 10*, 369–386.

Deci, E. L. (1975). *Intrinsic motivation*. New York: Plenum.

Deci, E. L., & Ryan, R. M. (1985). *Intrinsic motivation and self-determination in human behavior*. New York: Plenum.

Deci, E. L., & Ryan, R. M. (2000). The "what" and "why" of goal pursuits: Human needs and the self-determination of behavior. *Psychological Inquiry, 11*, 227–268.

Deci, E. L., & Ryan, R. M. (2002). Self-determination research: Reflections and future directions. In E. L. Deci & R. M. Ryan (Eds.), *Handbook of self-determination research* (pp. 431–441). Rochester, NY: University of Rochester Press.

Deci, E. L., Betley, G., Kahle, J., Abrams, L., & Porac, J. (1981a). When trying to win: Competition and intrinsic motivation. *Personality and Social Psychology Bulletin, 7*(1), 79–83. doi:10.1177/014616728171012.

Deci, E. L., Schwartz, A. J., Sheinman, L., & Ryan, R. M. (1981b). An instrument to assess adults' orientations toward control versus autonomy with children: Reflections on intrinsic motivation and perceived competence. *Journal of Educational Psychology, 73*, 642–650.

Deci, E. L., Spiegel, N. H., Ryan, R. M., Koestner, R., & Kauffman, M. (1982). Effects of performance standards on teaching styles: Behavior of controlling teachers. *Journal of Educational Psychology, 74*(6), 852–859.

Deci, E. L., Vallerand, R. J., Pelletier, L. G., & Ryan, R. M. (1991). Motivation and education: The self-determination perspective. *The Educational Psychologist, 26*, 325–346.

Deci, E. L., Eghrari, H., Patrick, B. C., & Leone, D. R. (1994). Facilitating internalization: The self-determination theory perspective. *Journal of Personality, 62*(1), 119–142. doi:10.1111/1467-6494.ep9406221281.

Dev, P. C. (1997). Intrinsic motivation and academic achievement: What does their relationship imply for the classroom teacher? *Remedial and Special Education, 18*(1), 12–19.

Dignath, C. C., Buettner, G. B., & Langfeldt, H. L. (2008). How can primary school students learn self-regulated learning strategies most effectively?: A meta-analysis on self-regulation training programmes. *Educational Research Review, 3*(2), 101–129.

Fisher, C. D. (1978). The effects of personal control, competence, and extrinsic reward systems on intrinsic motivation. *Organizational Behavior & Human Performance, 21*(3), 273–288.

Flavell, J. H. (1999). Cognitive development: Children's knowledge about the mind. *Annual Review of Psychology, 50*, 21–45.

Furtak, E. M., & Kunter, M. (2012). Effects of autonomy-supportive teaching on student learning and motivation. *The Journal of Experimental Education, 80*(3), 284–316.

Grolnick, W. S., & Ryan, R. M. (1987). Autonomy in children's learning: An experimental and individual difference investigation. *Journal of Personality and Social Psychology, 52*(5), 890–898.

Grolnick, W. S., & Ryan, R. M. (1989). Parent styles associated with children's self-regulation and competence in school. *Journal of Educational Psychology, 81*(2), 143–154.

Grolnick, W. S., Ryan, R. M., & Deci, E. L. (1991). Inner resources for school achievement: Motivational mediators of children's perceptions of their parents. *Journal of Educational Psychology, 83*, 508–517.

Harackiewicz, J. M., & Larson, J. R. (1986). Managing motivation: The impact of supervisor feedback on subordinate task interest. *Journal of Personality & Social Psychology, 51*(3), 547–556.

Jang, H., Reeve, J., Ryan, R. M., & Kim, A. (2009). Can self-determination theory explain what underlies the productive, satisfying learning experiences of collectivistically oriented korean students? *Journal of Educational Psychology, 101*(3), 644–661.

Jang, H., Reeve, J., & Deci, E. L. (2010). Engaging students in learning activities: It is not autonomy support or structure but autonomy support and structure. *Journal of Educational Psychology, 102*(3), 588–600.

Jelsma, B. M. (1982). Adult control behaviors: The interaction between orientation toward control in women and activity level in children. *Dissertation Abstracts International, 43*, 1892.

Katz, I., & Assor, A. (2007). When choice motivates and when it does not. *Educational Psychology Review, 19*, 429–442.

Kistner, S., Rakoczy, K., Otto, B., Dignath-van Ewijk, C., Büttner, G., & Klieme, E. (2010). Promotion of self-regulated learning in classrooms: Investigating frequency, quality, and consequences for student performance. *Metacognition and Learning, 5*(2), 157–171. doi:10.1007/s11409-010-9055-3.

Koh, C., Wang, C. J., Tan, O. S., Liu, W. C., & Ee, J. (2009). Bridging the gaps between students' perceptions of group project work and their teachers' expectations. *Journal of Educational Research, 102*(5), 333–348.

Kusurkar, R. A., Croiset, G., & Ten Cate, T. J. (2011). Twelve tips to stimulate intrinsic motivation in students through autonomy-supportive classroom teaching derived from self-determination theory. *Medical Teacher, 33*(12), 978–982.
Little, T. D., Hawley, P. H., Henrich, C. C., & Marsland, K. W. (2002). Three views of the agentic self: A developmental synthesis. In E. L. Deci & R. M. Ryan (Eds.), *Handbook of self-determination research* (pp. 389–404). Rochester: University of Rochester Press.
Little, T. D., Snyder, C. R., & Wehmeyer, M. (2006). The agentic self: On the nature and origins of personal agency across the life span. In D. K. Mroczek & T. D. Little (Eds.), *Handbook of personality development* (pp. 61–79). Mahwah: LEA.
Niemiec, C. P., & Ryan, R. M. (2009). Autonomy, competence, and relatedness in the classroom: Applying self-determination theory to educational practice. *Theory and Research in Education, 7*(2), 133–144.
Niemiec, C. P., Lynch, M. F., Vansteenkiste, M., Bernstein, J., Deci, E. L., & Ryan, R. M. (2006). The antecedents and consequences of autonomous self-regulation for college: A self-determination theory perspective on socialization. *Journal of Adolescence, 29*, 761–775.
Oga-Boldwin, W. L. Q., & Nakata, Y. (2015). Structure also supports autonomy: Measuring and defining autonomy-supportive teaching in Japanese elementary foreign language classes. *Japanese Psychological Research, 27*(3), 167–179.
Patrick, H., & Williams, G. C. (2009). Self-determination in medical education: Encouraging medical educators to be more like blues artists and poets. *Theory and Research in Education, 7*(2), 184–193.
Pelletier, L. G., Séguin-Lévesque, C., & Legault, L. (2002). Pressure from above and pressure from below as determinants of teachers' motivation and teaching behaviors. *Journal of Educational Psychology, 94*, 186–196.
Reeve, J., Deci, E. L., & Ryan, R. M. (2004). Self-determination theory: A dialectical framework for understanding sociocultural influences on student motivation. In D. M. McInerney & S. van Etten (Eds.), *Big theories revisited* (pp. 31–60). Greenwich: Information Age Publishing Inc.
Roth, G., Assor, A., Kanat-Maymon, Y., & Kaplan, H. (2007). Autonomous motivation for teaching: How self-determined teaching may lead to self- determined learning. *Journal of Educational Psychology, 99*, 761–774.
Ryan, R. M. (1982). Control and information in the intrapersonal sphere: An extension of cognitive evaluation theory. *Journal of Personality and Social Psychology, 43*, 450–461.
Ryan, R. M. (1991). The nature of the self in autonomy and relatedness. In G. R. Goethals & J. Strauss (Eds.), *Multidisciplinary perspectives on the self* (pp. 208–238). New York: Springer.
Ryan, R. M., & Brown, K. W. (2005). Legislating competence: High-stakes testing policies and their relations with psychological theories and research. In A. J. Elliot & C. S. Dweck (Eds.), *Handbook of competence and motivation* (pp. 354–372). New York: Guilford Publications.
Ryan, R. M., & Connell, J. P. (1989). Perceived locus of causality and internalization: Examining reasons for acting in two domains. *Journal of Personality and Social Psychology, 57*(5), 749–761.
Ryan, R. M., & Deci, E. L. (2000a). Intrinsic and extrinsic motivations: Classic definitions and new directions. *Contemporary Educational Psychology, 25*(1), 54–67. doi:10.1006/ceps.1999.1020.
Ryan, R. M., & Deci, E. L. (2000b). Self-determination theory and the facilitation of intrinsic motivation, social development, and well-being. *American Psychologist, 55*, 68–78.
Ryan, R. M., & Grolnick, W. S. (1986). Origins and pawns in the classroom: Self-report and projective assessments of individual differences in children's perceptions. *Journal of Personality and Social Psychology, 50*, 550–558.
Sierens, E. F., Vansteenkiste, M., Goossens, L., Soenens, B., & Dochy, F. (2009). The synergistic relationship of perceived autonomy support and structure in the prediction of self-regulated learning. *British Journal of Educational Psychology, 79*(1), 57–68.

Skinner, E. A., & Belmont, M. J. (1993). Motivation in the classroom: Reciprocal effects of teacher behavior and student engagement across the school year. *Journal of Educational Psychology, 85*(4), 571–581.

Swann, W. J., & Pittman, T. S. (1977). Initiating play activity of children: The moderating influence of verbal cues on intrinsic motivation. *Child Development, 48*, 1128–1132.

Szeto, A. C. H., Sorrentino, R. M., Yasunaga, S., Kouhara, S., & Lin, L. (2011). Motivation and performance: Uncertainty regulation in Canada and Japan. *Motivation and Emotion, 35*, 338–350.

Tsai, Y., Kunter, M., Lüdtke, O., Trautwein, U., & Ryan, R. M. (2008). What makes lessons interesting? The role of situational and individual factors in three school subjects. *Journal of Educational Psychology, 100*(2), 460–472. doi:10.1037/0022-0663.100.2.460.

Vallerand, R. J. (1983). Effect of differential amounts of positive verbal feedback on the intrinsic motivation of male hockey players. *Journal of Sport Psychology, 5*, 100–107.

Vallerand, R. J., & Reid, G. (1984). On the causal effects of perceived competence on intrinsic motivation: A test of cognitive evaluation theory. *Journal of Sport Psychology, 6*, 94–102.

Vallerand, R. J., Fortier, M. S., & Guay, F. (1997). Self-determination and persistence in a real-life setting: Toward a motivational model of high school dropout. *Journal of Personality and Social Psychology, 72*(5), 1161–1176.

Wang, Q., Pomerantz, E. M., & Chen, H. (2007). The role of parents' control in early adolescents' psychological functioning: A longitudinal investigation in the United States and China. *Child Development, 78*, 1592–1610.

White, R. W. (1959). Motivation reconsidered. *Psychological Review, 66*, 297–333.

Williams, G. C., & Deci, E. L. (1996). Internalization of biopsychosocial values by medical students: A test of self-determination theory. *Journal of Personality and Social Psychology, 70*, 767–779.

Williams, G. C., & Deci, E. L. (1999). The importance of supporting autonomy in medical education. *Annual of Internal Medicine, 129*, 303–308.

Ying Hwa, K., Wang, C. J., Lim, B. C., & Woon Chia, L. (2012). Secondary students' motivation and learning strategies profiles: The importance of an autonomy-supportive classroom structure. In J. N. Franco & A. E. Svensgaard (Eds.), *Handbook on psychology of motivation* (pp. 271–282). Inc: Nova Science Pubilishers.

Young, M. (2005). The motivational effects of the classroom environment in facilitating self-regulated learning. *Journal of Marketing Education, 27*(1), 25–40.

Zuckerman, M., Porac, J., Lathin, D., Smith, R., & Deci, E. L. (1978). On the importance of self-determination for intrinsically motivated behavior. *Personality and Social Psychology Bulletin, 4*, 443–446.

Chapter 9
Applications of the Self-Determination Construct to Disability

Michael L. Wehmeyer and Karrie A. Shogren

Abstract Causal Agency Theory grew out of research and intervention development with, primarily, youth with disabilities. Much of the self-determination research in the disability context has examined interventions to teach or promote skills such as problem solving, goal setting, self-advocacy, and such and was, often, not theory-driven. Causal Agency Theory, however, emerged from research and theory pertaining to self-determination in the broader context of personality psychology and within the context of adolescent development, and understanding of the self-determination construct, from the onset, was heavily influenced by and drew from work in the early stages of the development of SDT. This chapter provides an overview of research in special education and related disciplines, as driven by Causal Agency Theory. We then discuss the knowledge and information from this literature base that can inform knowledge pertaining to self-determination, in general.

As discussed in Chap. 5, Causal Agency Theory grew out of research and intervention development with, primarily, youth with disabilities. In a 2004 chapter on SDT and intrinsic motivation and people with intellectual disability, Deci noted that the literature pertaining to self-determination in the disability sphere differed from SDT in several ways, particularly around understandings of autonomy and control. One of the purposes of this text is to align Causal Agency Theory, which intends to explain how people become self-determined, with work in SDT and intrinsic motivation to form an overarching model for the development of causal action and self-determination. Much of the self-determination research in the disability context has examined interventions to teach or promote skills such as problem solving, goal setting, self-advocacy, and such and was, often, not theory-driven. Causal Agency Theory, however, emerged from research and theory pertaining to self-determination in the broader context of personality psychology and within the context of adolescent development, and our understanding of the self-determination construct, from the onset,

M.L. Wehmeyer (✉) • K.A. Shogren
Special Education, University of Kansas, Lawrence, KS, USA
e-mail: wehmeyer@ku.edu

M.L. Wehmeyer et al. (eds.), *Development of Self-Determination Through the Life-Course*, DOI 10.1007/978-94-024-1042-6_9

was heavily influenced by and drew from work by Deci and Ryan and colleagues in the early stages of the development of SDT (Deci 1980; Deci and Ryan 1985) and, later, from work by colleagues framing self-determination as a form of self-regulation (Mithaug 1993). This, in turn, resulted in a revised theoretical model, the first version of Causal Agency Theory (Wehmeyer and Mithaug 2006; Wehmeyer 2004) and, most recently, to a more fully formed and aligned version of Causal Agency Theory (Shogren et al. 2015a) as described in this volume.

The intent of this chapter is to provide the context in which the issue of promoting self-determination emerged within the disability sphere, and to elaborate on research and theory development that led to Causal Agency Theory and its alignment with SDT, and then to examine how research on self-determination within the disability context (that is aligned with Causal Agency Theory) informs knowledge and understanding about self-determination, more broadly.

The Emergence of a Focus on Self-Determination in the Disability Context

People with disabilities have, for centuries, been subject to societal discrimination and lived, through no choice of their own, on the margins of society (Wehmeyer 2013a). Disability itself has been (and continues to be) understood in the context of models of disease, deficits, and pathology, and people with disabilities were (and are) perceived to be broken, atypical, aberrant or, in some way, outside the norm of human functioning. It was into this context that the first usage of the term self-determination in reference to disability issues occurred, and, perhaps not surprisingly given the marginalized status of people with disability, that usage mixed the meanings of the term as a psychological construct emphasizing volition and will and the use of the term in its political sense, as referring to the right of marginalized people to self-governance. Bengt Nirje, mentioned briefly in Chaps. 1 and 5, was a Swedish philosopher and in 1972 wrote a chapter in an influential text in the disability field calling for the "right to self-determination" for people with intellectual and related disabilities. From the onset, then, these issues of self-determination in a disability context were framed within an empowerment focus; people with disabilities were denied opportunities to live self-determined lives, and the response was to call for action with regard to both personal opportunities to make decisions in their lives, be free from the control of others, and act based upon personal preferences and interests; but, also, to have legally protected rights to self-governance.

It is important to recognize why a focus on self-determination emerged in the disability context, in the first place, to understand why there were (and still are) differences in how the term is utilized when compared with SDT and related work in psychology. Nirje's chapter is illustrative for this purpose. He began with the following statement:

> One major facet … is to create conditions through which a [person with a disability] experiences the normal respect to which any human being is entitled. Thus the choices, wishes, desires, and aspirations of a [person with a disability] have to be taken into consideration as much as possible in actions affecting him (Nirje 1972, p. 177).

So, from the start, self-determination (as Nirje applies it in his chapter) was equated with *the normal respect to which any human being is entitled*. People with disabilities were not valued as human beings, not respected, and were subject to discrimination and abuse. Within a disability context, self-determination has always been equated with the right to basic human dignity. Of course, people with disabilities are not alone as marginalized peoples to emphasize self-determination in terms of rights and dignity. Day two of the African American celebration of Kwanzaa emphasizes Kujichagulia, a Swahili word roughly translating as self-determination, defined as the need for African-Americans to act in their own self-interest based upon their own needs and reflecting their own history and culture.

Nirje then emphasizes the importance of respecting the choices, wishes, desires, and aspirations of people, thus aligning, to a degree, this intent with the notion of self-determination as volitional action.

Nirje continued:

> To assert oneself with one's family, friends, neighbors, co-workers, other people, or vis-à-vis an agency is difficult for many persons. It is especially difficult for someone who has a disability or is otherwise perceived as devalued (p. 177).

Again, themes of dignity (*otherwise perceived as devalued*) are emphasized, and, to a degree, issues pertaining to agentic behavior (it should be noted that in Nirje's quote the "*vis-à-vis an agency*" mention refers, literally, to an agency or organization providing disability supports, not to agentic action), but in the form of self-assertion or, as is emphasized throughout the disability literature, self-advocacy. Again, this is not unique to people with disabilities: Kujichagulia is frequently described in terms of speaking out on one's own behalf, voicing one's own concerns (Anokye 2013).

Nirje's opening paragraph concluded:

> But, in the end, even the [person with a disability] has to manage as a distinct individual, and thus has his identity defined to himself and to others through the circumstances and conditions of his existence. Thus, the road to self-determination is indeed both difficult and all-important. (p. 177).

It is hard to say with any certainty how, exactly, Bengt Nirje understood the self-determination construct. As a philosopher, he would have certainly been knowledgeable about philosophical discussions about determinism and free will. As an advocate for people who were marginalized, he was clearly influenced by the notion of self-determination in a political sense, the right to self-governance. He talked about self-determination as the right to be heard, to express one's self, and, mostly, about human dignity and the lack of power and control held by people with intellectual disability.

From Nirje onward, the application of the self-determination construct to the disability context has, for reasons articulated above, heavily reflected the notion of a corporate or national self-determination. As noted in Chap. 1, Heater (1994) attributed much of the notoriety for self-determination and its relative importance in twentieth century politics to Woodrow Wilson's famous "Fourteen Points" speech to a joint session of Congress on January 8, 1918. In this speech, Wilson outlined fourteen points for a postwar settlement that would lead to world peace. Six of the fourteen referred specifically to ensuring that nations who were defeated in the war would be assured the opportunity for national self-determination. Heater noted that the twentieth century preference for national self-determination emerged from twin eighteenth century notions that the people, not monarchs, are sovereign and that the people are to be thought of as "the nation." Through the nineteenth century the belief that a people should have the right and opportunity to determine their own government spread and gained wide acceptance, and by the twentieth century became a principal of international justice.

As the twentieth century progressed, this sense of the 'right of a peoples of a nation to self-governance' was adapted by other groups of people who were not identified as being the citizens of a country, but instead were self-identified by some factor (racial identity, disability status) that, in turn, was seen to result in the loss of a corporate right to self-governance, as illustrated by Nirje and issues pertaining to disability and Kwanzaa and issues pertaining to African-American identity. The importance of this sense of the term in disability is captured best by Robert Williams (1989), a national leader in the disability rights effort and a man with a disability, who stated:

> But, without being afforded the right and opportunity to make choices in our lives, we will never obtain full, first class American citizenship. So we do not have to be told what self-determination means. We already know that it is just another word for freedom. We already know that self-determination is just another word for describing a life filled with rising expectations, dignity, responsibility, and opportunity. That it is just another word for having the chance to live the American Dream (p. 16).

It was almost 20 years before self-determination, as a construct, was applied broadly to the disability sphere, and when that occurred, it was in the context of efforts to enable young people with disabilities to 'transition' from school to adult life more successfully. Before elaborating slightly on this, it is worth noting that Deci and Chandler (1986) and Grolnick and Ryan (1990) published studies looking at aspects of intrinsic motivation and related constructs with students with learning disabilities. In the former, Deci and Chandler argued that "self-determination as a quality of behavior should be a goal of all education" (p. 589). The latter study found that students with learning disabilities were lower in perceived cognitive competence and academic self-regulation relative to nondisabled control groups.

These two studies notwithstanding, the ascendency of self-determination as a construct applied to the disability context in the early 1990s was attributable to the growth of the disability rights movement through the 1970s and 1980s, which emphasized empowerment and equity and the "right" to self-determination. By the late 1980s, there was a sense among policy makers in the discipline of special education that one of the things that was serving as a barrier to students with disabilities achieving more positive adult outcomes (e.g., employment, independent living, community integration, etc.) was that there was no real focus on active student involvement in the educational planning process, nor were existing efforts to prepare students for the transition to adulthood adequately accounting for student preferences and interests. Language was added to federal disability legislation, including special education legislation, that emphasized choice and independence and the importance of personal preferences and interests in designing services and supports. In fact, the by the mid-1990s, the opening section (Findings and Purposes) for almost all federal disability legislation contained language emphasizing choice and independence. For example, the Findings from Congress for the Americans with Disabilities Act state that "the Nation's proper goals regarding individuals with disabilities are to assure equality of opportunity, full participation, independent living, and economic self-sufficiency." The Findings and Purposes for the Individuals with Disabilities Education Act reauthorization of 2004 state that "Improving educational results for children with disabilities is an essential element of our national policy of ensuring equality of opportunity, full participation, independent living, and economic self-sufficiency for individuals with disabilities." The Findings from Congress for the Vocational Rehabilitation Act state that "the goals of the Nation properly include the goal of providing individuals with disabilities with the tools necessary to make informed choices and decisions; and achieve equality of opportunity, full inclusion and integration in society, employment, independent living, and economic and social self-sufficiency, for such individuals."

When, in 1989, the U.S. Department of Education's Office of Special Education Programs (OSEP) announced grant funding to fund the development of models to promote the self-determination of youth with disabilities, the construct's intent was construed in much the way that Nirje positioned it; as reflecting the importance of choice and control, as promoting independence, as a rights-based issue, and as requiring efforts to promote skills leading to these outcomes. Ultimately, there were 26 such projects funded, with total funding just under $10 million dollars. This federal investment provided a foundation for promoting self-determination as critical in educating learners with disabilities.

Precursors to Causal Agency Theory

Chapter 5 detailed the theoretical framework ("functional" model) that drove initial phases of our work. We will not revisit that early model in this chapter, other than to note that even at that early stage, the issue of causal agency was central to our understanding of the construct, an emphasis drawn from the same early theories from which SDT drew. In their 1985 text, Deci and Ryan quote deCharms (1968): "[man's] primary motivational propensity is to be effective in producing changes in his environment. Man strives to be a causal agent, to be the primary locus of causation for, or the origin of, his behavior; he strives for personal causation" (p. 269). The functional model defined self-determination as being the causal agent in one's life. Further, Deci and Ryan (1985) drew upon pioneering theoretical work by

Angyal (1941), noting in a discussion of his influence that "[t]o be self-determining one must have the skills to manage various elements of one's environment. Otherwise, one is likely to be controlled by them" (Deci and Ryan 1985, p. 30).

As discussed in Chap. 1, in his early text, *Foundations for a Science of Personality*, Angyal (1941) proposed that an essential feature of a living organism is its autonomy, where autonomous means self-governing or governed from inside. According to Angyal, an organism "lives in a world in which things happen according to laws which are heteronomous (e.g., governed from outside) from the point of view of the organism" and that "organisms are subjected to the laws of the physical world, as is any other object of nature, with the exception that it can oppose self-determination to external determination" (p. 33). Angyal suggested that the important task for developing a science of personality was the identification of principle(s) of the biological total process—the movement of organisms from undifferentiated parts to an organized whole. He defined the "biological total process" as a trend toward autonomy, and argued that the science of personality is, in essence, the study of two essential components or determinants to behavior, autonomous-determinism (or self-determination) and heteronomous-determinism (other-determined). He noted that "in the realm of 'organismic happenings' we find neither entirely autonomous nor entirely heteronomous determinants" (p. 21), and suggested a psychology of individual differences by noting that, within nature, there are marked variations in the importance and balance of autonomous and heteronomous determinants to behavior. Nonetheless, Angyal places primary importance for laying the foundation for a science of personality in the fact that a central process of an organism is the movement toward self-determination. He showed this by stating:

> It would probably be generally agreed that without autonomy, without self-government, the life process could not be understood. Selection, choice, self-regulation, adaptation, regeneration are phenomena which logically imply the autonomy of the organism. Selection, that is the search for certain environmental conditions, is only possible in a being capable of self-directed activity (p. 34).

So, the functional theory was heavily influenced by early formulations of SDT and by theoretical frameworks that had influenced SDT. As mentioned previously, differences in SDT and most of the applied research and model development in the disability realm involved understandings of self-determination as equated with control and in the use of (or understanding of) autonomy. With regard to the former, when—as was the case in the disability context—self-determination is understood in a rights-based frame, the notion of taking control over one's life becomes a logical theme. Wehmeyer (2005) addressed this misperception of self-determination, stating:

> Control may be a useful heuristic when rallying others to the cause, but it is not an accurate way to define self-determination and, I believe, its use represents the most consistent misuse of the self-determination construct and contributes significantly to the limited degree to which the field has focused on promoting the self-determination of people with severe disabilities (p. 116).

As reflected in that quote, not only was the conflation of self-determination and control incorrect, but it created a situation in which others perceived people with disabilities (and particularly, as was the issue being addressed in this quote, people with the most severe disabilities) as being unable to "control" their lives, and, as such, dismissed the relevance of self-determination to their lives. With regard to autonomy, the field emphasized autonomy as independence (again, logically when approaching these issues from a rights-based perspective) rather than as volitional or self-endorsed functioning, as emphasized in SDT (and the functional theory).

The application of the functional model within the disability context was not the sole theoretical frame within which self-determination was conceptualized in ways that more closely aligned with SDT. Mithaug et al. (2003) suggested that "self-determination is a form of self-regulation—one that is unusually effective and markedly free of external influence" (p. iii) in which people who are self-determined regulate their choices and actions more successfully than others. Mithaug and colleagues observed that individuals are often in flux between existing states and goal or desired states. When a discrepancy between what one has and wants occurs, an incentive for self-regulation and action may be operative. With the realization that a discrepancy exists, the individual may set out to achieve the goal or desired state.

The ability to set appropriate expectations is based on the individual's success in matching his or her capacity with present opportunity. Capacity is the individual's assessment of existing resources (e.g., skills, interests, motivation), and opportunity refers to aspects of the situation that allow the individual to achieve the desired gain. Mithaug (1996) referred to optimal prospects as just-right matches in which individuals are able to correctly match their capacity (i.e., skills, interests) with existing opportunities (e.g., potential jobs). The experience generated during self-regulation, then, becomes a function of the interaction between the person's capacity and opportunity (Mithaug 1996). As Mithaug noted, "the more competent we are, the fewer errors we make, and the less time we take, the greater the gain we produce" (p. 156).

Mithaug (1998) also suggested that self-determination always occurs in a social context and that the social nature of the concept is worth reviewing because the distinction between self-determination and other-determination is nearly always in play when assessing an individual's prospects for controlling their life in a particular situation.

In 2006, Wehmeyer and Mithaug proposed the first iteration of Causal Agency Theory to explain how people become self-determined. The chapter in which this was proposed, notably, was in the second of two volumes on personality and motivational systems in people with intellectual disability, published in 2004 and 2006 respectively. The first volume was led off by a chapter by Deci (2004), in which he specified how "the innate psychological needs for competence, autonomy, and relatedness are used as a basis for specifying how ongoing social contexts as well as intervention programs will affect self-determined motivation and, in turn, learning, adjustment, and life circumstances" (p. 1). After overviewing SDT and intrinsic motivation and issues pertaining to motivation, social contexts, and learning, Deci concluded with the statement that SDT maintains that people with intellectual disability "like all other individuals, whether disabled or non-disabled, will become more motivated and self-determined to the extent that teachers or caregivers are autonomy-supportive and involved" and that "healthy development and greater self-determination can be facilitated when interventions or educational programs are administered by involved and autonomy-supportive educators and providers" (p. 25). We return to the issue of interventions and educational programs that are autonomy supportive in a subsequent section.

The first iteration of Causal Agency Theory proposed by Wehmeyer and Mithaug was intended to conceptualize how people become self-determined and act as causal agents in their lives.

Causal Agency Theory posited that there are a number of 'operators' at work that lead to self-determined behavior. These operators involve the capability to perform causal actions or behaviors, subdivided into causal capacity and agentic capacity, and challenges to the organism's self-determination, through causal opportunities or causal threats, which serve as a catalyst to action.

These operators were discussed in Chaps. 5 and 6 and in Chap. 18 (goal setting and attainment).

The current version of Causal Agency Theory (Shogren et al. 2015a) moves this theoretical framework more closely in alignment with SDT, allowing us to propose a model of the development of self-determination that draws from both theoretical frameworks. What we believe Causal Agency Theory has to offer is both a theoretical framework to guide research as well as a means for practitioners to implement interventions that promote causal action and causal agency; fulfill basic psychological needs for competence, autonomy, and relatedness; further enhance autonomous motivation and, through this cycle, result in enhanced self-determination. The purpose of the next section is to examine what intervention research driven by the functional model and Causal Agency Theory tells us about such efforts.

What Does Research with Causal Agency Theory in Disability Tell Us About Promoting Self-Determination?

Research pertaining to self-determination was one of the earliest areas in which a strengths-based focus was brought to bear in a disability context. This is because of the pathology-focused issues discussed previously… for much of history, the notion of disability—as it was then defined and conceptualized—was incompatible with strengths-based approaches. For multiple reasons paralleling the reasons that contributed to the rise of positive psychology, the field has begun to shift toward positive, strengths-based models and, in many ways, research in self-determination provides a template for approaching disability within a strengths model (Wehmeyer 2013b). Shogren et al. (2006) conducted a content analysis of 30 years of literature in the field of intellectual disability to examine the degree to which research in the field emphasized the strengths and capacities of people with intellectual disability and the degree to which the literature base included constructs associated with positive psychology. Shogren and colleagues found a gradual progression of the implementation of constructs found in positive psychology across decades (beginning in 1975 through 2004), with only slightly more than 27% of articles that studied some aspect of human functioning identifying positive constructs from 1975 to 1984, slightly more than 44% from 1985 to 1994, and 63% from 1995 to 2004. From among all of these constructs, examinations of personal control (recalling the above discussion of the conflation of self-determination and control in the disability context), problem-solving, goal setting, and self-determination constituted the largest percentage of positive constructs studied (15% of the 27% total from 1975–1984, 19% of 44% total from 1985–1994, and almost 30% of the 63% total from 1995 to 2004).

Findings from this research (and, of course, research from 2005 onward) can, we believe, provide some information with regard to mediators and moderators of self-determination and the impact of promoting self-determination on more positive life outcomes. To begin with, research in SDT focuses on the contexts that result in autonomous motivation and one of the things that research in the disability context can confirm is this importance of context. Measurement issues have limited the measurement of self-determination to allow for comparisons between adolescents and adults with and without disabilities, but it is clear that people with disabilities are less (and probably much less) self-determined than their non-disabled peers. They live, learn, work, and play in environments and contexts that are controlling and dependency-creating (see discussion about outerdirectedness in Chap. 16). It stands to reason that they are less likely to develop autonomous motivation and intrinsic regulation, and the research is clear that people with disabilities have fewer opportunities to express preferences and make choices in their lives (Stancliffe and Wehmeyer 1995; Wehmeyer and Abery 2013; Wehmeyer and Metzler 1995). Such opportunities—and, consequently, self-determination—are directly related to the physical environments in which people live and work. Research has shown that congregate living or work environments (in which people with disabilities are disproportionally likely to receive disability services) restrict choice opportunity and self-determination (Wehmeyer and Bolding 1999) and that by simply moving to less congregate (and thus, less restrictive) work or living environments, choice opportunity and self-determination are enhanced (Wehmeyer and Bolding 2001).

Beyond the importance of context to self-determination, perhaps the area in which research in the disability sphere has the most to contribute to knowledge in the broader area of self-determination is the positive impact of interventions to promote causal action (and self-determination). Some of this was discussed in Chap. 5, so we will only summarize the knowledge base in this chapter. In considering this literature, we return to the comment by Deci (2004) that "healthy development and greater self-determination can be facilitated when interventions or educational programs are administered by involved and autonomy-supportive educators and providers" (p. 25). The issues (and practices) of autonomy-supportive educators are mentioned throughout this text, though particularly in Chap. 8. The intervention work we have done can be categorized as, in essence, putting methods, materials, and strategies into the hands of autonomy-supportive educators to enable them to facilitate the acquisition and development of component skills leading to causal action and self-determination. These are, in essence, *autonomy-supportive instructional strategies*.

Chapters 15, 16, 17, 18, 19, 20 and 21 describe the development of volitional and agentic action, and it is in these domains from which autonomy-supportive instructional strategies are developed. Some such domains, such as choice and preference, require only (or, at least, primarily) the types of interactions described with regard to autonomy-supportive education (Chap. 8). In other such domains—goal setting or problem solving, for example—students benefit not only from contextual supports and autonomy-supportive interactions, but direct instruction on how to set goals or solve problems.

There is, now, clear evidence from the special education intervention literature that providing instruction to promote component skills of causal action results in enhanced skills and greater self-determination. Algozzine et al. (2001) conducted group- and single-subject design meta-analyses of studies in which individuals with disabilities had received some intervention to promote component skills of causal action, specifically, decision-making, goal setting and attainment, self-advocacy, problem-solving, and self-awareness skills. The median effect size across 100 group intervention comparisons was 1.38, interpreted as a moderate effect (which is positive for education interventions, as a multitude of factors impact outcome effects). For the single-subject design studies, the median percentage of nonoverlapping data (PND) was 95%, with seven interventions with a PND of 100%. This is interpreted as a strong effect. Subsequently, Cobb et al. (2009) conducted a narrative metasynthesis—a narrative synthesis of multiple meta-analytic studies—covering seven existing meta-analyses examining causal action skills and concluded that there is sufficient evidence to conclude that interventions to teach or promote choice-making, problem-solving, decision-making, goal setting and attainment, and self-advocacy skills result in enhanced skills in these areas.

More recently, several studies provide causal evidence of the impact of autonomy-supportive interventions on self-determination and on valued life outcomes. For example, in a recent cluster randomized control group study of the effect of interventions to promote self-determination in high school students receiving special education services under the categorical areas of intellectual disability or learning disabilities, we found that over 3 years, students who received interventions to promote skills related to causal action and active involvement showed significant growth in their self-determination, at higher levels than students with disabilities who did not receive interventions to promote self-determination (Wehmeyer et al. 2012). In a follow-up study of the treatment and control group students from Wehmeyer et al. (2013), Shogren et al. (2015b) investigated adult outcomes 1 and 2 years after leaving school. The study measured employment, community access, financial independence, independent living, and life satisfaction outcomes. Results indicated that self-determination status at the end of high school predicted significantly more positive employment and community access outcomes. A recent randomized-trial study by Powers et al. (2012) also provided causal evidence of the effect of promoting self-determination on community inclusion, particularly for youth in foster care and special education.

The primary intervention we have developed and evaluated, the Self-Determined Learning Model of Instruction (SDLMI), provides teachers an autonomy-supportive instructional model to teach students a self-regulated problem-solving process that enables them to set goals, create action plans to achieve those goals, and revise their plans or goal to attain the goal. Specific studies pertaining to the SDLMI were discussed in greater detail in Chap. 5, so we will only summarize the findings from research with the SDLMI for this chapter. In essence, multiple randomized trial design studies have shown that instruction using the SDLMI results in enhanced self-determination, enhanced study and organization skills in the classroom, and better post-secondary outcomes. The research also shows that teachers change their perceptions (in essence, become more autonomy-supportive) after implementing the instructional model.

Finally, a focus in the special education research has been to promote more active student involvement in educational planning. Recall that the original intent of the OSEP self-determination initiative, discussed previously in this chapter, was to improve transition outcomes for youth with disabilities by promoting self-determination and active student engagement and involvement in the educational process. In a number of studies, research has found that students with disabilities can acquire skills to play a meaningful role in their educational planning process (Martin and Marshall 1996; Martin et al. 2006; Wehmeyer and Lawrence 1995) and, when they do, students achieve more positive school outcomes (Wehmeyer et al. 2011) and enhanced self-determination (Seong et al. 2015). In fact, research has shown a reciprocal relationship between student involvement and self-determination, in which students who are more involved in their educational planning process become more self-determined, and students who are more self-determined are more likely to be involved in their planning.

Conclusions

Although much of the research in self-determination within the disability context has approached the construct from its rights-based meaning, research within the context of Causal Agency Theory and its precursors has drawn heavily from SDT and related theories. This text provides an opportunity to explore a model of the development of self-determination that draws from SDT and Causal Agency Theory, and serves to align work in disability more closely with work with SDT. Further, there is clear evidence from special education research that autonomy-supportive interventions can enable teachers to support self-determination and to further the impact of autonomy-supportive education.

References

Algozzine, B., Browder, D., Karvonen, M., Test, D. W., & Wood, W. M. (2001). Effects of interventions to promote self-determination for individuals with disabilities. *Review of Educational Research, 71*(2), 219–277.

Angyal, A. (1941). *Foundations for a science of personality*. Cambridge, MA: Harvard University Press.

Anokye, A. D. (2013). Standard language ideology and African American Vernacular English. In C. A. Chapelle (Ed.), *The encyclopedia of applied linguistics* (pp. 1–3). London: Blackwell Publishing Ltd.

Cobb, B., Lehmann, J., Newman-Gonchar, R., & Morgen, A. (2009). Self-determination for students with disabilities: A narrative metasynthesis. *Career Development for Exceptional Individuals, 32*(2), 108–114.

deCharms, R. (1968). *Personal causation: The internal affective determinants of behavior*. New York: Academic Press.

Deci, E. L. (1980). *The psychology of self-determination*. Lexington: Lexington Books.

Deci, E. L. (2004). Promoting intrinsic motivation and self-determination in people with mental retardation. In H. Switzky, L. Hickson, R. Schalock, & M. Wehmeyer (Eds.), *Personality and motivational systems in mental retardation, International review of research in mental retardation* (Vol. 28, pp. 1–29). San Diego: Academic Press.

Deci, E. L., & Chandler, C. L. (1986). The importance of motivation for the future of the LD field. *Journal of Learning Disabilities, 19*, 587–594.

Deci, E. L., & Ryan, R. M. (1985). *Intrinsic motivation and self-determination in human behavior*. New York: Plenum.

Grolnick, W. S., & Ryan, R. M. (1990). Self-perceptions, motivation, and adjustment in learning disabled children: A multiple group comparison study. *Journal of Learning Disabilities, 23*, 177–184.

Heater, D. (1994). *National self-determination: Woodrow Wilson and his legacy*. New York: St. Martin's Press.

Martin, J. E., & Marshall, L. H. (1996). ChoiceMaker: Infusing self-determination instruction into the IEP and transition process. In D. J. Sands & M. L. Wehmeyer (Eds.), *Self-determination across the life span: Independence and choice for people with disabilities* (pp. 215–236). Baltimore: Paul H. Brookes.

Martin, J. E., Van Dycke, J., Christense, W. R., Greene, B. A., Gardner, J. E., & Lovett, D. L. (2006). Increasing student participation in IEP meetings: Establishing the self-directed IEP as an evidenced-based practice. *Exceptional Children, 72*, 299–316.

Mithaug, D. E. (1993). *Self-regulation theory: How optimal adjustment maximizes gain*. Westport: Praeger Books.

Mithaug, D. (1996). The optimal prospects principle: A theoretical basis for rethinking instructional practices for self-determination. In D. J. Sands & M. L. Wehmeyer (Eds.), *Self-determination across the life span: Independence and choice for people with disabilities* (pp. 147–165). Baltimore: Paul H. Brookes.

Mithaug, D. (1998). Your right, my obligation? *Journal of the Association for Persons with Severe Disabilities, 23*, 41–43.

Mithaug, D. E., Campeau, P. L., & Wolman, J. M. (2003). Assessing self-determination prospects among students with and without disabilities. In D. E. Mithaug, D. K. Mithaug, M. Agran, J. E. Martin, & M. L. Wehmeyer (Eds.), *Self determined learning theory: Construction, verification, and evaluation* (pp. 61–76). Mahwah: Lawrence Erlbaum Associates.

Nirje, B. (1972). The right to self-determination. In W. Wolfensberger (Ed.), *Normalization: The principle of normalization in human services* (pp. 176–193). Toronto: National Institute on Mental Retardation.

Powers, L. E., Geenen, S., Powers, J., Pommier-Satya, S., Turner, A., Dalton, L., et al. (2012). My life: Effects of a longitudinal, randomized study of self-determination enhancement on the transition outcomes of youth in foster care and special education. *Children and Youth Services Review, 34*, 2179–2187.

Seong, Y., Wehmeyer, M. L., Palmer, S. B., & Little, T. D. (2015). Effects of the self-directed individualized education program on self-determination and transition of adolescents with disabilities. *Career Development and Transition for Exceptional Individuals, 38*(3), 132–141.
Shogren, K. A., Lopez, S. J., Wehmeyer, M. L., Little, T. D., & Pressgrove, C. L. (2006). The role of positive psychology constructs in predicting life satisfaction in adolescents with and without cognitive disabilities: An exploratory study. *Journal of Positive Psychology, 1*, 37–52.
Shogren, K. A., Wehmeyer, M. L., Palmer, S. B., Forber-Pratt, A., Little, T., & Lopez, S. (2015a). Causal agency theory: Reconceptualizing a functional model of self-determination. *Education and Training in Autism and Developmental Disabilities, 50*(3), 251–263.
Shogren, K. A., Wehmeyer, M. L., Palmer, S. B., Rifenbark, G. G., & Little, T. D. (2015b). Relationships between self-determination and postschool outcomes for youth with disabilities. *Journal of Special Education, 53*, 30–41.
Stancliffe, R., & Wehmeyer, M. L. (1995). Variability in the availability of choice to adults with mental retardation. *The Journal of Vocational Rehabilitation, 5*, 319–328.
Wehmeyer, M. L. (2004). Beyond self-determination: Causal agency theory. *Journal of Developmental and Physical Disabilities, 16*, 337–359.
Wehmeyer, M. L. (2005). Self-determination and individuals with severe disabilities: Reexamining meanings and misinterpretations. *Research and Practice for Persons with Severe Disabilities, 30*, 113–120.
Wehmeyer, M. L. (2013a). *The story of intellectual disability: An evolution of meaning, understanding, and public perception*. Baltimore: Paul H. Brookes.
Wehmeyer, M. L. (2013b). *Handbook of positive psychology and disability*. Oxford: Oxford University Press.
Wehmeyer, M. L., & Abery, B. (2013). Self-determination and choice. *Intellectual and Developmental Disabilities, 51*(5), 399–411.
Wehmeyer, M. L., & Bolding, N. (1999). Self-determination across living and working environments: A matched-samples study of adults with mental retardation. *Mental Retardation, 37*, 353–363.
Wehmeyer, M. L., & Bolding, N. (2001). Enhanced self-determination of adults with mental retardation as an outcome of moving to community-based work or living environments. *Journal of Intellectual Disability Research, 45*, 371–383.
Wehmeyer, M. L., & Lawrence, M. (1995). Whose future is it anyway? Promoting student involvement in transition planning with a student-directed process. *Career Development for Exceptional Individuals, 18*, 69–83.
Wehmeyer, M. L., & Metzler, C. (1995). How self-determined are people with mental retardation? The National Consumer Survey. *Mental Retardation, 33*, 111–119.
Wehmeyer, M. L., & Mithaug, D. (2006). Self-determination, causal agency, and mental retardation. In L. M. Glidden (Series Ed.) & H. Swtizky (Vol. Ed.), *International review of research in mental retardation: Vol. 31 current perspectives on individual differences in personality and motivation in persons with mental retardation and other developmental disabilities* (pp. 31–71). San Diego: Academic Press.
Wehmeyer, M. L., Palmer, S. B., Lee, Y., Williams-Diehm, K., & Shogren, K. A. (2011). A randomized-trial evaluation of the effect of *Whose Future is it Anyway?* On self-determination. *Career Development for Exceptional Individuals, 34*(1), 45–56.
Williams, R. R. (1989). Creating a new world of opportunity: Expanding choice and self-determination in lives of Americans with severe disability by 1992 and beyond. In R. Perske (Ed.), *Proceedings from the national conference on self-determination* (pp. 16–17). Minneapolis: Institute on Community Integration.
Wehmeyer, M. L., Palmer, S., Shogren, K., Williams-Diehm, K., & Soukup, J. (2012). Establishing a causal relationship between interventions to promote self-determination and enhanced student self-determination. *Journal of Special Education, 46*(4), 195–210.

Chapter 10
The Role of Passion in Adult Self-Growth and Development

Robert J. Vallerand and Maylys Rapaport

Abstract This chapter introduces the concept of passion, and describes its relationship to self-growth and development. The Dualistic Model of Passion is highlighted, and two types of passion, harmonious and obsessive, defined. Research on passion is described, including work to identify the prevalence of passion, to develop a measure of passion, the Passion Scale, and to test the validity of passion constructs.

On the Role of Passion in Self-Growth and Development

People grow and develop into complex entities with a sense of self and identity, one part of which is the development of self-determination. Such development is not limited to childhood. Quite the contrary, people evolve and grow throughout the life span. Such self-development can take various forms and shapes but does not take place haphazardly. Engagement in activities that reflect our sense of self and identity follow a certain logic that provides a chartered course of who we are to become. Activities that we are passionate about represent one type of activity with high potential for self-growth and development and have obvious links to the development and expression of self-determination. Indeed, when passionate about something, people do not merely engage in the activity, they embrace it to the fullest as it reflects who they are deeply. Accordingly, such high-involvement in the activity can influence psychological experiences and outcomes in important ways. Such experiences, however, are not fleeting but when recurrent can be internalized, thereby helping shape further the person that people become. As we'll see, however, not all passions are equivalent. Some types of passion involve more self-determination

R.J. Vallerand (✉)
Laboratoire de Recherche sur le Comportement Social, Université du Québec à Montréal, Montréal, QC, Canada

Australian Catholic University, Sydney, NSW, Australia
e-mail: vallerand.bob@gmail.com

M. Rapaport
Laboratoire de Recherche sur le Comportement Social, Université du Québec à Montréal, Montréal, QC, Canada

M.L. Wehmeyer et al. (eds.), *Development of Self-Determination Through the Life-Course*, DOI 10.1007/978-94-024-1042-6_10

than others and therefore lead to high quality outcomes that translate into self-growth and development of better quality than others.

The purpose of this chapter is to address this issue. The present chapter starts with a presentation of the passion construct and our theory of passion, the Dualistic Model of Passion (Vallerand 2015). Second, we make a case for the role of passion in self-growth and development. Third, we briefly review research on passion that shows that passion does matter with respect to outcomes and processes that foster self-growth. Finally, we conclude with some thoughts on the role of passion in self-growth.

On the Psychology of Passion: A Dualistic Model of Passion

Historically, the concept of passion has been portrayed in various ways (see Vallerand 2015, Chapters 1 and 2). For instance, philosophers could not agree on its role in human functioning, seeing as either an uncontrollable force to be afraid of (e.g., Plato, 427–348 BC) or an adaptive source of high energy (Hegel, 1770–1831). Psychologists have typically neglected the construct until recently (for reviews, see Vallerand 2010, 2015). Those who have studied passion, however, have either limited themselves to romantic passion (e.g., Hatfield and Walster 1978) or as an emotional goal (Frijda and Mesquita 1994).

Vallerand and colleagues (Vallerand 2010, 2015; Vallerand et al. 2003; Vallerand and Houlfort 2003) proposed the Dualistic Model of Passion that, as of the writing of this chapter, represents the most detailed and validated model on passion. As we'll see in this chapter, the Dualistic Model of Passion has much to say in a discussion on self-growth and self-development across the lifespan. The Dualistic Model of Passion defines passion as a strong inclination toward a self-defining activity that one likes (or even loves), finds important, and in which one invests time and energy. One can become passionate for activities, objects, causes, and even persons (see Vallerand 2015). Typically, although people may be motivated for several activities, they are passionate for only a few, sometimes only one. These activities, however, come to be so self-defining that they represent central features of identity. Such internalization will be the case to the extent that the activity is highly valued by the person (Aron et al. 1992), thereby leading to a passion toward that activity. Thus, through the development of a passion for a given activity or object, one grows as the self and identity expand as well.

The Dualistic Model of Passion further posits the existence of two types of passion, harmonious and obsessive passion depending how the activity has been internalized in self and identity. Research on Self-Determination Theory (SDT; Deci and Ryan 1985; Ryan and Deci 2000) has revealed that the internalization of non-interesting activities will take place to the extent that these are highly valued and meaningful for the person. Similarly, the model posits that activities that people love but that are highly valued will also be internalized. Further, in line with SDT, such internalization can take place through either a controlled or an autonomous process (see Deci et al. 1994; Sheldon 2002; Vallerand 1997, 2001, 2007; Vallerand et al. 1997). It is these two types of internalization processes that determine the two types of passion mentioned previously, harmonious and obsessive passion.

Harmonious passion results from an autonomous internalization of the activity into the person's identity and self. An autonomous internalization occurs when individuals have freely accepted the activity as important for them without any contingencies attached to it. This type of internalization emanates from the intrinsic and integrative tendencies of the self (Deci and Ryan 2000; Ryan and Deci 2003) and produces a motivational force to willingly engage in the activity that one loves and engenders a sense of volition and personal endorsement about pursuing the activity. When harmonious passion is at play, individuals freely choose to engage in the activity that they love. With this type of passion, the activity occupies a significant but not overpowering space in the person's identity and is in harmony with other aspects of the person's life. In other words, with harmonious passion the authentic integrating self (Deci and Ryan 2000) is at play allowing the person to fully partake in the passionate activity in a mindful (Brown and Ryan 2003) and open way (Hodgins and Knee 2002) that is conducive to positive experiences.

In line with the above, engaging in an activity with a harmonious passion should allow people to fully focus on the task at hand and to experience positive outcomes and pleasure both during task engagement (e.g., positive affect, concentration, flow etc.) as well as after (general positive affect, life satisfaction etc.). Such a harmonious integration should prevent conflict between the person's passionate activity and his or her other life activities. Furthermore, when prevented from engaging in their passionate activity, with a harmonious passion people should be able to adapt well to the situation and focus their attention and energy on other tasks that need attention. Finally, because with harmonious passion the person is in control of the activity, he or she can then decide when to and when not to engage in the activity. For instance, if a university professor who has a harmonious passion for playing the guitar is being asked to go for a music jam session with friends even though she has to complete a research grant due the next day, she should be able to resist playing music with her friends so as to complete the research grant that still needs work. Thus, she should readily tell her friends that she'll take a rain check on the music jam and proceed to be fully immersed in the grant without thinking about music. With harmonious passion, people are able to decide not to play on a given day if needed or even to eventually terminate the relationship with the activity if they decide that it has become a permanent negative factor in their life. Thus, behavioral engagement in the passionate activity can be seen as flexible.

Conversely, obsessive passion, results from a controlled internalization of the activity that one loves into identity. Such an internalization process leads the activity representation, and values and regulations associated with the activity, to be at best partially internalized in the integrative self (Ryan and Deci 2000), and, at worse, to be internalized completely outside the identity. A controlled internalization originates from intra and/or interpersonal pressure typically because certain contingencies are attached to the activity, such as feelings of social acceptance or self-esteem (Mageau et al. 2011), or because the sense of excitement derived from activity engagement is uncontrollable. With obsessive passion people can thus find themselves in the position of experiencing an uncontrollable urge to partake in the activity they view as important and enjoyable. They cannot help but to engage in the passionate activity. Consequently, they risk experiencing conflict and other negative affective, cognitive, and behavioral consequences during and after activity engagement.

For instance, if the university professor who needs to work on a research grant due the next day has a predominant obsessive passion for playing the guitar, she might not be able to resist the invitation to play music with her friends that evening. During the jam session, she might feel upset with herself for playing music instead of working on the grant. She might therefore have difficulties focusing on the task at hand (playing the guitar), may not experience much positive affect and flow while playing the guitar, and may experience guilt and anxiety as she should be doing something else instead (i.e., working on her research grant). Furthermore, if she says no to the invitation to play music, she may find it difficult to focus on the research grant as she may ruminate about the lost opportunity to play music. It is thus proposed that when obsessive passion is operative, people display a rigid persistence toward the activity, leading one to feel that he or she can't help it and has to engage in the passionate activity. This is so because ego-invested, rather than integrative, self-processes (Hodgins and Knee 2002) are at play with obsessive passion leading the person to eventually becoming dependent on the activity. While such persistence may lead to some benefits (e.g., improved performance at the activity), it may also come at a cost for the individual, potentially leading to less than optimal functioning within the confines of the passionate activity because of the lack of flexibility that it entails, and eventually less self-growth overall in the person's life outside of the passionate activity.

On Passion and Self-Growth

The Dualistic Model of Passion rests on the firm assumption that people have a natural tendency toward self-growth that is experienced throughout life. That is, people seek to master both their outside and inside worlds (e.g., Deci and Ryan 1985; Maslow 1954; Rogers 1963). In so doing, they grow and develop psychologically. It is posited that one of the key variables that contributes to self-growth is engaging in activities that reflect our identity (Waterman 1993) and especially those about which we are passionate (Vallerand 2015). In life, we engage in a number of activities. Typically, we are motivated for most of them and passionate only for one or two. For instance, we are motivated to go to school and to do chores at home but may be passionate about playing a musical instrument or playing basketball or soccer. We would like to suggest that those activities that people are passionate about have the best potential for self-growth. This is not to say that other activities that people are non passionate about do not lead to self-growth. Clearly, everything we do in life has such a potential. We posit, however, that everything being equal in terms of activity complexity, and thus self-growth potential, activities that we are passionate about should contribute the most to self-growth.

There are a number of reasons why activities about which we are passionate should lead to higher levels of self-growth than those engaged in without passion. We will only mention three here (see Vallerand 2015, Chapter 3 for a more detailed discussion). First, passion entails a powerful motivational force that is conducive to fully engaging in the activity with high levels of energy and enthusiasm. You do not have to push or force people to do the activity that they are passionate about. Quite the contrary, sometimes you may even be tempted to restrain people from engaging in their activity as they just can't get enough of it and may sometimes overdo it. Thus, when passionate about an activity, people engage in their beloved activity with full energy, persistence, and regularity, several hours weekly (on average 8 h per week for non-work passionate activities; Vallerand et al. 2003, Study 1). They put in lots of hours with a high quality engagement that is likely to promote self-growth within the purview of the activity.

A second reason why passion can maximize self-growth is that it fosters mastery goals (Elliot and Church 1997). Mastery goals entail focusing on improving and mastering the various aspects of the activity itself. Much research reveals that mastery goals foster a variety of adaptive outcomes such as positive affect, persistence, and enjoyment (see Elliot et al. 2007 for reviews), as well as sustained engagement in deliberate practice that is known to foster high performance on the activity (see Bonneville-Roussy et al. 2011; Vallerand et al. 2008a; Vallerand et al. 2007). Over time, people come to know just about everything there is to know about the activity; they become experts at their activity, thereby allowing them to psychologically grow at least within the realm of the activity. Thus, research reveals that harmonious passion, and obsessive passion to a lesser degree, contributes to mastery goals, and therefore indirectly to self-growth and development.

A third and final reason why passion may lead to the highest levels of self-growth is that one's passion for a given activity can facilitate the experience of a number of recurrent positive experiences and processes during activity engagement that, in turn, can promote adaptive outcomes (and self-growth) within the sphere of the activity as well as outside of it in one's life in general. Some of these adaptive processes include flow and positive emotions. Flow and emotions are important because they are hypothesized to serve several adaptive functions. For instance, Csikszentmihalyi (1990) has proposed that because it necessitates having one's abilities matching the challenge of the activity, flow can lead people to work hard so as to improve and face challenges in the passionate activity. During this process, self-growth consistently increases. Similarly, positive emotions (especially, joy, interest, contentment, and love) are proposed to serve to broaden the momentary thought –action repertoire (Fredrickson 2001). Thus, when repeatedly experiencing positive emotional states, people will broaden their scope of attention and show an expanded use of information and strategies at their disposal that, in turn, leads to a more permanent building of physical and psychological skills and tools that can be made available in the future when needed and that can contribute to self-growth.

To return to our example of the university professor who has a passion for playing the guitar, such passion (both harmonious passion and obsessive passion) would lead her to spend a lot of time learning how to play new chords, melodies, and arrangements on the guitar, thereby leading to self-growth and development in the musical sphere. Furthermore, with harmonious passion, our professor would experience flow and positive emotions during her music gigs and sessions that should also lead to self-growth not only within music but also in the rest of the person's life. Indeed, flow and positive emotions experienced regularly in the music realm persist over time and can lead the professor to engage in teaching and research with a happy mood leading her to adopt a more open frame of mind, potentially leading to better performance and creativity, and thus to self-growth in the person's life outside of music. Such should not be the case with obsessive passion. Quite the contrary, because of the contingences attached to music, with obsessive passion people should not welcome engaging in other activities as much and, in fact, just can't wait until the next time that they will play music. Thus, self-growth attained in music would come with a price as it would be limited to the music activity, and not as much in the rest of the person's life, if it takes place at all.

Research on Passion

As seen above, the position of the Dualistic Model of Passion is that harmonious passion leads to self-growth and development both within the area of one's passion (e.g., music) as well as in other areas of the person's life as well (e.g., work, relationships). It will be seen that such self-growth and development takes place in part through the effects that adaptive processes and outcomes produce during and after activity engagement. Conversely, the effects of obsessive passion should be much less adaptive. This is because obsessive passion entails outcomes and processes of lower levels of self-determination and psychological quality than harmonious passion. Although some self-growth may take place with obsessive passion, it should be limited to the area of one's passion and even it should be of lower quality than with harmonious passion. In this section, we review research that addresses these issues. First, we address initial research that took place with respect to passion. Then, we focus on the role of passion as pertains to a number of adaptive outcomes reflecting self-growth that are cognitive, affective, behavioral, and interpersonal nature that reflect self-growth. These are divided in two sections depending if such self-growth takes place within the activity one is passionate about or if such outcomes generalize and take place in the person's life outside the passionate activity. Let us start with some initial passion research that provides support for the concept of passion and its methodology.

Initial Passion Research

There were three major purposes to the initial work on passion (Vallerand et al. 2003): (1) to determine the prevalence of passion for an activity; (2) to develop the Passion Scale; and (3) to test the validity of some of the elements of the passion constructs. In this regard, Vallerand et al. (2003, Study 1) had over 500 university students complete the Passion Scale with respect to an activity that they loved, that they valued, and in which they invested time and energy (i.e., the passion definition), as well as other scales leading to testing predictions derived from the Dualistic Model of Passion. The following results were obtained.

Who Becomes Passionate and for Which Type of Activity?

Using the criteria reflecting the definition of passion (love and valuation of the activity, time spent on the activity, and the activity being part of identity), several studies show that a majority of the population is either highly passionate (75%) or moderately passionate (84%) for at least one activity in their lives. Further, research has found the same findings with participants ranging in age from 8 to 90 years (Philippe et al. 2009, Vallerand 2015). Thus, there is a rather high level of prevalence with respect to passion (for similar results in other countries, see Lecoq 2012; Liu et al. 2011; Stenseng 2008). Such a high prevalence of passion is exactly what would be expected if passion contributes to self-growth and development: it should be present in most individuals. Further, people can become passionate for a number of activities. Of importance, such passion is not fleeting but rather persistent as people typically engage in their passionate activity on average 8 h per week and have been doing so for several years (for over 6 years, on average, in the Vallerand et al. 2003).

It appears that most activities that include some interesting elements have the potential to become passionate for a given individual. Indeed, Vallerand et al. (2003) found that their sample of over 500 university students reported having a passion for one of over 100 different activities ranging from individual and team sports, passive leisure (e.g., listening to music and movies), reading, active arts (e.g., painting), education, work, and relationships. Similar findings have been obtained in different countries. These results underscore the highly idiosyncratic person-activity interface with respect to passion. While most people are passionate for something, this "something" may vary depending on the specific individual. Thus, passion is not a "trait" but rather targeted toward one specific activity. Finally, other research reveals that a passion for a given activity typically develops in the teen years as people seek to develop their identity and self-growth and development on the activity continues well into adulthood. The social environment plays an important part in the development of passion by making available certain types of activities, providing models as to how to perform the activity, underscoring the importance of the activity, and by providing autonomy support vs control when one engages in the activity (see Mageau et al. 2009; Vallerand 2015, Chapter 5).

The Passion Scale

Second, it should be underscored that the Passion Scale, Vallerand et al. (2003, Study 1), has gone through extensive development and validation procedures. The Passion Scale consists of 2 subscales of 6 items each reflecting Obsessive (e.g., "I almost have an obsessive feeling toward this activity") and harmonious passion (e.g., "This activity is in harmony with other activities in my life"). Results from confirmatory factor analysis provide strong support for its bi-factorial structure in over 20 studies dealing with a number of activities and languages (see Vallerand 2015, Chapter 4 for a review). In addition, in a study with over 3500 participants, Marsh et al. (2013) have shown that the scale is invariant (or equivalent) both in English and French, for both men and women, across various age groups, and for a number of different activities. Furthermore, internal consistency analyses have shown that both subscales are reliable (typically .75 and above). Finally, test-retest correlations over periods ranging from four to 6 weeks revealed moderately high stability values (in the .80s, Rousseau et al. 2002), thereby supporting the reliability of the scale. Thus, overall, the Passion Scale can be readily used for most if not all types of activities and populations and in several languages.

Construct Validity

Finally, with respect to the third purpose, a series of critical findings with partial correlations (controlling for the correlation between the two types of passion) revealed that both harmonious passion and obsessive passion were positively associated with the passion criteria thereby providing support for the definition of passion (see Vallerand et al. 2003, Study 1; Marsh et al. 2013). In addition, both types of passion were found to relate to one's identity and obsessive passion was found to more strongly relate to a measure of conflict with other life activities than harmonious passion. These findings support the view that both harmonious and obsessive passions are indeed a "passion" as each one reflects the definition of the passion construct. Furthermore, other studies in this initial research (Vallerand et al. 2003) have also shown that obsessive (but not harmonious) passion correlated with rigid persistence in ill-advised activities such as cycling over ice and snow in winter (Vallerand et al. 2003, Study 3) and pursuing one's engagement in activities that have become negative for the person such as pathological gambling (Vallerand et al. 2003, Study 4).

In sum, initial research provided support for the concept of harmonious and obsessive passion. Since then, over 200 studies have been conducted on the role of passion in a variety of outcomes. Such research has been conducted in both our lab as well as other laboratories (see Curran et al. 2015; Vallerand 2010, 2015 for reviews). Such research has been typically conducted in field settings with a variety of real-life participants such as athletes, musicians, actors, dancers, painters, teachers, nurses, administrators, video gamers, and others of various ages across the lifespan. In most studies, participants are asked to complete the Passion Scale with respect to their favorite activity (e.g., basketball) and scales assessing various outcomes experienced both while engaging in the passionate activity (e.g., flow, positive affect, performance, creativity, etc.) and in one's life in general (e.g., relationships outside the activity, well-being, health, contributions to society etc.). Such research also used a variety of methodological designs (e.g., cross-sectional, longitudinal, diary study, and even experimental) and has been conducted in a variety of countries. Further, it also deals with a variety of outcomes highly relevant for self-growth. Below, we briefly summarize such research in two areas depending if outcomes pertain to activity self-growth or more global self-growth that takes place outside the passionate activity. It will be shown that passion matters greatly. The reader is referred to Vallerand (2008, 2010, 2015) for recent reviews that include a wider larger variety of outcomes and Curran et al. (2015) for a recent meta-analysis of such research within the intra-personal sphere.

Passion and Self-Growth Within the Purview of the Activity

As mentioned previously, the position of the Dualistic Model of Passion is that harmonious passion leads to self-growth and development both within the area of one's passion, as well as in the rest of the person's life. It is also hypothesized that such self-growth takes place in part through the effects of passion on adaptive processes and cognitive, affective, and interpersonal outcomes that take place during activity engagement. Conversely, the effects of obsessive passion are much less adaptive because it entails outcomes and processes of lower levels of self-determination and psychological quality than harmonious passion. Although some self-growth may take place with obsessive passion, it should be limited to the area of one's passion and of lower quality than with harmonious passion.

Let's look at the empirical evidence. Research on passion and outcomes has looked at a number of on-task cognitive outcomes. Such research reveals that harmonious passion leads to positive cognitions such as attention, concentration, task absorption, and flow during task engagement (e.g., Forest et al. 2011; Vallerand et al. 2003, Study 1). For instance, in a study with adult workers, Ho et al. (2011) found that harmonious passion predicts better attention on the job. Similarly, much research reveals that harmonious passion (but not obsessive passion) leads to experiencing higher levels of flow in a variety of contexts that include sports (e.g., Philippe et al. 2009) and work (e.g., Forest et al. 2011). Research also reveals that obsessive passion is either negatively or unrelated to positive forms of cognitions such as concentration (see Curran et al. 2015). Furthermore, it should be noted that not only does obsessive passion typically yield less adaptive cognitions than harmonious passion but it can also lead to some maladaptive ones as well. For instance, research reveals that obsessive passion positively predicts ruminations about the activity (e.g., Vallerand et al. 2003, Study 1; Vallerand 2010, Studies 1–2) and cognitive conflict between the passionate activity and other activities in the person's life (e.g., Caudroit et al. 2011).

A lot of research has focused on affective outcomes, such as positive and negative affect and task satisfaction, with harmonious passion leading to more positive affect and typically less negative affect than obsessive passion (see Curran et al. 2015 for a meta-analysis of such effects). For instance, in a study with basketball players, Vallerand et al. (2006, Study 2) showed that harmonious passion positively predicted positive, but negatively predicted negative, affect following a game. Conversely, obsessive passion positively predicts negative affect and is either unrelated or negatively related to negative affect. These findings have been replicated in a number of studies conducted in a variety of settings such as sports, work, and school (e.g., Philippe et al. 2010; see Curran et al. 2015; Vallerand 2015, Chapter 7, for reviews).

Research has also assessed the link between passion and interpersonal outcomes. It is often assumed that passionate people are charismatic and should make more friends within the purview of the activity. Research reveals that it is indeed true, but only for harmonious passion (e.g., Philippe et al. 2010). For instance, in a short longitudinal study, Philippe et al. (2010, Study 3) showed that over the course of a 1-week basketball camp, harmonious passion for basketball predicted making more new friends over the course of the week. Such was not the case for obsessive passion. Further, once developed, friendships are maintained much more with harmonious passion than with obsessive passion (Philippe et al. 2010).

Passion has also been found to predict behavioral engagement. In this case, however, both harmonious passion and obsessive passion have been typically found to positively predict sustained engagement in the passionate activity. For instance, in a study with Greek exercisers, Parastatidou et al. (2012) showed that both types of passion for exercise leads one to engage in exercise several hours weekly and to do so for years. In addition, both harmonious passion and obsessive passion have been found to positively predict engagement in highly demanding task activities (i.e., deliberate practice) aimed at improving on the activity (e.g., Vallerand et al. 2007, 2008a). It is through such regular engagement in deliberate practice activities that long-term improvement in performance takes place (see Bonneville-Roussy et al. 2011; Vallerand et al. 2007, Studies 1 and 2; Vallerand et al. 2008a Studies 1 and 2). Thus, because both harmonious passion and obsessive passion lead one to engage in deliberate practice to similar extent, they both facilitate long-term performance. Although the long-term performance effects of the two types of passion may be similar, the process would appear to be quite different. Specifically, because harmonious passion also facilitates the experience of more adaptive on-task cognitive and affective as well as life outcomes (see below), the harmonious road to excellence would appear to be much more adaptive than the obsessive road that is devoid of such a positive process (see Vallerand 2015) and may include emotional suffering along the way (Vallerand 2015).

In sum, research on outcomes and experiences that are experienced during task engagement reveals that harmonious passion leads to positive advantages relative to obsessive passion, except as pertains to performance. Because such outcomes are experienced in a recurrent fashion, they are conducive to self-growth, and much more so for harmonious passion than obsessive passion.

Passion and Self-Growth in the Person's Life

The research briefly mentioned in the previous section is important in that it underscores the fact that passion matters with respect to self-growth. Indeed, one does not need to elaborate to make it clear that remaining enthusiastically engaged in a given activity for years will allow one to develop knowledge and proficiency in this activity relative to people who don't engage in the activity or who are not passionate about it. Thus, people who are passionate about an activity will experience increased self-growth with respect to the activity. They will perform better, know much more about the activity (an expert so to speak), and the activity will be more central in their lives. The self has expanded and self-growth at the activity level has taken place.

As seen above, however, the quality of such self-growth at the activity level differs as a function of the type of passion involved. For instance, with harmonious passion, people come to experience more flow and positive emotions than those with obsessive passion. Furthermore, there should be a ripple effect as these adaptive outcomes and experiences contribute to the presence of additional positive outcomes outside the realm of the passionate activity. In other words, positive on-task experiences facilitate optimal functioning in other areas of the person's life and self that goes beyond activity self-growth and takes place at the global level (Vallerand 1997). For instance, recall our university professor who, because of harmonious passion experienced positive emotions and flow that led to better performance at work. Below, we briefly review some research that supports this claim both at the intra and the interpersonal levels.

Research has looked at the role of passion in cognitions experienced outside the realm of the passionate activity (see Curran et al. 2015). Such research also reveals strong advantage of harmonious passion over obsessive passion. For instance, research reveals that harmonious passion for one's favorite activity (e.g., playing the guitar) positively contributes to experiencing flow in a second activity, such as when studying, whereas such is not the case with obsessive passion (Mageau et al. 2011). In fact, with obsessive passion, ruminations about the passionate activity conflict with the second activity and prevent flow from being experienced when studying! A series of studies by Belanger and colleagues, went one step further. In this research, Bélanger et al. showed that being led to unconsciously think about the passionate activity when engaging in a non passionate activity leads to conflicts with the activity that one is currently doing thereby preventing smooth performance on this other activity. In the long run, self-growth in these other activities will be curtailed by the conflict induced by obsessive passion about the passionate activity. It should be underscored, however, that this "goal-shielding" effect only takes place with obsessive passion. With harmonious passion, no conflict takes place and the person can think about the passionate activity and still be efficient on what the person is doing! Thus, one can be passionate about a given activity without suffering in other areas in one's life. Thus, harmonious passion can facilitate self-growth in the person as a whole.

We have seen in the previous section that harmonious passion leads to experiencing more positive, and obsessive passion to more negative, affect during task engagement. Furthermore, research has also shown that these effects affect what people experience after task engagement as well as later on that evening in other areas of their lives. Of interest is a diary study conducted by Mageau and Vallerand (2007) that revealed that over a two-week period, each day that one engaged in the passionate activity, harmonious passion led to an increase of positive affect over baseline level, whereas failing to engage in the passionate activity led obsessive passion to predict a decrease in positive affect over baseline days. These findings were basically replicated in a 2-week diary study with women passionate about physical exercise (Guérin et al. 2013). Even better, research by Vallerand et al. (2003, Study 2), followed collegiate football players over the course of an entire football season and showed that harmonious passion and obsessive passion predicted increases in general positive and negative affect, respectively, that took place over the course of an entire football season. Furthermore, these findings were obtained while controlling for intrinsic and extrinsic motivation toward football. Thus, passion can trigger affect that can be long lasting.

Other research has looked at the role of passion in psychological wellbeing. Once more research reveals that having harmonious passion for an activity has some positive effects on one's psychological wellbeing (Rousseau and Vallerand 2003, 2008). No such benefits take place with obsessive passion. In fact, research reveals that obsessive passion can predict various forms of psychological ill-being such as generalized anxiety and depression (Rousseau and Vallerand 2003). Of major interest, longitudinal research also reveals that obsessive passion for work can predict several years down the road being unable to psychologically adjust following retirement whereas harmonious passion protects from such psychological problems and leads to a highly fulfilling state of retirement (Houlfort et al. 2015). Research has also shed light on some of the mediating processes of such effects and reveals that on-task experiences mediate some of the observed effects of passion on well and ill-being. For instance, positive affect experienced during exercise (Rousseau and Vallerand 2008) and flow at work (Lavigne et al. 2012) mediate the positive and preventive effects of harmonious passion on life satisfaction and burnout, respectively.

Finally, it should be underscored that the adaptive outcomes engendered by harmonious passion are experienced on a recurrent basis because people engage in the activity that they are passionate several hours weekly. Thus, contrary to the belief that such gains are not sustained and that people return to baseline after a while (the so-called "thread mill effect"), the positive effects due to harmonious passion are indeed "sustainable" and long lasting (see Vallerand 2012, 2015). Once more, this is not the case with obsessive passion.

Passion for an activity can also have important effects on interpersonal outcomes outside the passionate activity. For instance, research reveals that having a harmonious passion for the Internet and Facebook can even promote friendships outside the passionate activity, whereas obsessive passion does not (Utz et al. 2012). In fact, contrary to harmonious passion, with obsessive passion there is a risk of losing one's friends due to over engagement in Facebook or other activities that they do not engage with us. Similarly, obsessive passion for a highly-involving activity such as being a soccer fan in the UK, undermines the quality of one's romantic relationship whereas harmonious passion has no such ill effects (Vallerand et al. 2008b, Study 3). Finally, obsessive passion leads to negative intergroup behavior such as verbally provoking others (Vallerand et al. 2008b, Study 2) and being ready to physically hurt others (Donahue et al. 2009; Rip et al. 2012; Vallerand et al. 2008b, Study 2) who do not share our beliefs or worse, who dare provoke us. Such is not the case with harmonious passion. Once more, processes experienced while engaging in the passionate activity have been identified as a mediator of the effects of passion. For instance, experiencing hatred toward others who attack one's faith mediates the impact of obsessive passion on intended violent behavior toward these other individuals (Rip et al. 2012, Study 2).

So with obsessive passion, people seem to lose twice: self-growth at the task level is limited at best and it contributes to further curtailing self-growth in other areas of the person's life. Thus, with obsessive passion, self-growth and development are not optimal but rather limited in scope. With harmonious passion, however, a recurrent series of micro-moments of self-growth take place where those positive moments experienced in the passionate activity contributes to the next one outside of it, and so on. Passion does matter!

Caveats and Limitations

While these findings provide strong support for the Dualistic Model of Passion, one may question the fact that these findings have been mostly obtained in a string of different studies that seem to mostly come from our lab. So do these findings generalize? Further, these studies used mostly correlational designs. This raises the causality issue. To this end, a few issues need to be underscored. First, there is now more research coming out of other labs than from ours (see Vallerand 2015). Second, a recent meta-analysis involving more than 94 studies and over 1300 independent effect sizes coming from a number of different laboratories provide strong support for the Dualistic Model of Passion (see Curran et al. 2015). Third, as pertains to the causality issue it is true that most studies used correlational designs. Research using cross-lagged panel designs in which both outcomes and the two types of passion are measured at two points in time reveals that passion leads to outcomes and not the other way around (see Carbonneau et al. 2008; Lavigne et al. 2012). Furthermore, research employing experimental inductions of the two types of passion (and random assignment to conditions) has led to the same findings as those using the Passion Scale. For instance, Lafrenière et al. (2013, Study 2) showed that inducing harmonious passion led to increases of life satisfaction relative to the induction of obsessive passion or that of a control group (see also Bélanger et al. 2013b for similar findings in several studies). In sum, overall, there is strong support for the validity of the findings reported in this chapter.

Another important issue to address deals with the fact that the above findings paint a picture in which harmonious passion is "good" and obsessive passion "bad". Let us qualify this conclusion in three ways. First, obsessive passion can predict some adaptive outcomes such as positive emotions in the form of self-related affect (e,g., hubristic pride) and high excitement (feeling "high"). While these types of emotions have not been found to be conducive to well-being (see Vallerand 2015, Chapter 8), they nevertheless seem more adaptive than emotional suffering. Second, obsessive passion provides one with high energy *during* engagement in the passionate activity just as much as harmonious passion (see Lafrenière et al. 2009; Przybylski et al. 2009). Such energy is important in overcoming obstacles and in achieving high performance when engaging in the activity, for sure. It should be noted, however, that obsessive passion leaves one with less energy than harmonious passion *following* task engagement. Such a difference in post-task energy may be crucial to ensure that positive growth takes place in other life activities besides the passionate activity (to this end, see Rapaport et al. 2016). Indeed, if obsessive passion leaves one burned out after engaging in the passionate activity, one can understand why very little positive outcomes can be derived outside the passionate activity. Finally, third, obsessive passion does not lead to lower levels of performance than harmonious passion. In fact, in the short term, obsessive passion may even lead to higher performance under conditions of ego-threat. One will then expend high energy to display high performance and thus superiority to others. Such expenditure may explain, at least in part, the loss of energy following task engagement that may undermine self-growth outside of the passionate activity in the person's life. Clearly future research on this issue and the others above is warranted.

Conclusion

The purpose of the present chapter was to introduce the concept of passion and show how it comes into play with respect to self-growth and development into adulthood. In so doing, we have presented the Dualistic Model of Passion (e.g., Vallerand 2010, 2015; Vallerand et al. 2003). The research reviewed in this chapter leads to three major conclusions. First, there is an overwhelming support for the Dualistic Model of Passion. The model defines passion as a strong inclination toward a self-defining activity that one loves, finds important, and devotes significant amount of time and energy. Furthermore, two types of passion are proposed depending on how the activity representation has been internalized in one's identity. While harmonious passion entails control of the activity and a harmonious coexistence of the passionate activity with other activities of the person's life, obsessive passion entails the relative lack of control over the passionate activity, rigid persistence, and conflict with other life activities. Research reviewed provided strong support for the existence of the two types of passion as well as for the processes that the Dualistic Model of Passion posits that they entail.

The second major conclusion is that passion matters with respect to self-growth and development into adulthood. We have seen that being passionate for a given activity leads to two types of self-growth, one that pertains to the activity one is passionate about and the other that deals with other life pursuits. Clearly, being passionate for a given activity leads to some self-growth and development with respect to the activity, irrespective of the type of passion at play. Being passionate for playing a musical instrument, for instance, leads one to become skills and knowledge (a kind of expert) in music relative to people who do not engage in these activities. We have also seen that there is evidence that harmonious passion leads to both types of self-growth and development (inside the realm of the activity as well as in the person's life as a whole) whereas obsessive passion leads to an impoverished and limited growth within the purview of the passionate activity as well as outside of it. Of importance, such self-growth takes place across the life span. Indeed, research has found the same findings with participants ranging in age from 8 to 100 years of age (Philippe et al. 2009; Vallerand 2015). In other words, passion, and especially harmonious passion, contributes to self-growth across the life span. It should be noted that no research has yet looked at the longitudinal contribution of passion in self-growth. Such research is clearly necessary in order to confirm the role of passion in changes in self-growth and identity.

In sum, as individuals, we evolve through life and become increasingly complex, while retaining our identity: "change in sameness" (Haan and Day 1974). The passion we develop for some activities determine in part if such change will be fully internalized in our identity and self or if it will lead us astray and stall or even limit such potential for growth. Future research on the construct of passion and its impact on self-growth would therefore appear as not only important but as crucial for a better understanding of our own psychological development into adulthood.

References

Aron, A., Aron, E. N., & Smollan, D. (1992). Inclusion of other in the self scale and the structure of interpersonal closeness. *Journal of Personality and Social Psychology, 63*, 596–612.

Baum, J. R., & Locke, E. A. (2004). The relationship of entrepreneurial traits, skill, and motivation to subsequent venture growth. *Journal of Applied Psychology, 89*, 587–598.

Bélanger, J., Lafrenière, M.-A., Vallerand, R. J., & Kruglanski, A. W. (2013a). When passion makes the heart grow colder: The role of passion in alternative goal suppression. *Journal of Personality and Social Psychology, 104*, 126–147.
Bélanger, J., Lafrenière, M.-A., Vallerand, R. J., & Kruglanski, A. W. (2013b). Driven by fear: The role of failure in passionate individuals' performance. *Journal of Personality and Social Psychology, 104*, 180–195.
Bonneville-Roussy, A., Lavigne, G. L., & Vallerand, R. J. (2011). When passion leads to excellence: the case of musicians. *Psychology of Music, 39*, 123–138.
Brown, K. W., & Ryan, R. M. (2003). The benefits of being present: Mindfulness and its role in psychological well-being. *Journal of Personality and Social Psychology, 84*, 822–848.
Carbonneau, N., Vallerand, R.J., Fernet, C., & Guay, F. (2008). The role of passion for teaching in intra and interpersonal outcomes. *Journal of Educational Psychology, 100*, 977–987.
Carpentier, J., Mageau, G., & Vallerand, R. J. (2012). Ruminations and flow: Why do people with a more harmonious passion experience higher well-being? *Journal of Happiness Studies, 13*, 501–518.
Caudroit, J., Boiche, J., Stephan, Y., Le Scanff, C., & Trouilloud, D. (2011). Predictors of work/family interference and leisure-time physical activity among teachers: The role of passion towards work. *European Journal of Work and Organizational Psychology, 20*(3), 326–344.
Csikszentmihalyi, M. (1990). Literacy and intrinsic motivation. *Daedalus, 119*, 115–140.
Curran, T., Hill, A. P., Appleton, P. R., Vallerand, R. J., & Standage, M. (2015). The psychology of passion: A meta-analytical review of a decade of research on intrapersonal outcomes. *Motivation and Emotion, 39*, 631–655.
Deci, E. L., & Ryan, R. M. (1985). The general causality orientations scale: Self-determination in personality. *Journal of Research in Personality, 19*(2), 109–134.
Deci, E. L., & Ryan, R. M. (2000). The "what" and "why" of goal pursuits: Human needs and the self-determination of behavior. *Psychological Inquiry, 11*, 227–268.
Deci, E. L., Egharri, H., Patrick, B. C., & Leone, D. R. (1994). Facilitating internalization: The self-determination perspective. *Journal of Personality, 62*, 119–142.
Donahue, E. G., Rip, B., & Vallerand, R. J. (2009). When winning is everything: On passion, identity, and aggression in sport. *Psychology of Sport and Exercise, 10*(5), 526–534.
Elliot, A. J., & Church, M. A. (1997). A hierarchical model of approach and avoidance achievement motivation. *Journal of personality and social psychology, 72*(1), 218.
Elliot, A. J., Maier, M. A., Moller, A. C., Friedman, R., & Meinhardt, J. (2007). Color and psychological functioning: the effect of red on performance attainment. *Journal of experimental psychology: General, 136*(1), 154.
Forest, J., Mageau, G. A., Sarrazin, C., & Morin, E. M. (2011). "Work is my passion": The different affective, behavioural, and cognitive consequences of harmonious and obsessive passion toward work. *Canadian Journal of Administrative Sciences/Revue Canadienne des Sciences de l'Administration, 28*(1), 27–40.
Fowler, J. H., & Christakis, N. A. (2008). Dynamic spread of happiness in a large social network: longitudinal analysis over 20 years in the Framingham Heart Study. *BMJ: British medical journal, 337*, 1–9.
Fredrickson, B. L. (2001). The role of positive emotions in positive psychology: the Broaden-and Build theory of positive emotions. *American Psychologist, 56*, 218–226.
Fredrickson, B. L. (2009). *Positivity*. New York: Three Rivers Press.
Fredrickson, B. L., & Branigan, C. (2005). Positive emotions broaden the scope of attention and thought-action repertoires. *Cognition and Emotion, 19*, 313–332.
Fredrickson, B. L., & Joiner, T. (2002). Positive emotions trigger upward spirals toward emotional well-being. *Psychological Science, 13*, 172–175.
Frijda, N. H., & Mesquita, B. (1994). The social roles and functions of emotions. In S. Kitayama & H. R. Markus (Eds.), *Emotion and culture: Empirical studies of mutual influence* (pp. 51–87). Washington, DC: American Psychological Association.
Gousse-Lessard, A.-S., Vallerand, R. J., Carbonneau, N., & Lafrenière, M.-A. K. (2013). The role of passion in mainstream and radical behaviors: A look at environmental activism. *Journal of Environmental Psychology, 35*, 18–29.

Guérin, E., Fortier, M. S., & Williams, T. (2013). "I just NEED to move...": examining women's passion for physical activity and its relationship with daily affect and vitality. *Psychology of Well-Being: Theory, Research and Practice, 3*(1), 1–24.

Haan, N., & Day, D. (1974). A longitudinal study of change and sameness in personality development: Adolescence to later adulthood. *The International Journal of Aging and Human Development, 5*(1), 11–39.

Haidt, J. (2003). The moral emotions. In R. J. Davidson, K. R. Scherer, & H. H. Goldsmith (Eds.), *Handbook of affective sciences* (pp. 852–870). New York: Oxford University Press.

Hatfield, E., & Walster, G. W. (1978). *A new look at love*. America: University Press of America.

Ho, V. T., Wong, S. S., & Lee, C. H. (2011). A tale of passion: Linking job passion and cognitive engagement to employee work performance. *Journal of Management Studies, 48*(1), 26–47.

Hodgins, H. S., & Knee, R. (2002). The integrating self and conscious experience. In E. L. Deci & R. M. Ryan (Eds.), *Handbook on self-determination research: Theoretical and applied issues* (pp. 87–100). Rochester: University of Rochester Press.

Houlfort, N., Vallerand, R.J., Laframboise, A., Fernet, C., & Koestner, R. (2015). The role of passion for work and need satisfaction in post-retirement psychological adjustment. *Journal of Vocational Behavior, 88*, 84–94.

Huta, V. (2013). Pursuing eudaimoniaVersus hedonia: Distinctions, similarities, and relationships. In A. S. Waterman (Ed.), *The best within us: Positive psychology perspectives on eudaimonic functioning* (pp. 139–158). Washington, DC: APA books.

Isen, A. M. (1987). Positive affect, cognitive processes, and social behavior. In L. Berkowitz (Ed.), *Advances in experimental social psychology* (Vol. 20, pp. 203–253). New York: Academic.

Johnson, K. J., Waugh, C. E., & Fredrickson, B. L. (2010). Smile to see the forest: Facially expressed positive emotions broaden cognition. *Cognition and Emotion, 24*(2), 299–321.

Joussain, A. (1928). *Les passions humaines (The human passions)*. Ernest Flammarion.

Jowett, S., Lafrenière, M.-A. K., & Vallerand, R. J. (2013). Passion for activities and relationship quality: A dyadic approach. *Journal of Social and Personal Relationship, 30*, 734–749.

Lafrenière, M.-A. K., Vallerand, R. J., Donahue, R., & Lavigne, G. L. (2009). On the costs and benefits of gaming: The role of passion. *CyberPsychology and Behavior, 12*, 285–290.

Lafrenière, M.-A. K., Vallerand, R. J., & Sedikides, C. (2013). On the relation between self-enhancement and life satisfaction: The moderating role of passion. *Self and Identity, 12*, 516–530.

Lavigne, G., Forest, J., & Crevier-Braud, L. (2012). Passion at work and burnout: A two-study test of the mediating role of flow experiences. *European Journal of Work and Organizational Psychology, 21*, 518–546.

Lecoq, J. (2012). *La passion: Aspects émotionnels, sociaux et existentiels* [The passion: Emotional, social, and existential aspects]. Doctoral thesis, Université Catholique de Louvain, Belgique.

Liu, D., Chen, X. P., & Yao, X. (2011). From autonomy to creativity: a multilevel investigation of the mediating role of harmonious passion. *Journal of Applied Psychology, 96*, 294–309.

Mageau, G., & Vallerand, R. J. (2007). The moderating effect of passion on the relation between activity engagement and positive affect. *Motivation and Emotion, 31*, 312–321.

Mageau, G. A., Vallerand, R. J., Charest, J., Salvy, S., Lacaille, N., Bouffard, T., & Koestner, R. (2009). On the development of harmonious and obsessive passion: The role of autonomy support, activity valuation, and identity processes. *Journal of Personality, 77*, 601–645.

Mageau, G. A., Carpentier, J., & Vallerand, R. J. (2011). The role of self-esteem contingencies the distinction between obsessive and harmonious passion. *European Journal of Social Psychology, 41*, 720–729.

Marsh, H. W., Vallerand, R. J., Lafreniere, M. A. K., Parker, P., Morin, A. J. S., Carbonneau, N., et al. (2013). Passion: Does One Scale Fit All? Construct Validity of Two-factor Passion Scale and Psychometric Invariance over Different Activities and Languages. *Psychological Assessment, 25*, 796–809.

Maslow, A. H. (1954). *Motivation and personality*. Oxford, England: Harpers.

Parastatidou, I. S., Doganis, G., Theodorakis, Y., & Vlachopoulos, S. P. (2012). Exercising with passion: Initial validation of the Passion Scale in Exercise. *Measurement in Physical Education and Exercise Science, 16*(2), 119–134.

Philippe, F. L., Vallerand, R. J., & Lavigne, G. L. (2009). Passion does make a difference in people' s lives: A look at well-being in passionate and non-passionate individuals. *Applied Psychology: Health and Well-Being, 1*, 3–22.

Philippe, F. L., Vallerand, R. J., Houlfort, N., Lavigne, G. L., & Donahue, E. G. (2010). Passion for an activity and quality of interpersonal relationships: The mediating role of emotions. *Journal of Personality and Social Psychology, 98*, 917–932.

Przybylski, A. K., Ryan, R. M., & Rigby, C. S. (2009). The motivating role of violence in video games. *Personality and Social Psychology Bulletin, 35*(2), 243–259.

Rapaport, M., Vallerand, R.J., & Verner-Fillion, J. (2016). *On overcoming obstacles: The role of passion.* Manuscript submitted for publication.

Ribot, T. (1907). *Essai sur les passions* (Essay on passions). Paris : Alcan.

Rip, B., Vallerand, R. J., & Lafrenière, M.-A. K. (2012). Passion for a cause, passion for a creed: On ideological passion, identity threat, and radicalization. *Journal of Personality, 80*, 573–602.

Rogers, C. (1963). The actualizing tendency in relation to "motives" and to consciousness. In M. R. Jones (Ed.), *Nebraska Symposium on Motivation*. Lincoln: University of Nebraska Press.

Rousseau, F. L., & Vallerand, R. J. (2003). Le rôle de la passion dans le bien-être subjectif des aînés [The role of passion in the subjective well-being of the elderly]. *Revue Québécoise de Psychologie, 24*, 197–211.

Rousseau, F. L., & Vallerand, R. J. (2008). An examination of the relationship between passion and subjective well-being in older adults. *International Journal of Aging & Human Development, 66*, 195–211.

Rousseau, F. L., Vallerand, R. J., Ratelle, C. F., Mageau, G. A., & Provencher, P. (2002). Passion and gambling: On the validation of the Gambling Passion Scale (GPS). *Journal of Gambling Studies, 18*, 45–66.

Ryan, R. M., & Deci, E. L. (2000). Self-determination and the facilitation of intrinsic motivation, social development, and well-being. *American Psychologist, 55*, 68–78.

Ryan, R. M., & Deci, E. L. (2001). On happiness and human potentials: A review of research on hedonic and eudaimonic well-being. *Annual Review of Psychology, 52*, 141–166.

Ryan, R. M., & Deci, E. L. (2003). On assimilating identities to the self: A Self-Determination Theory perspective on internalization and integrity within cultures. In M. R. Leary & J. P. Tangney (Eds.), *Handbook of self and identity* (pp. 253–272). New York: Guilford.

Ryff, C. D., & Keyes, C. L. (1995). The structure of psychological well-being revisited. *Journal of Personality and Social Psychology, 69*, 719–727.

Seligman, M. E. P., & Csikscentmihalyi, M. (2000). Positive psychology: An introduction. *American Psychologist, 55*, 5–14.

Sheldon, K. M. (2002). The Self-Concordance Model of healthy goal-striving: When personal goals correctly represent the person. In E. L. Deci & R. M. Ryan (Eds.), *Handbook of self-determination research* (pp. 65–86). Rochester, NY: The University of Rochester Press.

Stenseng, F. (2008). The two faces of leisure activity engagement: Harmonious and obsessive passion in relation to intrapersonal conflict and life domain outcomes. *Leisure Sciences, 30*, 465–481.

Sternberg, R. J. (1986). A triangular theory of love. *Psychological Review, 93*, 119–153.

St-Louis, A. C., Carbonneau, N., & Vallerand, R. J. (in press). Passion for a cause: How it affects health and well-being. *Journal of Personality, 83*(3), 263–273.

Utz, S., Jonas, K. J., & Tonkens, E. (2012). Effects of passion for massively multiplayer online role-playing games on interpersonal relationships. *Journal of Media Psychology: Theories, Methods, and Applications, 24*, 77–86.

Vallerand, R. J. (1997). Toward a hierarchical model of intrinsic and extrinsic motivation. *Advances in Experimental and Social Psychology, 29*, 271–360.

Vallerand, R. J. (2001). A hierarchical model of intrinsic and extrinsic motivation in sport and exercise. In G. Roberts (Ed.), *Advances in motivation in sport and exercise* (pp. 263–319). Champaign, IL: Human Kinetics.
Vallerand, R. J. (2008). On the psychology of passion: In search of what makes people's lives most worth living. *Canadian Psychology, 49*, 1–13.
Vallerand, R. J. (2010). On passion for life activities: The Dualistic Model of Passion. In M. P. Zanna (Ed.), *Advances in Experimental Social Psychology* (pp. 97–193). New York: Academic.
Vallerand, R. J. (2012). The role of passion in sustainable psychological well-being. *Psychological Well-Being: Theory, Research, and Practice, 2*, 1–21.
Vallerand, R. J. (2013). Passion and optimal functioning in society: A eudaimonic perspective. In A. S. Waterman (Ed.), *The best within us: Positive psychology perspectives on eudaimonic functioning* (pp. 183–206). Washington, DC: APA books.
Vallerand, R. J. (2015). *The psychology of passion: A dualistic model*. Oxford: New York.
Vallerand, R. J., & Houlfort, N. (2003). Passion at work: Toward a new conceptualization. In S. W. Gilliland, D. D. Steiner, & D. P. Skarlicki (Eds.), *Emerging perspectives on values in organizations* (pp. 175–204). Greenwich, CT: Information Age Publishing.
Vallerand, R. J., Fortier, M. S., & Guay, F. (1997). Self-determination and persistence in a real-life setting: Toward a motivational model of high school dropout. *Journal of Personnality and Social Psychology, 72*, 1161–1176.
Vallerand, R. J., Blanchard, C. M., Mageau, G. A., Koestner, R., Ratelle, C. F., & Léonard, M. (2003). Les passions de l'âme: On obsessive and harmonious passion. *Journal of Personality and Social Psychology, 85*, 756–767.
Vallerand, R. J., Rousseau, F. L., Grouzet, F. M. E., Dumais, A., & Grenier, S. (2006). Passion in sport: A look at determinants and affective experiences. *Journal of Sport & Exercise Psychology, 28*, 454–478.
Vallerand, R. J., Salvy, S. J., Mageau, G. A., Elliot, A. J., Denis, P. L., Grouzet, F. M. E., & Blanchard, C. (2007). On the role of passion in performance. *Journal of Personality, 75*, 505–533.
Vallerand, R. J., Mageau, G. A., Elliot, A. J., Dumais, A., Demers, M. A., & Rousseau, F. (2008a). Passion and performance attainment in sport. *Psychology of Sport and Exercise, 9*, 373–392.
Vallerand, R. J., Ntoumanis, N., Philippe, F. L., Lavigne, G. L., Carbonneau, N., Bonneville, A., et al. (2008b). On passion and sports fans: A look at football. *Journal of Sports Sciences, 26*, 1279–1293.
Vitterso, J. (2013). Feelings, meaning, and optimal functioning: Some distinctions between hedonic and eudaimonic well-being. In A. S. Waterman (Ed.), *The best within us: Positive psychology perspectives on eudaimonic functioning* (pp. 39–55). Washington, DC: APA books.
Waterman, A. S. (1993). Two conceptions of happiness: Contrasts of personal expressiveness (eudaimonia) and hedonic enjoyment. *Journal of Personality and Social Psychology, 64*(4), 678–691.
Waterman, A. S. (2013). *The best within us: Positive psychology perspectives on eudaimonia*. Washington, DC: APA Books.
Waugh, C. E., & Fredrickson, B. L. (2006). Nice to know you: Positive emotions, self-other overlap, and complex understanding in the formation of new relationships. *Journal of Positive Psychology, 1*, 93–106.

Chapter 11
Understanding, Supporting and Safeguarding Self-Determination as We Age

Philip McCallion and Lisa A. Ferretti

Abstract The proportion of the population who is aging or elderly is rapidly growing. The health of older adults has improved over the past 30 years with declines in mortality and late onset disability and with disease in old age less likely to result in death or loss of physical or mental functions. However, improved ability to treat diseases and chronic conditions also means increased prevalence of chronic conditions challenging the very independence that medical improvement was designed to increase. Understandings of quality of life concerns and markers of success or decrements in aging or successful aging are increasingly expressed in terms of independence and self-determination. This chapter considers theoretical perspectives on independence and self-determination as people age by examining the positive support of aging in place and the challenges experienced when dementia, self-neglect or abuse, and the approaching of end of life become part of older age. A particular consideration will be both the compromises and the opportunities presented by being the recipient of caregiving.

As of 2011, the year the oldest baby boomers started to turn 65, 40 million people in the United States were ages 65 and older and this number is projected to double to more than 89 million by 2050 with those aged 85 and older projected to rise even more rapidly. Such rapid changes in the age structure are already having major and somewhat unanticipated social and economic consequences straining, in past decades, local hospital, public school, and postsecondary education systems and the labor force. Greater impact from the baby boom generation is now expected as they age with changes in health and disability status, living arrangements, kinship networks, and economic well-being.

The health of older adults has improved over the past 30 years with declines in mortality and late onset disability and with disease in old age less likely to result in death or loss of physical or mental functions. However, improved ability to treat diseases and chronic conditions also means increased prevalence of chronic

P. McCallion (✉) • L.A. Ferretti
University of Albany, Albany, NY, USA
e-mail: pmccallion@albany.edu

M.L. Wehmeyer et al. (eds.), *Development of Self-Determination Through the Life-Course*, DOI 10.1007/978-94-024-1042-6_11

conditions challenging the very independence that medical improvement was designed to increase (Jacobsen et al. 2011). Half of all adults have one or more chronic conditions, one in four have two or more and rates are highest among those over 65 and among the 53 million with Arthritis, almost half report difficulties with daily activities (Barbour et al. 2013; Ward et al. 2014). Already increases in late onset disability, often associated with increased chronic conditions (Hootman et al. 2012), are being highlighted with further rapid expansion anticipated in coming decades. There are particular concerns that this expansion will particularly occur among older women, African-Americans and Latinos and those living in poverty, i.e., populations who often have the least resources to be able to support their own decision-making around care (He and Larson 2014).

Quality of life is now an increasing consideration for older adults (McCallion et al. 2013) in terms of (1) *Material well-being* – ability (often financial) to meet needs for basics such as food and shelter. (2) *Physical well-being* – the ability to perform basic activities of daily living and to live independently. (3) *Social engagement* – involvement with and support received from family, peers, community members, and community organizations, and (4) *Emotional well-being* – mental and psychological wellness often tied to physical health and social support (Jacobsen et al. 2011). Each of these domains, therefore, is an area where self-determination may or may not be present with implications for experienced quality of life.

Understandings of quality of life concerns and markers of success or decrements in aging or successful aging are increasingly expressed in terms of independence and self-determination. For example, Rowe and Kahn (1998) in describing successful aging articulated three critical components: absence or avoidance of disease and risk factors for disease, maintenance of physical and cognitive functioning, and active engagement with life. The definition of active engagement with life includes maintenance of autonomy (Bowling and Dieppe 2005), a core component of self-determination. Consideration of these issues begin from a belief that independence and self-determination are largely expressed and experienced in the middle adult and early aging years but because of changes in older years they come increasingly under threat. The continued expression of independence and self-determination in older years is both valued and expressed in the person's choices about where to live and in the management of major decisions about one's life and care when care is needed. A fundamental tenet is that one's successful aging is best determined by individual actions (Rubenstein and de Medeiros 2015), implying active management and self-determination of one's aging roadmap.

This chapter considers theoretical perspectives on independence and self-determination as people age by examining the positive support of aging in place and the challenges experienced when dementia, self-neglect or abuse, and the approaching of end of life become part of older age. A particular consideration will be both the compromises and the opportunities presented by being the recipient of caregiving.

Self-Determination

Within the literature on persons with developmental disabilities there is a strong belief in the value of self-determination and a range of opinions on its components. Most arrive at that self-determination occurs when the person is the primary agent making the decisions that cause things to happen in their lives (Wehmeyer 2011) and functional theories of self-determination have emerged outlined in four characteristics: (1) actions by the individual are autonomous, (2) behaviors are self-regulated, (3) it is the empowered person who initiates/responds to an event and (4) the actions of the individual are self-realizing (Wehmeyer and Abery 2013). These are ideas that also have relevance for older adults.

More fundamentally, as described throughout this book, self-determination begins with personal motivation. Motivation may be considered on a continuum involving amotivation, extrinsic motivation, and intrinsic motivation. Intrinsic motivation is described as highly self-determined (Ryan and Deci 2000), as "the inherent tendency to seek out novelty and challenges, to extend and exercise one's capacities, to explore, and to learn" (p.70). There is a need for both supportive conditions and for three psychological needs to be met: competency, autonomy, and relatedness. A sense of competency comes from receiving positive feedback regarding performance, autonomy from determining one's own behavior and relatedness from feelings of security and relational support. When all three needs are met, individuals experience high levels of well-being (Ryan and Deci 2000). These three constructs form an important value criteria framework for considering best practices for working with older adults.

Most attention in the literatures on aging is focused on the relationship between autonomy and competence. People are autonomously motivated when they experience choice in their behaviors as opposed to pressure or coercion, believe their own actions will improve their situation (health or otherwise) and perceive themselves to have competence (the skills, knowledge and ability) to control important outcomes (Williams and Deci 1996; Williams et al. 1998). In this view concerns about one's autonomy when initiating behaviors and perceived competence directly influences one's feelings about achieving the outcome. As older adults experience increases in chronic conditions and their consequences and in other challenges to their independence, effectiveness in self-management of health, healthcare and other aspects of daily living is seen as requiring both the experience of autonomy and feelings of competence (Williams et al. 2004).

Self-Determination Theory also contends that extrinsic motivation can be internalized and integrated with sufficient support. Initial extrinsic motivation is often initiated by health and other practitioners. There is growing recognition that the attitudes and behaviors of practitioners may support or hinder autonomy, competence and motivation. For example, acknowledgement of patients' perspectives, support for activities and decisions patients initiate, offering choices among treatment options, and the provision of relevant information have all been shown to support patients' motivation and health-relevant behaviors (Williams et al. 2004).

While self-determination is clearly influenced by individual motivation and abilities to think, choose, and act, often encapsulated in ideas of autonomy (Elander and Hermeren 1989), it is more complex; there are additional elements of knowledge, level of control, organization/ community/family context, free will and legal and ethical rights (Ekelund et al. 2014). In the aging literature there is concern that reductions in the ability to exercise self-determination whether initiated by self or others (professionals, caregivers and society at large) has consequences for:

1. reducing one's sense of and actual experience of health and well-being (Flick et al. 2003),
2. exacerbating the stressfulness of situations,
3. increasing dependence
4. contributing to deterioration in the ability to perform tasks (Breitholtz et al. 2013).

Some reductions in independence/ performance are related to aging, increased disability and the consequences of chronic disease, but increasingly the idea is being challenged that growing dependence in old age is necessarily directly linked to reductions in opportunities for and actual exercise of self-determination (Hammar et al. 2014). On the one hand, the ability to independently perform daily activities naturally deteriorates in advanced age (Holstein et al. 2007). On the other hand, reduced possibilities to exercise self-determination will also increase dependence (Breitholtz et al. 2013). When increased dependence is unavoidable, there remains for many a desire for continued self-determination. Success in supporting self-determination in older age is increasingly influenced by the commitment of professionals and caregivers, concerns about safety (both the person's concerns and the beliefs of carers), purposeful efforts to provide opportunities for involvement in decision-making, and evidence/experience that the views of the aging person matter (Breitholtz et al. 2013; Ekelund et al. 2014).

For older adults the realization of these ideas will occur in the arenas of (1) Health and Healthcare, (2) Aging in Place, (3) Self-neglect and Abuse, (4) Dementia, (5) End of Life, and (6) Caregiving.

Health and Health Care

Much of the effort in managing the consequences of chronic diseases is focused upon ensuring patient adherence to recommended protocols and on the pursuit of health behavior change (McCallion and Ferretti 2015). An absence of consideration of self-determination often means frustration for practitioners as adherence is poor and there are concerns that this is an expensive approach which should not be expected to be effective (Frieden 2010). More recent models such as the Chronic Care Model (Wagner et al. 2001) argue for approaches that build upon proactive patients actively managing their conditions in collaboration with thoughtful, energized and collaborative care practice teams of healthcare professionals who also interact with community-based providers able to support the patient actions outside of healthcare services and support ongoing self-management success (Wagner et al. 2001).

At an individual level, frameworks such as the Chronic Care Model have an intent to build upon a person's long standing desires for self-determination and proactively support the building of activation around self-management (McCallion and Ferretti 2015). Initial behavior change and on-going maintenance requires beliefs both that a given behavior will lead to the desired outcome and that one is capable of performing the behavior (Bandura 1977). Such beliefs have been built up over a life time but with the changes experienced in independence/ dependence in older age beliefs about capability are often under threat. Interventions are therefore needed that respect, encourage and support individual self-determination despite the challenges of chronic conditions and late onset disability.

There are also external changes in healthcare that will advance such supports for self-determination in the face of increased chronic conditions and late onset disability. The transformations in the delivery of health care desired in the Affordable Care Act to support better health, better care and lower cost are moving health care from an acute to a chronic disease management perspective, are advancing holistic, person in environment and patient as partner emphases and encouraging greater self-management of their conditions by patients. Change rarely happens simply from stated intent; instead there is a need for sustained and committed action. Hibbard et al. (2010) in their promotion of strategies to raise the levels of activation to undertake self-management among patients have also raised that while healthcare professionals are overwhelmingly supportive of patients taking and following through on their instructions and advice, they are less enthusiastic about treating patients as partners in care, and in patients independently seeking information, making decisions and taking actions to advance their care (cornerstones of self-management and potentially products of self-determination). This leads to questions as to how well codes of professional conduct, educational and continuing education programs and provider procedures actively support and prepare/require professionals to support such advances. A readiness to acknowledge the centrality of self-determination seems critical.

Aging in Place

It is well established that a majority of older adults wish to remain in their own homes and communities throughout their aging years (Pynoos et al. 2009). Diminished and declining health and functioning, unavailability of family members [due to death or moving away] and increasing costs make aging in place more difficult (McCallion 2014). Planning to remain often results in investment both in physical modifications to the home and in building community connections that will benefit the aging individual as well as the community in which he or she is located. Such steps reflect a process of active self-determination. Social connectedness within a neighborhood and community increases informal supports likely to be critical to remaining there (Sabia 2008).

Most considerations of aging in place emphasize the importance of the fit between one's home and the individual. Moss and Lawton (1982) argued that as people get older they spend more time in their home and less time in work and social activities but they have the ability to increase competence in finding resources in the environment to improve the fit (Lawton 1989). Therefore as well as the physical housing environment and neighborhood the person's subjective impressions and coping style will advance new understandings of "fit". The Wald and Oswald Conceptual Framework (2003) extends our understanding of "fit." Person environment exchanges involve both subjective (housing-related identity) and objective (housing related autonomy) outcomes mediated by the individual's changing levels of independence, increases in needs and challenges to connectedness to others (Oswald et al. 2003). Two key concepts of the framework are belonging and agency. There are three aspects to the concept of belonging:

1. satisfaction with one's living space (why would I leave, I like it here)
2. attachments to that location on behavioral, cognitive and emotional levels;
3. the meaning the home has.

In an update to the model Wahl et al. (2012) make explicit that sense of belonging is "driven" by experience. These ideas then contribute significantly to housing related identity (this house is part of who I am) and a sense of housing related autonomy (I will be able to maintain quality of life if I remain here). More directly related to housing related autonomy (but also to identity) are ideas of agency; the extent to which the home itself is perceived by the older adult to compensate for declines in ways that maintain independence. There are three considerations: (1) environmental press (changing circumstances and declining functional abilities make independence and remaining in place more difficult); (2) environmental richness (people acquiring personal and technological supports to increase their ability to remain within the home); and (3) person-environment fit (the congruence between needs and the capacity of the home to support those needs). As well as being influenced by experience-driven belonging, outcomes are enhanced by behavior-driven agency or older adults being active participants in shaping their older age. (Fig. 11.1).

The other aspect of aging in place is social relationships and community connections which gives value to ideas of social capital. Social capital represents a benefit to an individual (both psychosocial and tangible in terms of reciprocal support) that emerges from connecting with others both from volunteerism and from participation in supportive community activities (Cannuscio et al. 2003).

Staying connected with one's communities and supports and engaging in roles that contribute to community building have positive effects, including raising the significance for individuals of the experience of later life and contributing to the individual's better health (Martinson and Minkler 2006; Scharlach et al. 2012; Vladeck and Segel 2010; Yen et al. 2012). The resulting social capital both has resulted from the self-determined acts of older adults and offers older adults further opportunities for independent, fulfilling and self-determined aging in place (Tang and Lee 2011).

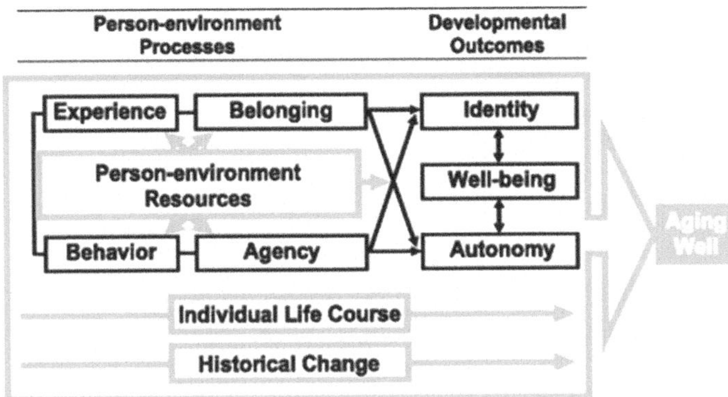

Fig. 11.1 Revised conceptual framework – housing in later life (Wahl et al. 2012)

Self-Neglect and Abuse

An unfortunate consequence, for some, in determined pursuit of aging in place is the potential for self-neglect and/or abuse or exploitation by others. Elder abuse is defined as intentional actions that cause or create risk for harm (whether or not intended) for vulnerable older adults by caregivers or others including failures by caregivers to meet the person's basic needs or to protect them from harm (Bonnie and Wallace 2003). Self-neglect is behavior by an older person that threatens his/her own health or safety such as refusal or failure to address adequate food, water, clothing, shelter, personal hygiene, medication (when indicated), and safety precautions (ACL 2016). A characteristic of self-neglect is that the person's capacity to make decisions may be intact; the challenge is around capacity to extract one's self from harmful situations, circumstances and/or relationships (Naik et al. 2008).

Statistics are incomplete but females appear to be twice as likely to be abused; abuse and self-neglect increase with age and significant numbers of cases go unreported (Bonnie and Wallace 2003). Major financial exploitation has been self-reported at a rate of 41 per 1000 surveyed, i.e., at rates higher than self-reported rates of emotional, physical, and sexual abuse or neglect (Lifespan et al. 2011).

Underreporting of cases in general and "acceptance" of financial exploitation is widely reported as emanating from (1) an inability because of frailty or access to assistance to report, (2) embarrassment at admitting that those they love and/or trusted exploited or abused them and (3) the victim's concerns that pursuit of the complaint will result in negative consequences either because abuse will not be substantiated and they will experience greater abuse or the victim will be without support and therefore placed outside their home and the life they are trying to preserve. As may be seen in Fig. 11.2, looking specifically at the issue of financial abuse there is a complex web of relationships and decisions with both perpetrator and victim characteristics, issues of inequality and power and the consequences of self-determined decisions about linkages to social networks and perceptions, in this case, of financial vulnerability that then influence abuse outcomes.

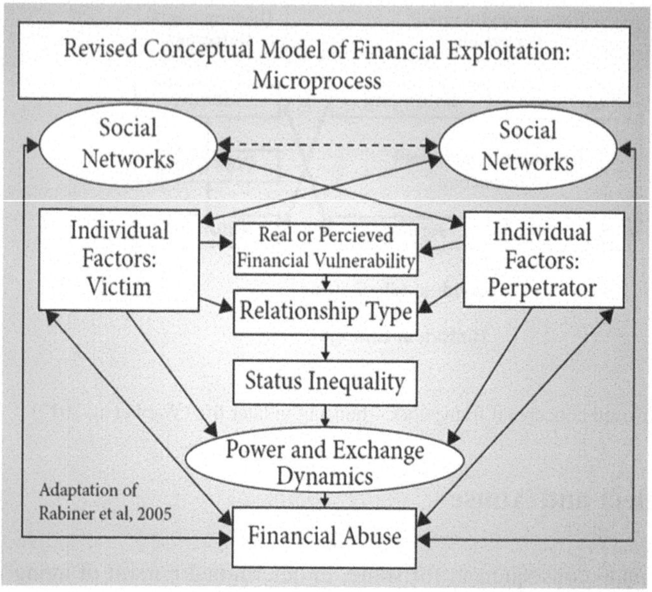

Fig. 11.2 Revised conceptual model of financial exploitation

The availability of adult protective workers in most states represents a resource to pursue cases of abuse, completing investigations, supporting prosecutions and providing needed supports to restore independence. The provision of such services varies by state and is not as well supported legislatively as child protective services but there is widespread support for a series of principles laid out by the National Adult Protective Services Association to underpin those services.

1. A right to self-determination
2. The least restrictive alternative
3. Family unit should be maintained where possible
4. Use of community based over institutional services
5. Blaming the victim should be avoided
6. Failure to provide adequate or appropriate services is worse than no services.

Such is the respect for self-determination that there is also agreement that older adults may refuse services and may make choices that adult protective services workers may not themselves recommend (Kosberg et al. 2006), with examples often cited around hoarding, living situations, and persons lived with (Dennis et al. 2012; Tompkins 2011). Most critically in the absence of a formal adjudication that the person does not have decision-making capacity or is in need for guardianship, there is no basis on which to deny continuing self-determination (Dennis et al. 2012). There is perhaps no other area of aging where the challenges of respecting, valuing and advancing self-determination are as starkly highlighted. In the terms previously highlighted, the individual's desire for autonomy and feelings of competence directly clashes with the values and appraisals of practitioners, making more difficult the delivery of positive feedback which is at the core of building an appraisal of personal competence at a moment when the person has been abused or neglected and reinforcement of a sense of competence is probably most desired.

Dementia

The experience of dementia is a moment in an aging life where loss of independence and reduction in opportunities for self-determination often occurs. With figures of 5.2 million people in the United States experiencing Alzheimer's disease and other dementias and risk increasing with age (Alzheimer's Association 2014), the challenge is growing. Dementia in any form is a progressive and degenerative disease diminishing the most recent memories first and progressively effecting judgement and ability to manage one's household first and then one's self care while care needs mount and the ability to express those needs declines. Yet there are many people in the early stages of dementia continuing to live alone and seeking to continue to manage their own affairs (McCallion 2014). Dementia introduces both issues of self-determination in decline and a temporal aspect to the collection of information to support such decision-making. A majority of nursing home residents have dementia. Findings that (1) empowerment approaches such as the culture change movement where residents and direct care staff are facilitated to be the major decision-makers about care and (2) nursing homes meeting of individual autonomy and relatedness needs result in improved outcomes in terms of nursing inspections outcomes and measured psychological need satisfaction and wellbeing (Grabowski et al. 2014; Mitty 2005) point to the value of continuing to advance self-determination.

Similarly, efforts to gather information before dementia advances on the desires and preferences of the person with dementia offers opportunities to continue to respect the autonomy of the person and to advance and support the person's remaining competency for which there is some evidence to support the potential to slow if not the progression of the disease at least the changes it produces in a person's life (McCallion 2005).

End of Life

Much of the discussion about self-determination and end of life is focused upon euthanasia, expressed as the exercise of a choice to end suffering. However, the larger movement in end of life and palliative care is around both the expression of choice not just in the last months of life but as disease progresses. Hospice care is viewed as being about care as dying approaches. The World Health Organization (2002) defines palliative care as an approach to improving the quality of life of patients and families facing life-threatening illnesses, by preventing and relieving suffering through identification, assessment and treatment of pain and other problems. Palliative care:

- provides relief from pain and distressing symptoms;
- affirms life with dying as a normal process;
- neither hastens nor postpones death;
- integrates with psychological and spiritual aspects of patient care;
- offers support to patients to live as actively as possible until death;
- offers supports to help family cope during illness and bereavement;
- uses a team approach;
- enhances quality of life, and positively influences the course of illness;
- may be used in conjunction with other therapies intended to prolong life and with investigations to better understand and manage clinical complications.

This last point of using palliative care in conjunction with other interventions points up a critical area of choice for patients, often older adults, to include comfort care with curative care. Going further, through advanced directives, instructions to proxy decision-makers and discussions with physicians and other practitioners, individuals have the opportunity to exercise autonomy. A challenge is the feeling of competency when decisions are complex, e.g., to ensure not to become machine dependent or otherwise artificially prolong life and yet give instructions that reflect an informed understanding of medical procedures. Increasingly end of life decision-making is being supported by professions. For social workers in this role Csikai and Raymer (2003) argue that the key skills are

- assessment of complex needs of patients and families;
- communication of psychosocial needs of patients and families to team members;
- facilitation of effective family and team communication;
- provision of crisis intervention.

However, the support of self-determination is also critical. When people are at perhaps the most dependent moment of their lives supporting the expression of autonomy and behavior by professionals in ways that reinforce a patient's sense of competence are critical.

Caregiving (or Managing Being Cared for)

In 2015 there was an estimated 43.5 million adults in the United States who had provided unpaid care to an adult or a child in the prior 12 months with an estimated prevalence of caring for an adult at 16.6%, or 39.8 million Americans with 34.2 million Americans providing unpaid care to an adult age 50 or older. The majority of caregivers are female (60%), eight in 10 take care of one person (82%), a further majority provide care for a relative (85%), with 49% caring for a parent or parent-in-law and the one in 10 providing care for a spouse/partner are four times as likely to be a higher-hour caregiver. On average, caregivers spend 24.4 h a week providing care with 23% providing 41 or more hours of care a week (NAC & AARP 2015).

Caregiving suggests increased dependence of the person cared for, the caregiver may be stressed and experiencing their own health issues and there is little training for family caregivers (Toseland et al. 2001). Also the caregiver is not a practitioner and may have poor understanding both of the value of self-determination and the role they may play in its support.

In being cared for, the experience of self-determination is influenced by the effects on independence of the person's aging or ill body, and by caregivers with the experience further varying by activity, *who* is helping, and *how* extensive the help is. Deterioration in health and abilities increases frustration and further reduces feelings of autonomy and competence.

Decision-making in caregiving is also relational, meaning the exercise of self-determination is also influenced by the relationship between the person receiving, and the person offering help. To the extent there is respect and consideration in the caregiving relationship this will facilitate more active participation in decision-making and the experience of personal needs being met as desired may increase the care recipient's confidence, further enhancing the exercise of self-determination (Hammar et al. 2014). The view of caregiving must also be modified so that the person receiving care is not seen simply as a passive recipient but instead as a person interested in maintaining independence. Recommended strategies include only accepting or offering the minimum amount of help needed for each caregiving activity. So much of the caregiving literature is focused upon the welfare and support of the caregiver and the physical care needed by and offered to the care recipient. There is less but needed attention to the support of self-determination and the measurement of its impact on the health and wellbeing of the care recipient.

Conclusions

To return to themes explored at the beginning of this chapter, the intent of self-determination focused efforts for people with developmental disabilities are to increase the opportunity for personally motivated and directed decisions that advance the day to day realization of their desired daily lives, often something that was not previously a part of the person's life experience. For older adults, aspects of self-determination were always a part of the person's adult life but in older age, with the onset of chronic conditions and reduced social networks and resources, the exercise of self-determination becomes more difficult. What work on self-determination with older adult populations adds to the overall discussion of self-determination are ideas on the importance of environmental modifications and active efforts to link to others to improve self-determination opportunities as was illustrated in the discussion of aging in place; the active involvement of practitioners in the healthcare arena and in family caregiving will help sustain or rebuild the senses of autonomy and competence at the core of self-determination; and advance planning and reconnection with past values and preferences may help overcome the barriers to self-determination when dementia symptoms are present or the individual is approaching end of life. Finally, the consideration of abuse and neglect issues points out the challenging aspects of the exercise of self-determination; actively shaping and managing one's life through one's own decisions may include steps and actions that place the person at risk but the denial of self-determination should be a last resort step when lack of safety is demonstrated rather than anticipated. All in all the ideas reviewed emphasize the importance of both the opportunity for and the support of self-determination and their direct linkage with successful aging, improved health and a quality life.

References

ACL. (2016). Elder abuse statistics/Data. http://www.ncea.aoa.gov/Library/Data/

Alzheimer's Association. (2014). *Alzheimer's disease facts and figures*. Chicago: Author.

Bandura, A. (1977). Self-efficacy: Toward a unifying theory of behavioral change. *Psychological Review, 84*, 191–215.

Barbour, K. E., Helmick, C. G., Theis, K. A., Murphy, L. B., Hootman, J., & Brady, T. J. (2013). Prevalence of doctor-diagnosed arthritis and arthritis-attributable activity limitation — United States, 2010–2012. *Morbidity and Mortality Weekly Report (MMWR), 62*(44), 869–873.

Bonnie, R., & Wallace, R. (Eds.). (2003). *Elder mistreatment: abuse, neglect and exploitation in an aging America*. Washington, DC: National Academies Press.

Bowling, A., & Dieppe, P. (2005). What is successful aging and who should define it? *BMJ, 331*(7531), 1548–1551.

Breitholtz, A., Snellman, I., & Fagerberg, I. (2013). Older people's dependence on caregivers' help in their own homes and their lived experiences of their opportunity to make independent decisions. *International Journal of Older People Nursing, 8*, 139–148.

Cannuscio, C., Block, J., & Kawachi, I. (2003). Social capital and successful aging: The role of senior housing. *Annals of Internal Medicine, 139*(Suppl 2), 395–399.

Csikai, E. L., & Raymer, M. (2003). *The Social Work End of Life Care Education Project*. http://www.nhpco.org/files/public/InsightsIssue2_2003Social_Worker_pp8-9.pdf.

Dennis, C., McCallion, P., & Ferretti, L. (2012). Understanding implementation of best practices for working with the older homeless through the lens of self-determination theory. *Journal of Gerontological Social Work, 55*(4), 352–366.

Ekelund, C., Dahlin-Ivanoff, S., & Eklund, K. (2014). Self-determination among older people – A concept analysis. *Scandinavian Journal of Occupational Therapy, 21*, 116–124.

Elander, G., & Hermeren, G. (1989). Autonomy and paternalistic behaviour in care. *Scandinavian Journal of Caring Sciences, 3*, 153–159.

Flick, U., Fischer, C., Neuber, A., Schwartz, F. W., Walter, U. (2003). Health in the context of growing old: Social representations of health. *Journal of Health Psychology, 8*(5), 539–556.

Frieden, T. R. (2010). A framework for public health action: The health impact pyramid. *American Journal of Public Health, 100*(4), 590–595.

Grabowski, D. C., O'Malley, A. J., Afendulis, C. C., Caudry, D. J., Elliot, A., & Zimmerman, C. (2014). Culture change and nursing home quality of care. *The Gerontologist, 54*, S35–s45.

Hammar, I. O., Dahlin-Ivanoff, S., Wilhelmson, K., & Eklund, K. (2014). Shifting between self-governing and being governed: A qualitative study of older persons' self-determination. *BMC Geriatrics, 14*, 126.

He, W., & Larson, L. J. (2014). *Older Americans with a disability: 2008–2012*. Washington, DC: U.S. Dept. of Health & Human Services.

Hibbard, J. H., Collins, P. A., Mahoney, E., & Baker, L. H. (2010). The development and testing of a measure assessing clinician beliefs about patient self-management. *Health Expectations, 13*, 65–72.

Holstein, B. E., Due, P., Almind, G., & Avlund, K. (2007). Eight-year change in functional ability among 70- to 95-year-olds. *Scandinavian Journal of Public Health, 35*, 243–249.

Hootman, J. M., Helmick, C. G., & Brady, T. J. (2012). A public health approach to addressing arthritis in older adults: the most common cause of disability. *American Journal of Public Health, 102*, 426–433.

Jacobsen, L. A., Kent, M., Lee, M., & Mather, M. (2011). America's aging population. *Population Bulletin, 66*(1), 1–16.

Kosberg, J., Rothman, M., & Dunlop, B. (2006). Advocacy and protection of older adults. In B. Berkman (Ed.), *Handbook of social work in health and aging* (pp. 355–362). New York: Oxford University Press.

Lawton, M. P. (1989). Environmental proactivity in older people. In V. L. Bengtson & K. W. Schaie (Eds.), *The course of later life* (pp. 15–23). New York: Springer.

Lifespan of Greater Rochester, Inc., Weill Cornell Medical Center of Cornell University. & New York City Department for the Aging. (2011). *Under the radar: New York state elder abuse prevalence study*. New York: Author.

Martinson, M., & Minkler, M. (2006). Civic engagement and older adults: A critical perspective. *The Gerontologist, 46*, 318–324.

McCallion, P. (2005). Supporting families of persons with dementia in nursing homes: The family visit education program. In J. E. Gaugler (Ed.), *Promoting family involvement in nursing homes: making programs work* (pp. 123–140). Baltimore: Health Professions Press.

McCallion, P. (2014). Aging in place. In K. Whitfield & T. Baker (Eds.), *Handbook of minority aging* (pp. 277–290). NY: Springer.

McCallion, P., & Ferretti, L. A. (2015). Building capacity for self-management interventions: The challenges. *The Journal of Nursing Care, 4*(6), 1–2.

McCallion, P., Ferretti, L., & Park, J. (2013). Financial issues and an aging population: Responding to an increased potential for financial abuse and exploitation. In J. Birkenmaier, J. Curley, & M. Sherraden (Eds.), *Financial education & capability: Research, education, policy and practice* (pp. 129–155). New York: Oxford University Press.

Mitty, E. L. (2005). Culture change in nursing homes: An ethical perspective. *Annals of Long Term Care, 13*(3), 1–2.

Moss, M. S., & Lawton, M. P. (1982). Time budgets of older people: A window of four lifestyles. *Journal of Gerontology, 37*, 115–123.

Naik, A. D., Lai, J. M., Kunik, M. E., & Dyer, C. B. (2008). Assessing capacity in cases of self-neglect. *Geriatrics, 63*(2), 24–31.

National Alliance for Caregiving (NAC) and AARP. (2015). *Caregiving in the U.S*. Bethesda/Washington, DC: AARP Public Policy Institute.

Oswald, F., Wahl, H. W., Martin, M., & Mollenkopf, H. (2003). Physical environments and aging: Critical contributions of M. Powell Lawton to theory and practice. *Journal of Housing for the Elderly, 17*, 135–155.

Pynoos, J., Caraviello, R., & Cicero, C. (2009). Lifelong housing: The anchor in aging-friendly communities. *Generations, 33*(2), 26–32.

Rowe, J. W., & Kahn, R. L. (1998). *Successful aging*. New York: Pantheon Books.

Rubenstein, R. L., & de Medeiros, K. (2015). "Successful aging," gerontological theory and neoliberalism: A qualitative critique. *The Gerontologist, 55*(1), 34–42.

Ryan, R. M., & Deci, E. L. (2000). Self-determination theory and the facilitation of intrinsic motivation, social development, and well-being. *American Psychologist, 55*(1), 68–78.

Sabia, J. J. (2008). There's no place like home. A hazard model analysis of aging in place among older homeowners. *Research on Aging, 30*, 3–35.

Scharlach, A., Graham, C., & Lehning, A. (2012). The "Village" model: A consumer-driven approach for aging in place. *The Gerontologist, 52*, 418–427.

Tang, F., & Lee, Y. (2011). Social support networks and expectations for aging in place and moving. *Research on Aging, 33*, 444–464.

Tompkins, M. (2011). *Clinician's guide to hoarding: A harm reduction approach*. New York: Springer.

Toseland, R. W., Smith, G., & McCallion, P. (2001). Helping family caregivers. In A. Gitterman (Ed.), *Handbook of social work practice with vulnerable populations* (pp. 548–581). New York: Columbia University Press.

Vladeck, F., & Segel, R. (2010). Identifying risks to healthy aging in New York city's varied NORCs. *Journal of Housing for the Elderly, 24*, 356–372.

Wagner, E. H., Austin, B. T., Davis, C., Hindmarsh, M., Schaefer, J., et al. (2001). Improving chronic illness care: translating evidence into action. *Health Affairs (Millwood), 20*, 64–78.

Wahl, H. W., Iwarsson, S., & Oswald, F. (2012). Aging well and the environment: Toward an integrative model and research agenda for the future. *The Gerontologist, 52*(3), 306–316.

Ward, B. W., Schiller, J. S., & Goodman, R. A. (2014). Multiple chronic conditions among US adults: A 2012 update. *Preventing Chronic Disease, 11*, E62.

Wehmeyer, M. L. (2011). Empowerment. In A. Michalos (Ed.), *Encyclopedia of quality of life research*. Heidelberg: Springer.

Wehmeyer, M. L., & Abery, B. H. (2013). Self-determination and choice. *Intellectual and Developmental Disabilities, 51*(5), 399–411.

Williams, G. C., & Deci, E. L. (1996). Internalization of biopsychosocial values by medical students: A test of self-determination theory. *Journal of Personality and Social Psychology, 70*, 767–779.

Williams, G. C., Freedman, Z. R., & Deci, E. L. (1998). Supporting autonomy to motivate glucose control in patients with diabetes. *Diabetes Care, 21*, 1644–1651.

Williams, G. C., McGregor, H. A., Zeldman, A., Freedman, Z. R., & Deci, E. L. (2004). Testing a self-determination theory process model for promoting glycemic control through diabetes self-management. *Health Psychology, 23*, 58–66.

World Health Organization (WHO). (2002). *National cancer control programmes: Policies and managerial guidelines* (2nd ed.). Geneva: World Health Organization.

Yen, I. H., Shim, J. K., Martinez, A. D., & Barker, J. C. (2012). Older people and social connectedness: How place and activities keep people engaged. *Journal of Aging Research*, 1–10.

Chapter 12
Culture and Self-Determination

Karrie A. Shogren and Michael L. Wehmeyer

Abstract This chapter explores the impact of context, namely cultural factors, on the development of self-determination. The influence of one's personal culture and cultural norms and beliefs on the development of self-determination are reviewed. The role of Causal Agency Theory in understanding influence of culture on the development of self-determination, and research on the operationalization of self-determined action in diverse cultures is presented. Implications for the development of self-determination across cultural contexts is discussed.

As described throughout this text, we define self-determination as a general psychological construct that refers to self- (vs. other-) caused action. Self-determined people act volitionally, based on their own will. In other chapters in this text, we describe theoretical frameworks for understanding the self-determination construct, including Self-Determination Theory and Causal Agency Theory. A commonality across theoretical frameworks is an understanding that the development of self-determination is influenced by contextual factors, which includes one's personal culture. While as a *psychological construct* self-determination means the same thing for every person; that is, the notion that self-determination is self- (vs. other-) caused action is universal, the theories reviewed throughout this text also illuminate that the operationalization of self-determined action varies across contexts and cultures. Thus, the construct of self-determination has relevance across contexts and cultures, but the actions and outcomes of self-determined action look different and will vary across contexts and cultures and over time.

Given this, the present chapter will describe the role of context, and specifically cultural factors, in the development of self-determination. Research that has explored the operationalization of self-determination in other cultures will be reviewed, and implications for the development of self-determination across cultural contexts discussed.

K.A. Shogren (✉) • M.L. Wehmeyer
Special Education,University of Kansas, Lawrence, KS, USA
e-mail: shogren@ku.edu

M.L. Wehmeyer et al. (eds.), *Development of Self-Determination Through the Life-Course*, DOI 10.1007/978-94-024-1042-6_12

Culture and Self-Determination

Frameworks for understanding the influence of contextual factors on human development and functioning describe context as encompassing the personal and environmental factors that influence a person's life and functioning (Shogren et al. 2014; World Health Organization 2001). These frameworks suggest that there are multiple levels of influence, and to understand the relationship between contextual factors, such as culture, and human development and functioning, the interrelated ecological systems that influence human functioning must be considered. Brofenbrenner (Bronfenbrenner 1979) operationalized several interrelated systems that influence human functioning with the individual at the center and the systems that shape the individual's experiences moving out from the center. These systems include: (a) the microsystem (i.e., the immediate social setting, including the person, family and social networks), (b) the mesosystem (i.e., the school and community environment that influence the individual), and (c) the macrosystem (i.e., the overarching patterns of culture and society). It is also asserted that the various systems change and interact in diverse ways over time (chronosystem). Specific to culture, one's personal culture as well as cultural norms and beliefs adopted by organizations, communities and societies that a person exists in over time influences functioning, including the development and expression of self-determination.

Personal Culture

Culture provides the lens through which we view, interpret, and find meaning in the world in which we live. Culture structures perceptions, shapes behaviors, and defines our sense of reality. Cultural theorists assert that one's personal culture or cultural identify is shaped by multiple factors that interact across contexts and institutions (Triandis and Suh 2002). Given this complexity, researchers have proposed the adoption of an ecological framework to understand cultural identities (Suarez-Balcazar et al. 2014) acknowledging the "inclusive and interacting nature" (Trainor et al. 2008, p. 57) of multiple factors in shaping cultural identities. Trainor et al. highlight that multiple personal factors contribute to cultural identity, including gender, disability, race/ethnicity, language, and socioeconomic background and that these factors are embedded in communities and society. Further, they describe how certain cultural identities have shared experiences of oppression, exclusion, and discrepant education and postsecondary opportunities that necessitate specific attention to reduce oppression and exclusion and support culturally valued outcomes. Relatedly, understanding of self-determination at a group or national level, rather than as a psychological construct, highlights the role of self-determination in struggles for equity, equality, and empowerment. The term self-determination (referring to group or national self-determination) has been used in a political context, often referring to the rights of people of a given country to determine their own political status and to self-governance, and, subsequently, by groups of people defined by features other than geographic boundaries who adopted the theme of the right to self-determination regarding self-governance. For example, one principle of the celebration of Kwanzaa, observed in the U.S. to honor African-American heritage, is Kujichagulia. Kujichagulia, when translated, means self-determination and is used to refer to the principle of self-rule and self-governance in support of the importance of African people in culture, philosophy, and history in the context of the American civil rights movement (Robinson 2002).

Research in cross-cultural psychology also suggests that values differ not only inter-culturally, but also intra-culturally. Thus, an individual's cultural identity is not static and is shaped by many factors, which can vary across contexts, environments and over time. In recent years increased attention has been directed towards the interaction between culture and situational or contextual factors. Research has found that individuals can, and often do, hold more than one cultural belief system (e.g., an individual may endorse both individualist and collectivist values) and may draw on the different systems based on situational demands or characteristics (Hong and Chiu 2001). This complexity suggests the critical importance of examining the degree to which one's personal culture across contexts and times influences the development of self-determination, and the role of motivation and goal directed behavior in varying contexts.

Cultural Norms and Beliefs

In additional to, and influencing, one's personal culture, researchers have also suggested broader community and societal beliefs and values shape the experiences of people from varying cultures, and as a result of the development of self-determination. Researchers have suggested, for example, that cultural norms and beliefs can shape the manner in which we recognize, understand, and accept disability (Goode and Maloof 2011), as well as influence how we respond to others and how others respond to us (Nelson 2016). For example, with regard to youth with disabilities researchers have found that cultural beliefs about disability can shape employment opportunities. Carter et al. (2009) examined perceptions of members of community employment networks, including Chamber of Commerce members. They found that community members were significantly less likely to rate an employment activity as "feasible" if "youth with disabilities" were referenced as opposed to simply "youth" (p. 148). Relatedly, expectations related to one's gender or race/ethnicity can shape how people's actions are perceived, and detrimentally impact performance in conditions where negative stereotypes are held (Nelson 2016).

Research on Culture and Self-Determination

There have been critiques of theories of self-determination, linking the emphasis on the motivation for autonomy and on self- (vs. other-) caused action with Western values. However, self-determination theorists have responded and emphasized that such critiques confound autonomy with acting independently without any external influences (Ryan and Deci 2006). Autonomy, however, does not mean acting independently in human agentic theories. Acting with autonomy involves acting in ways consistent with one's personal culture and values. A person's motivation for acting autonomously can be influenced by individualistic values, collectivist values, or both. The key issue is whether a person is acting in ways that are concordant with their values, rather than being controlled by others. As Ryan and Deci ask, "if people truly valued and endorsed collectivism, would they not be autonomous when acting in accord with these values? Conversely, if they felt controlled to act collectively, would this not have psychological costs for them" (p. 1577).

Supporting the notion that self-caused action and acting autonomously can and do vary across cultural contexts, researchers have suggested that when autonomy is understood as self-caused action in accordance with one's personal cultural identity, the theoretical tenants of Self-Determination Theory and Causal Agency Theory are not confounded with Western values (Chirkov et al. 2011; Shogren 2011). For example, researchers have found, with regard to SDT, that the strong relationship between higher levels of autonomy and motivation and interest in samples of U.S. children holds when examining these relations in samples from other countries including South Korea, Japan, Brazil, Russia, and India, all of which tend to more strongly endorse collectivistic values (Chen et al. 2014; Chirkov and Ryan 2001; Chirkov et al. 2003; Sheldon et al. 2009; Yamauchi and Tanaka 1998). This body of work suggests the importance of supporting self-caused action consistent with personal culture in promoting desired outcomes related to the development of self-determination across cultures.

Ewalt and Mokuau (1995) highlighted how self-determination can be operationalized in collectivist or family-centered cultures, in an analysis of self-determination from the Pacific Islander perspective. Pacific Island culture tends to be defined by values of collective affiliation and family decision-making. Ewalt and Mokuau highlight the experiences of a Hawaiian woman, who chose her work and living trajectory based on congruence with her value for her family and community.

> Debra, a Hawaiian woman, was interested in practicing medicine in the community in which she had recently completed her medical education. Here she was offered a physician's position with a reputable family clinic and a good salary. Combined with her comfortable living quarters and her network of friends, remaining in this community was an attractive option for Debra. However, her family, and in particular her parents, wished for Debra to establish her practice in the community in which she was raised. To do so would require her to move from the city back to her native community. Although there were a few moments of hesitation, Debra quickly adjusted and aligned her values with those of her family. She reasoned that by returning to her native community she would be reunited with

her family and be available to provide medical care to members of her family and a community with severe health problems (p. 170).

When interpreting Debra's actions from a SDT and Causal Agency Theory perspective, Debra identified multiple pathways that would enable her to achieve her goal of practicing medicine, taking into account the needs of the larger group within which she was situated and highly valued (family and community) as well as her psychological needs for autonomy, competence, and relatedness. By adopting a family-centered approach to decision-making Debra considered the mutual responsibilities she shared with her community, and engaged in self-caused action consistent with her value for relatedness to her family and community. Such an approach was motivating and empowering for Debra, and enabled her to act in a self-determined manner, meeting her need for autonomy, and situating her within her community and culture which emphasized (a) collective affiliation and the affiliative nature of relationships; (b) cooperation rather than individual achievement; (c) unity of the group by defined assignments for each member of the family; and (d) the family as the focal point, not the individual (Ewalt and Mokuau 1995).

Shogren (2012) explored the perspectives of Hispanic mothers of adolescents with disabilities in the United States. As with Pacific Islander culture, Hispanic families, generally, tend to engage in higher levels of family-oriented decision making. Using the framework of Causal Agency Theory, Shogren explored the perspectives of these mothers on the universality of the self-determination construct, as well as differences in its operationalization with a particular emphasis on conflicts that emerged between family values and school systems that were attempting to emphasize the promotion of self-determination for students with disabilities. The themes of the study found that the mothers strongly endorsed the importance of self-determination when definitions consistent with those introduced in this and other chapters (i.e., self- [vs. other] caused action) were adopted. As one mother noted: "She needs to learn [to solve problems] because we are not always going to be around her, to fix things, to guide her all the time" (p. 173). The mothers, however, also felt that the way schools operationalized this was associated with "mainstream" culture and often in direct conflict with their family values. The mothers described how goals within their families and culture were influenced by family considerations, and that these considerations were equally as important as personal considerations. And, it went beyond simply considering family needs, the family connections were so deep and ingrained in so many aspects of the family's life, that goals or decisions could not be made without considering the family and involving them in the process. As one mother said "when she sets goals, you see a little bit of her cousins, her grandma and grandpa and all of that like a network…" (p. 181). However, when schools emphasized goals related to independence and excluded family members from decisions, this became difficult and in direct conflict with self-determination for the child and their family members.

This work, as well as the work of others exploring the perspectives of families (Zhang 2005; Zhang et al. 2005) and of the operationalization of self-determination in school and community contexts (Goff et al. 2007; Trainor 2005) suggests that the construct of self-determination has relevance and is valued across cultures, but that conflicts often emerge when community or organizational norms or beliefs are not flexible and supportive of diverse operationalizations of the construct. Cultures that emphasize more collective or family-oriented values see the importance of self- (vs. other) caused action, but also want the deep and ingrained family connections and decision-making process to be valued. Thus efforts to support the development of self-determination must adopt a flexible self-determination perspective (Shogren 2011), that recognizes the universal nature of the construct, the need to understand and embed cultural considerations in efforts to support the development of self-determination.

To further understand self-determination across diverse cultural contexts, Shogren (2011) engaged in a thematic review of published studies on the application of Causal Agency Theory across cultures. Ten theoretical, review, and research articles were found. All articles highlighted the multiple factors that influenced one's personal culture, and the expression of self-determination varied based on each of these factors and the context within which self-determined action was expressed. For example, one article discussed self-determination in Diné (Navajo) culture, highlighting the high value placed on autonomy, but in the context of fulfilling family and clan roles, not individual roles (Frankland et al. 2004). Frankland et al. assert that the self-determination was highly relevant in Diné culture, stating that engaging in actions to advance the family and the tribe are self-determining, as long as the person is making the decision to apply his or her skills to familial goals. Across articles, a consistent theme was the value of self- (vs. other) caused action, but the need to embed this in the context the operationalized of self-determination in family-centered cultures, or high context cultures, that tend to emphasize interdependence and relationships with others having a present-time orientation. This is compared to low context cultures which tend to value individual rights and choice, and a future-time orientation (Hall 1981).

Developing supports for the development of self-determination that address issues of high and low context cultures and individualist vs. collectivist values is a critical need particularly of communities and organizations that influence the development of self-determination. Valenzuela and Martin (2005) provided a framework for how to include opportunities for cultural sharing and individualist and collectivist values in curricular materials used in schools to promote self-determination. They explored how skills and attitudes that can be fostered to enhance self-determination (i.e., self-awareness, decision making, self-advocacy, independent performance, and time) are traditionally operationalized in individualist cultures, as well as how these skills could be operationalized in collectivist cultures. They also explored how additional values, such as interdependence, group decision-making, and developing a family/group identify, could be embedded in the process of supporting students and their families to enhance outcomes for all students based on their personal cultural identity.

Ohtake and Wehmeyer (2004) explored the application of self-determination in Japanese culture, suggesting the importance of both individualistic and collectivist values in the Japanese context. They developed a four step process to consider when applying theories like Causal Agency Theory across cultures: (a) develop a deep understanding of the theory; (b) explore cultural values embedded in practices associated with the theory; (c) focus on similarities and overlap with existing theories and practices; and (d) identify and address possible negative influences of different value systems and address these influences. Similarly, Lee and Wehmeyer (2004) and Bae and Wehmeyer (2003) explored self-determination and Korean culture and again found that the construct had relevance, and was increasingly being considered within systems, such as the education system highlighting how self-determination may be operationalized differently in the home and school environment. Relatedly, other studies highlighted how cultural identities shifted across contexts (e.g., school and home), and the need for the infusion of culturally responsive practices in schools, communities, and other contexts that influence the development of self-determination (Leake and Boone 2007; Trainor 2002).

In addition, researchers have also validated measures associated with self-determination theory and Causal Agency Theory across cultural contexts, providing further support for the universal elements of the self-determination construct, as well as the presence of cultural and contextually-moderated differences (Wehmeyer et al. 2011). Researchers have validated scales associated with self-determination theory in the context of work motivation across multiple languages and countries (Gagné et al. 2015) as well as measures of exercise motivation and psychological need satisfaction across cultures (Vlachopoulos et al. 2013). These studies suggest that measures of psychological needs associated with self-determination theory can be used and have relevance across cultures, but that cultural and contextual factors impact the relationship between need satisfaction and outcomes, highlighting the importance of understanding and assessing these factors when structuring environments to support need satisfaction across domains (e.g., employment, education, exercise) associated with self-determination theory.

Additionally, researchers have explored the universality of assessments derived from Causal Agency Theory. For example, Ginevra et al. (2013) had Italian and American adolescents complete The Adolescent Self-Determination Assessment (ASDA; Wehmeyer et al. 2007), an assessment of self-determination aligned with Causal Agency Theory. They found that there were universal aspects of the self-determination construct across the cultures (i.e., the same items were endorsed at similar levels), but that there also differences suggesting variability in the operationalization of self-determination. For example, for the Autonomy subscale, Italian adolescents scored higher on items associated with self-direction in the home environment, but lower than American adolescents on items related to freedom outside the home when they are away from parents' supervision. Italian researchers have suggested that Italian parents may promote greater family direction prior to adolescents coming of age than American parents (Soresi et al. 2004), which may influence the expression of self-determination and its development across cultures.

Implications for the Development of Self-Determination

As we described at the beginning of this chapter, and as the research reviewed in the previous section highlights, as a *psychological construct* there is clear support for the notion that self-determination has universal applicability across cultures and contexts. As Zhang and Benz (2006) note, when diverse cultural operationalizations are accounted for, self-determination is "a universally accepted phenomenon" (p. 10), As described in Chapter 2, with regard to human agentic theories generally, when acting agentically, people respond to opportunities and threats in their environment. The opportunities and threats present in the environment and the responses to these threats and opportunities are shaped by personal cultural identities and cultural norms and beliefs that are embedded in the family, community, and societal systems within which people live their lives. When opportunities for congruence in the operationalization of self-determination are available across systems aligned with one's personal cultural identity and framework for engaging in self-determined action, people are able to meeting their psychological need for autonomy, competence, and relatedness as described by self-determination theory and respond to challenges (opportunities or threats) to their self-determination by employing volitional and agentic actions, supported and mediated by action-control beliefs as described by Causal Agency Theory. This enables people to initiate and direct their action toward goals aligned with their personal cultural identities, enhancing the development of self-determination.

References

Bae, S. J., & Wehmeyer, M. L. (2003). Perceptions of self-determination on transitional outcomes: A study of Korean students, parents, and teachers. *Korean Journal of Special Education, 10*, 123–141.

Bronfenbrenner, U. (1979). *The ecology of human development: Experiments by nature and design*. Cambridge: Harvard University Press.

Carter, E. W., Trainor, A. A., Cakiroglu, O., Cole, O., Swedeen, B., Ditchman, N., & Owens, L. (2009). Exploring school-employer partnerships to expand career development and early work experiences for youth with disabilities. *Career Development for Exceptional Individuals, 32*, 145–159.

Chen, Y., Yao, M., & Yan, W. (2014). Materialism and well-being among Chinese college students: The mediating role of basic psychological need satisfaction. *Journal of Health Psychology, 19*, 1232–1240. doi:http://dx.doi.org/10.1177/1359105313488973

Chirkov, V. I., & Ryan, R. M. (2001). Parent and teacher autonomy-support in Russian and U. S. Adolescents: Common effects on well-being and academic motivation. *Journal of Cross-Cultural Psychology, 32*, 618–635. doi:http://dx.doi.org/10.1177/0022022101032005006

Chirkov, V. I., Ryan, R. M., Kim, Y., & Kaplan, U. (2003). Differentiating autonomy from individualism and independence: A self-determination theory perspective on internalization of cultural orientations and well-being. *Journal of Personality and Social Psychology, 84*, 97–110. doi:http://dx.doi.org/10.1037/0022-3514.84.1.97

Chirkov, V. I., Ryan, R. M., & Sheldon, K. M. (2011). *Human autonomy in cross-cultural context: Perspectives on the psychology of agency, freedom, and well-being*. New York: Springer Science + Business Media.

Ewalt, P. L., & Mokuau, N. (1995). Self-determination from a Pacific perspective. *Social Work, 40*, 168–175.

Frankland, H. C., Turnbull, A. P., Wehmeyer, M. L., & Blackmountain, L. (2004). An exploration of the self-determination construct and disability as it relates to the Dine (Navajo) culture. *Education and Training in Developmental Disabilities, 39*, 191–205.

Gagné, M., Forest, J., Vansteenkiste, M., Crevier-Braud, L., van den Broeck, A., Aspeli, A. K., et al. (2015). The multidimensional work motivation scale: Validation evidence in seven languages and nine countries. *European Journal of Work and Organizational Psychology, 24*, 178–196. doi:10.1080/1359432X.2013.877892.

Ginevra, C., Nota, L., Soresi, S., Shogren, K. A., Wehmeyer, M. L., & Little, T. D. (2013). A cross-cultural comparison of the self-determination construct in Italian and American adolescents. *International Journal of Adolescence and Youth*. doi:10.1080/02673843.2013.808159.

Goff, C., Martin, J. E., & Thomas, M. K. (2007). The burden of acting white: Implications for transition. *Career Development for Exceptional Individuals, 30*, 134–146. doi:10.1177/08857288070300030301.

Goode, T., & Maloof, P. (2011). End of life through a cultural lens. In S. A. Friedman & D. T. Helm (Eds.), *End of life care for children and adults with intellectual and developmental disabilities* (pp. 147–159). Washington, DC: American Association on Intellectual and Developmental Disabilities.

Hall, E. (1981). *Beyond culture*. New York: Doubleday.

Hong, Y.-Y., & Chiu, C. (2001). Toward a paradigm shift: From cross-cultural differences in social cognition to social-cognitive mediation of cultural differences. *Social Cognition, 19*, 181–196.

Leake, D., & Boone, R. (2007). Multicultural perspectives on self-determination from youth, parent, and teacher focus groups. *Career Development for Exceptional Individuals, 30*, 104–115.

Lee, S. H., & Wehmeyer, M. L. (2004). A review of the Korean literature related to self-determination: Future directions and practices for promoting the self-determination of students with disabilities. *Korean Journal of Special Education, 38*, 369–390.

Nelson, T. D. (Ed.) (2016). *Handbook of prejudice, stereotyping, and discrimination* (2nd ed.). New York: Psychology Press.

Ohtake, Y., & Wehmeyer, M. L. (2004). Applying the self-determination theory to Japanese special education contexts: A four-step model. *Journal of Policy and Practice in Intellectual Disabilities, 1*, 169–178.

Robinson, E. G. (2002). Quilomboos, black nationalism, and self-determination for persons with intellectual disabilities: A psychohistorical perspective. *Mental Retardation, 40*, 81–83. doi:10.1352/0047-6765(2002)040<0081:QBNASD>2.0.CO;2.

Ryan, R. M., & Deci, E. L. (2006). Self-regulation and the problem on human autonomy: Does psychology need choice, self-determinaiton, and will? *Journal of Personality, 74*, 1557–1585.

Sheldon, K. M., Abad, N., & Omoile, J. (2009). Testing self-determination theory via nigerian and indian adolescents. International Journal of Behavioral Development, *33*, 451–459. doi:http://dx.doi.org/10.1177/0165025409340095

Shogren, K. A. (2011). Culture and self-determination: A synthesis of the literature and directions for future research and practice. *Career Development for Exceptional Individuals, 34*, 115–127. doi:10.1177/0885728811398271.

Shogren, K. A. (2012). Hispanic mothers' perceptions of self-determination. *Research and Practice for Persons with Severe Disabilities, 37*, 170–184.

Shogren, K. A., Luckasson, R., & Schalock, R. L. (2014). The definition of context and its application in the field of intellectual disability. *Journal of Policy and Practice in Intellectual Disabilities, 11*, 109–116. doi:10.1111/jppi.12077.

Soresi, S., Nota, L., & Ferrari, L. (2004). Autodeterminazione e scelte scolastico-professionali: Uno strumento per l'assessment (Selfdetermination and career choices: An assessment instrument). *Giornale Italiano di Psicologia dell'Orientamento, 5*, 26–42.

Suarez-Balcazar, Y., Balcazar, F., Garcia-Ramirez, M., & Taylor-Ritzler, T. (2014). Ecological theory and research in multicultural psychology: A community psychology perspective. In *APA handbook of multicultural psychology, Vol. 1: Theory and research* (pp. 535–552). Washington, DC: American Psychological Association.

Trainor, A. A. (2002). Self-determination for students with learning disabilities: Is it a universal value? *International Journal of Qualitative Studies in Education, 15*, 711–725.

Trainor, A. A. (2005). Self-determination perceptions and behaviors of diverse students with LD during the transition planning process. *Journal of Learning Disabilities, 38*, 233–248.

Trainor, A. A., Lindstrom, L., Simon-Burroughs, M., Martin, J. E., & Sorrells, A. M. (2008). From marginalized to maximized opportunities for diverse youths with disabilities: A position paper of the division on career development and transition. *Career Development for Exceptional Individuals, 31*, 56–64.

Triandis, H. C., & Suh, E. M. (2002). Cultural influences on personality. *Annual Review of Psychology, 53*, 133–160.

Valenzuela, R. L., & Martin, J. E. (2005). Self-directed IEP: Bridging values of diverse cultures and secondary education. *Career Development for Exceptional Individuals, 28*, 4–14.

Vlachopoulos, S. P., Asci, F. H., Cid, L., Ersoz, G., González-Cutre, D., Moreno-Murcia, J. A., & Moutão, J. (2013). Cross-cultural invariance of the basic psychological needs in exercise scale and need satisfaction latent mean differences among Greek, Spanish, Portuguese and Turkish samples. *Psychology of Sport and Exercise, 14*(5), 622–631. doi:http://dx.doi.org/10.1016/j.psychsport.2013.03.002

Wehmeyer, M. L., Lopez, S. J., & Shogren, K. A. (2007). *The adolescent self-determination assessment*. Lawrence: Kansas University Center on Developmental Disabilities.

Wehmeyer, M. L., Abery, B. H., Zhang, D., Ward, K., Willis, D., Hossain, W. A., et al. (2011). Personal self-determination and moderating variables that impact efforts to promote self-determination. *Exceptionality, 19*, 19–30. doi:10.1080/09362835.2011.537225.

World Health Organization. (2001). *International classification of functioning, disability, and health*. Geneva: Author.

Yamauchi, H., & Tanaka, K. (1998). Relations of autonomy, self-referenced beliefs and self-regulated learning among Japanese children. *Psychological Reports, 82*, 803–816.

Zhang, D. (2005). Parent practices in facilitating self-determination skills: The influences of culture, socioeconomic status, and children's special education status. *Research and Practice for Persons with Severe Disabilities, 30*, 154–162. doi:10.2511/rpsd.30.3.154.

Zhang, D., & Benz, M. R. (2006). Enhancing self-determination of culturally diverse students with disabilities: Current status and future directions. *Focus on Exceptional Children, 38*(9), 1–12.

Zhang, D., Wehmeyer, M. L., & Chen, L.-J. (2005). Parent and teacher engagement in fostering the self-determination of students with disabilities: A comparison between the United States and the Republic of China. *Remedial and Special Education, 26*, 55–64. doi:10.1177/07419325050260010701.

Part III
Self-Determination Theory and Healthy Psychological Development

Synthesis

Chapters in this part explore the role of self-determination in healthy psychological development. Chapter 13 explores how parental supports or thwarts for children's basic psychological needs either promote or diminish the children's mental health, social adjustment, and psychological growth. Chapter 14 discusses the nature of self-determination in the context of adolescent identity development. The chapter reviews definitions of adolescence and the many factors that contribution to the onset and offset of this critical developmental period. Then, two theoretical perspectives for understanding adolescence are introduced: Identity development and the nature of self-determination development during this epoch. The chapter closes with some thoughts on future directions for research on self-determination development during adolescence.

Chapter 13
How Parents Contribute to Children's Psychological Health: The Critical Role of Psychological Need Support

Bart Soenens, Edward L. Deci, and Maarten Vansteenkiste

Abstract Although different determinants, including genetics, temperament, and a variety of social-contextual influences, play roles in young people's development, the role of parents is paramount to healthy psychosocial adjustment. When children's psychological needs are satisfied, children report more well-being, engage in activities with more interest and spontaneity (intrinsic motivation), more easily accept guidelines for important behaviors (internalization), display more openness in social relationships, and are more resilient when faced with adversity and distress. This chapter will focus on how parental supports or thwarts for children's basic psychological needs either promote or diminish the children's mental health, social adjustment, and psychological growth.

Anyone observing young children in a playground will easily notice remarkable differences among them. Some of the children explore the playground with curiosity and have a great time; others are more withdrawn and feel uncomfortable with other children around. At home some children may accept parental rules or negotiate constructively with the parents; others may feel forced to comply with parental rules or even react defiantly against them. Later, in adolescence, some youngsters willingly share their thoughts and feelings with parents; others disclose much less and may even be secretive. How can these differences among the children's and adolescents' emotional, social, and behavioral adjustments be explained? Although different determinants, including genetics, temperament, and a variety of social-contextual influences, play roles in young people's development, this chapter will focus on the role of parents. Specifically, we address how parental supports or thwarts for

B. Soenens (✉)
Ghent University, Ghent, Belgium
e-mail: Bart.Soenens@ugent.be

E.L. Deci
University of Rochester, Rochester, NY, USA

M. Vansteenkiste
Ghent University, Ghent, Belgium

M.L. Wehmeyer et al. (eds.), *Development of Self-Determination Through the Life-Course*, DOI 10.1007/978-94-024-1042-6_13

children's basic psychological needs either promote or diminish the children's mental health, social adjustment, and psychological growth.

Basic Psychological Needs and Children's Psychosocial Adjustment

Self-Determination Theory (SDT; Deci and Ryan 2000; Ryan and Deci 2000) argues that children's psychosocial adjustment depends to a substantial degree on satisfactions of three basic psychological needs, namely, the needs for autonomy, competence, and relatedness (see also Chap. 4, this volume). Satisfaction of the *need for autonomy* manifests in experiences of volition, psychological freedom, authenticity, and ownership of one's behaviors and choices. When the *need for competence* is satisfied, children feel efficacious and able to deal with optimally challenging tasks. The *need for relatedness* is satisfied when children feel appreciated by and closely connected to important others, especially their parents during infancy and childhood. In SDT, psychological need satisfactions are considered essential and universal nutrients for healthy psychological development (Deci and Ryan 2000). When children's psychological needs are satisfied, the children report more well-being, engage activities with more interest and spontaneity (intrinsic motivation), more easily accept guidelines for important behaviors (internalization), display more openness in social relationships, and are more resilient when faced with adversity and distress (Vansteenkiste and Ryan 2013).

While much of the research on psychological need satisfaction has involved university students and adults (e.g., Chen et al. 2015), recent research has also demonstrated the importance of the psychological needs for children's and adolescents' adjustment. For example, Veronneau et al. (2005) found among 3rd and 7th graders that satisfaction of each of the three needs was related to positive affect. Satisfaction of the need for competence in particular predicted decreases in depressive symptoms across a 6-week interval. Luyckx et al. (2009) found psychological need satisfaction to be critical for adolescents' thorough exploration of identity options and stronger commitments to identity choices.

Recent work has also focused on people's dark sides resulting from psychological need frustration (e.g., Bartholomew et al. 2011). When social-contextual factors are thwarting of children's needs, the needs are likely to be frustrated, leaving the children feeling controlled (autonomy frustration), inferior (competence frustration), and lonely (relatedness frustration). In SDT, need frustration is not equated with an absence of need satisfaction. Rather, frustration ensues when the psychological needs are actively undermined rather than merely unsatisfied. Because frustration results from intruding on the children's sense of self, it is a serious threat that renders the children vulnerable to ill-being and psychopathology (Ryan et al. 2016). Research increasingly supports the notion that psychological need frustration is particularly predictive of maladaptive developmental outcomes. It has been shown, for instance, that need frustration is related to physiological indicators of stress (Bartholomew et al. 2011), interpersonal problems (Costa et al. 2015), and eating-disorder symptoms (Boone et al. 2014).

The Nurturing Role of Parents in Children's Development

Given the pivotal role of the basic psychological needs in children's and adolescents' well-being and adjustment, a key developmental question is how socializing agents—and parents in particular—affect psychological need satisfaction and psychological need frustration. SDT argues that parents, in interaction with other key individuals (i.e., the children's teachers and peers), play a crucial role in the nurturing versus thwarting of children's psychological needs. Paralleling the distinctions among the three needs, differences in parents' styles of interacting with children are conceptualized with three concepts (Grolnick et al. 1997; Joussemet et al. 2008a): (a) relatedness supports or *involvement* (e.g., respect and warmth), (b) competence supports or *structure* (e.g., offering clear expectations, adequate help, and non-critical feedback), and (c) *autonomy support* (e.g., acknowledging the children's perspective, providing choice, and encouraging exploration).

Each of these contextual, need-supportive concepts has a need-thwarting dark side just as each of the need satisfactions has a need-frustration dark side. For instance, relatedness thwarts are characterized by parental behaviors that are cold, neglectful, and rejecting; competence thwarts are demeaning and chaotic; and autonomy thwarts include pressuring demands and coercion. Importantly, being low in need supports does not necessarily mean that parents will be actively and intrusively thwarting of children's needs (Skinner et al. 2005), and similarly, being low in need thwarting does not necessarily mean that parents will be actively and happily supportive of children's needs. However, when parents are actively need supportive, it has been shown that they will foster experiences of need satisfaction (and subsequent well-being and positive adjustment), and when parents are actively need thwarting it has been shown to bring about experiences of need frustration (and subsequent ill-being and maladjustment).

We do note that there is not a simple one-to-one association between one of the parental need-supportive dimensions and satisfaction of the children's corresponding need (Grolnick et al. 1997), or between a parental need-thwarting dimension and frustration of the children's corresponding need. Each of the dimensions of need-supportive parenting is to some extent relevant to satisfaction to each of the three needs. For example, when parents take their children's perspective in a conversation, thus supporting the children's autonomy need, the children are likely to feel some relatedness satisfaction and also some indication of parental trust in their capabilities. In this regard, the graphical representation in Fig. 13.1, in which each need support and need thwart predicts only the corresponding need satisfaction and need frustration, is a simplification of reality, for there could be an arrow from each support to each need satisfaction, and from each thwart to each need frustration.

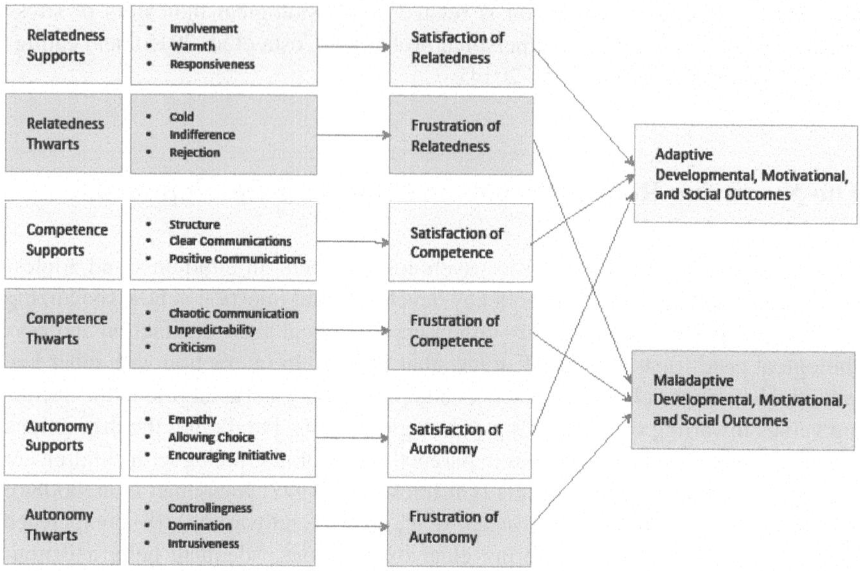

Fig. 13.1 Conceptual model showing: (1) Examples of each of the three basic psychological need supports and each of the need thwarts; (2) Relations from each of these supports and thwarts to the corresponding need satisfactions and frustrations; and relations from the satisfactions and frustrations to adaptive and maladaptive outcomes

In the remainder of this chapter we focus on the three dimensions of need-supportive parenting for our primary goal is to facilitate greater self-determination. [Those interested in further discussion of need-thwarting parenting are referred to Assor et al. (2014); Grolnick (2003); and Soenens and Vansteenkiste (2010)]. In discussing need-supportive parenting we describe the basic attitude underlying each dimension as well as their more specific manifestations (Vansteenkiste and Soenens 2015). We also provide a selective discussion of research relevant to each dimension.

Relatedness Support

The basic attitude behind relatedness-support is characterized by love, care and a genuine desire to support the child (Vansteenkiste and Soenens 2015). Parents supporting their child's need for relatedness deeply care about the child's well-being and enjoy being in the child's company (Deci and Ryan 2014). These parents engage in warm and sensitive interactions with the child, interactions that build a child's sense of attachment security (Bowlby 1988). As a consequence, a child feels protected and learns to trust and rely on the parent when experiencing distress. This supportive orientation can be contrasted with a cold parental orientation, where parents are largely unavailable, unresponsive to the child's requests, or even rejecting.

A basic requirement for all need-supportive parenting is parental presence and involvement. Parents who support children's need for relatedness spend a sufficient amount of time in the presence of their children and get at least minimally involved in the children's activities (e.g., Grolnick et al. 1999). However, parental involvement and investment of time is not a sufficient condition for children to feel deeply connected to their parents. Research shows that there is no straightforward association between the amount of time parents spend with their children and the children's well-being (Milkie et al. 2015), nor between parental involvement in the child's activities and the children's motivation for and performance in these activities (e.g., homework: Pomerantz et al. 2007).

For children to really benefit from their parents' involvement and presence, the *quality* of parents' involvement needs to be sufficiently high. In this regard, it is important for parents to be mentally present, to be alert to the children's feelings, and to proactively consider the impact of situations on the children's feelings. For instance, parents can try to anticipate how the children will respond to an episode of separation (e.g., leaving the children with a babysitter) or to a potentially painful situation (e.g., a doctor's visit). By announcing what will happen, these situations may become less emotionally unpredictable and overwhelming and parents can proactively help children to regulate their emotions. When children actually experience emotional distress or physical pain, parents high on relatedness need-support react in a responsive fashion. They offer comfort, and they are available for help. In doing so, they provide a safe haven for the children to turn to when feeling upset (Bowlby 1988).

In addition to being involved, alert, and responsive, parents high on relatedness need-support are warm and affectionate. This warmth can be expressed emotionally, through friendly, humorous, and positive interactions with their children as well as physically (e.g., through hugs, kisses, or embraces). A final element of parental relatedness need-support is engagement in joint activities. Parents can engage in enjoyable and interesting activities with their children one-on-one (e.g., father and son playing basketball or playing a board game) or with the family as a whole (e.g., taking a trip, going to a music festival, or having a family picnic beside a lake). While activities with an individual child can strengthen the parent-child bond, activities with the family can build a sense of family cohesion and collective identity.

There is a longstanding tradition of research, some of which is rooted in attachment theory, demonstrating the importance of parents' relational need support for children's healthy development. Relatedness need support has been shown to predict a plethora of adaptive outcomes, including secure attachment representations (Van IJzendoorn 1995), self-worth (Brummelman et al. 2015), social competence (Barber et al. 2005), and social skills contributing to social competence such as adequate emotion regulation (Davidov and Grusec 2006) and empathy (Soenens et al. 2007a). In contrast, cold and rejecting parenting has been found to predict a host of developmental problems, including internalizing and externalizing behaviors (Putnick et al. 2015).

Structure (Competence Support)

Parents who provide structure assist their children in building a sense of competence. Their basic attitude involves a focus on development of the children's skills and emerging abilities. These parents are process-oriented, meaning that they are interested in discovering the children's talents and in providing support to nurture the talents (Farkas and Grolnick 2010; Reeve 2006; Vansteenkiste and Soenens 2015). They are aware that children learn through trial and error and that substantial individual differences exist in the timing and rhythm of children's developing capacities. Parents who provide structure take into account these individual differences and try to provide a level of support and help that is attuned to the children's developmental levels and possibilities. Structure can be contrasted with chaos, which is characteristic of parents who do not match their level and type of involvement to what the children need. They provide unclear or confusing guidelines for adequate behavior, and they are inconsistent in the feedback they provide. They give unwanted help and irrelevant information, and, at times, they may become explicitly critical of the children's behavior and achievements.

The components of structure can be organized in terms of whether they are operative before, during, or after the children's engagement in competence-relevant activities (Reeve 2006). Two important elements are particularly relevant prior to children's engagement. When a child is about to begin an activity, parents high on structure provide clear guidelines at whatever level of specificity is needed. If needed, they communicate limits about what behaviors are allowed and what are not, and they may discuss the consequences of not following guidelines. Of course that needs to be done in an informative rather than controlling fashion. Further, they provide the necessary help for the child to set goals and, if needed, offer a step-by-step script so children know how to achieve the target goals. Parents who provide structure also attend to the kinds of activities their children engage in. Specifically, they try to stimulate activities and create conditions that are optimally challenging to the children. Activities that slightly exceed the children's developmental level but are still within reach (i.e., activities in the children's zones of proximal development) stimulate the children to learn new skills (Vygotsky 1978). For parents to create these optimally challenging conditions, they need to be aware of the children's abilities and present the activities in ways that do not overwhelm the children. It is also important for parents to openly convey their trust in the children's abilities to do well and master new skills.

Parents can also provide structure during the children's engagement by monitoring the children's progress in a process-oriented fashion. When parents and children have agreed upon a rule, parents high on structure are consistent in following up on the rule. They signal to the children in non-intrusive but consequent ways when agreements are not respected. Further, parents high on structure provide adequate help during children's engagement in the tasks. They are available in case the children ask for help. When their help is solicited, parents give advice or they break down the task into smaller units to make the task more feasible to the children. There is a thin line between providing appropriate and inappropriate help—that is, providing information and instruction—with inappropriate help being unwanted or excessive, such that the parents are essentially taking over the task and precluding a possible learning opportunity for the children. Yet, parents may also provide too little help such that children feel like they are left helpless. The provision of help in a way that meaningfully contributes to the children's competence thus requires an accurate parental assessment of the children's abilities and need for assistance.

Both during and after the children's engagement in an activity, the appropriate form of structure involves giving informational feedback. Ideally, this feedback is process-oriented and focused on the children's efforts and strategies (e.g., "You seem to have found a good way of studying for this course") rather than on the person's worth (e.g., "You are so smart") (Kamins and Dweck 1999). Even when children do not do well at a task, parents can be supportive. To encourage self-reflection, prior to the parents giving their own take on the situation, they may invite the children to reflect on what happened, and perhaps whether they see different ways they might try the task next time. This will allow the feedback interchanges to be learning experiences and allow the children to feel a sense of ownership. That is, when children are able to identify their own strengths and weaknesses, they are likely to develop a stronger willingness to improve their skills and to build a sense of mastery and a feeling of control over their own development. During the interchange, parents may need to provide some informational feedback by pointing out things that went well that the children did not notice. They may also formulate suggestions and hints in specific and constructive ways.

In sum, there is more to structure than rule setting and the communication of expectations. Clear expectations and rules are necessary, but not sufficient, for children to develop a sense of competence (Mouratidis et al. 2013). Children are more likely to feel competent when parents also provide adequate help, give process-oriented feedback, and assist the children in reflecting upon their learning process. Further, structure is relevant not only to activities that involve learning (e.g., homework) and play (e.g., games) but also to rule-compatible behavior. Also when teaching children to behave well (according to moral, conventional, or prudential standards), parents can provide structure by communicating clear guidelines, by giving advice about how to respond in challenging situations, and by giving constructive feedback on the children's behavior.

Compared to research on supports for relatedness and autonomy, there is less research on parental structure, although a relevant study on teachers providing structure to adolescents did predict more student behavioral engagement (Jang et al. 2010). Further, a few studies have shown that parental structure is related to important motivational and developmental outcomes in different life domains, including academic competence, engagement, and performance (e.g., Farkas and Grolnick 2010; Grolnick et al. 2015), feelings of competence during unsupervised time (e.g., activities with friends in the absence of parents; Grolnick et al. 2014), and engagement and positive experiences during parent-child conversations about sensitive topics such as sexuality (Mauras et al. 2013). In contrast, parental chaos has been found to relate to problem behaviors such as substance use and delinquency (Skinner et al. 2005).

Autonomy-Support

Parental autonomy-support is the parenting concept that is most unique and most central to SDT. Autonomy-supportive parents tend to focus on their children's perspectives. Rather than prioritizing their own personal agendas, the parents are interested in the children's point of view (Deci et al. 1994; Vansteenkiste and Soenens 2015). Also, they unconditionally accept the children as they are (Rogers 1961) so the children experience a sense of volition and feel able to be who they want to be. Autonomy-supportive parents are confident that children are naturally inclined to grow and develop in a positive direction (Landry et al. 2008), so they do not feel a constant need to intervene in the children's development. Instead, they are patient, they respect the children's pace of development, and they display a sincere curiosity for what happens in the children's lives. Autonomy support can be contrasted with a more controlling approach, where parents impose their own frame of reference and evaluate or judge the children in light of whether they meet expectations and standards held by the parents (Grolnick 2003; Grolnick and Pomerantz 2009).

A first important feature of autonomy-support is parental fostering of task enjoyment. As much as possible, autonomy-supportive parents try to emphasize the intrinsic value of activities, they capitalize on children's interest or they add fun elements to promote the children's enjoyment of the activities (Reeve 2009). Even seemingly uninteresting activities, such as brushing teeth and cleaning up, can be more fun by making games out of them, by telling stories, or by appealing to children's fantasies. This appeal to the children's inner motivational resources is profoundly different from an approach that relies on external contingencies such as rewards and threats of punishment.

Autonomy-supportive parents allow input from their children and encourage dialogue. They leave room for negotiation, offer choices, and encourage initiative (Soenens et al. 2007b). Such a participative approach allows children to explore possibilities and to have a say in important decisions. Of course, parents cannot always allow their children to make decisions freely. Sometimes they introduce rules that set limits to the children's behavior. But even in these instances parents can be autonomy-supportive by providing a meaningful rationale and hearing the children's point of view. Rather than simply imposing a rule, they give explanations that are relevant to the children. Doing so helps the children internalize the personal importance of the rule (Deci et al. 1994; Koestner et al. 1984).

When autonomy-supportive, parents are attuned to the children's rhythms and pace of development. If a child gets stuck on a task (e.g., homework), they help patiently and leave room for the child to try to come up with a solution rather than taking over the learning process. This requires parents to trust the child's natural capacity to develop skills (Landry et al. 2008). Parental support for autonomy also entails an open attitude towards children's negative emotions, oppositional behaviors, and diverging opinions. Rather than minimizing negative emotions, suppressing undesirable behavior, or invalidating different opinions, autonomy-supportive parents show an active interest in these "deviant" feelings, behaviors, and opinions. Rather than perceiving those as irritating, they curiously explore their meaning or role to fully understand the children's perspectives. For instance, even when children defy parental rules, autonomy-supportive parents pay attention to children's reasons for doing so and to the feelings that elicited reactance. Having heard the children's opinions, they acknowledge the children's perspective and perhaps flexibly adjust the rule or, if the rule cannot be changed, explain why the rule is meaningful.

Finally, autonomy-supportive parents rely on inviting rather than coercing or pressuring language. They say things such as "You can try to …", "I suggest that you. ", and "I propose that you …" instead of "You have to …", "You must …", and "I expect you to …". Pressuring language can be quite overt and explicit but also more subtle. Psychologically controlling parents (Soenens and Vansteenkiste 2010) or parents relying on conditional regard (Assor et al. 2014) in particular tend to pressure children in insidious ways by expressing disappointment non-verbally or by appealing to feelings of shame and guilt.

Autonomy-supportive parenting has been found to predict need satisfaction and high-quality motivation in different domains of life, including school (Grolnick et al. 1991), sports (Gagné et al. 2003), and friendships (Soenens and Vansteenkiste 2005). When children perceive their parents as autonomy-supportive, they engage in activities with a sense of volition, because they want to rather than because they have to. Autonomy support is also related to high-quality motivation in the context of adherence to parental rules. Children of autonomy-supportive parents display deeper internalization of parental rules (Vansteenkiste et al. 2014). They follow these rules because they accept and understand them rather than because they feel compelled to do so. Relatedly, autonomy-support fosters open and honest communication in parent-child relationships (Bureau and Mageau 2014; Wuyts et al. 2015). Possibly because of these beneficial effects of parental autonomy support on children's need satisfaction and motivation, autonomy-support is related to adjustment in specific domains of life and to children's and adolescents' overall well-being (Joussemet et al. 2005). Parental autonomy-support also contributes to key developmental skills, such as adequate emotion regulation (Brenning et al. 2015), cognitive self-regulation (Bindman et al. 2015), and altruism and moral development (Roth 2008).

In contrast, controlling parenting has been shown to predict need frustration (Mabbe et al. 2016), secrecy in parent-child relationships (Tilton-Weaver et al. 2010), maladaptive motivational orientations such as amotivation (Garn and Jolly 2015), oppositional defiance (Vansteenkiste et al. 2014), and developmental problems such as internalizing distress (Soenens et al. 2008) and externalizing behaviors (Joussemet et al. 2008b).

The Interplay Among the Three Dimensions of Parental Need Support

To fully understand the role of parents supports for children's satisfaction of the three basic psychological needs, it is important to consider the interplay of these three dimensions. Of particular relevance is the interplay between structure and autonomy-support. Some developmental scholars tend to confuse autonomy-support with parental permissiveness, leniency, and an absence of rules (Baumrind 2012). However, autonomy-support can be (and often is) combined with structure, in which case parents provide clear guidelines for behavior and at the same time respect the children's perspectives (e.g., by providing a rationale and leaving room for the children's voices). Autonomy-supportive parents are more likely to provide structure in ways that fosters competence and autonomy because their communication of expectations and their provision of assistance are better attuned to the children's abilities, preferences, and interests. In line with this reasoning, Sher-Censor et al. (2015) showed that maternal communication of expectations for behavior (a feature of structure) was related to fewer externalizing problems in adolescents only when mothers also scored high on perspective taking (a feature of autonomy-support). The combination of structure and autonomy support seemed to help adolescents understand the importance of the expectations and to experience more self-endorsement while enacting the behaviors.

While the combination of structure and autonomy-support gives rise to harmonious satisfaction of multiple needs, other parental behaviors give rise to a conflicting interaction between needs. A case in point is conditional regard, a parenting practice characteristic of parents who provide more love and affection than usual when a child meets their expectations and who withdraw their affection and appreciation when the child fails to meet the standards (Assor et al. 2004). While this parental practice may yield a short-term and superficial satisfaction of the need for relatedness, it is a controlling practice that not only undermines children's feelings of autonomy and competence but also leaves the children feeling like they are not really loved for who they are. Research even shows that the detrimental effects of conditional regard are more pronounced when it is combined with parental warmth (Kanat-Maymon and Assor 2010). This combination of conditional regard and warmth may create a loyalty conflict, where children strongly feel that they need to choose between having a close bond with their parent and preserving a sense of autonomy. Such internal conflicts ultimately give rise to feelings of resentment towards parents and to emotional costs in for the children (Assor et al. 2004, 2014).

The Role of Cultural, Developmental, and Individual Differences

The SDT-based argument that need-supportive parenting appeals to basic and fundamental needs that universally foster children's growth is a strong statement that may lead one to wonder whether in this perspective on parenting there is room for contextual and individual differences in effects of need-supportive parenting. An important concept in SDT that speaks to this issue is *functional significance* (Deci and Ryan 1985). This notion refers to differences in the way people appraise and interpret events. Most things that happen to people can be interpreted somewhat differently by different of the people. For instance, a reward to one child for doing homework might have an informational value indicating a job well done, but, if given to another child, it might be interpreted it as a control to get more homework done (Deci et al. 1999). Depending on factors such as age, culture, personality, and developmental experiences, different children may interpret practices differently.

For example, Pomerantz and Eaton (2000) found that with increasing age elementary school children were more likely to view parental involvement in homework as signaling incompetence and as a threat to their autonomy. As regards culture, several studies have shown that children and adolescents living in collectivist societies may have more benign interpretations of potentially autonomy-suppressing parenting practices than children from individualist societies (Miller et al. 2011; Rudy et al. 2014). Finally, to capture personality-based differences in the way social events are appraised, SDT distinguishes between autonomous and controlled causality orientations (Deci and Ryan 1985), although as a general orientation this typically emerges clearly only in later adolescence. Research shows that individuals high on the autonomous orientation are inclined to see the informational value of interpersonal (e.g., parental) behaviors, whereas individuals high on the controlled orientation tend to more easily experience interpersonal behaviors as pressuring and intrusive. As an example, a study by Hagger and Chatzisarantis (2011) showed that individuals who were high in autonomy interpreted rewards as informational and those high in controlled orientation interpreted them as controlling.

The fact that there are contextual and individual differences in children's appraisal and perception of parental behavior does not contradict SDT's claims about the universal importance of the psychological needs. The universality claim in SDT concerns the consequences of individuals' experiences of need satisfaction and need frustration. While children may differ in the way they interpret potentially autonomy-supportive practices, subjectively felt autonomy is said to be beneficial for all children. Indeed, SDT argues that children's perceptions of parental behavior in terms of need support or need thwarting ultimately affect the children's developmental outcomes. When parental practices are experienced as supportive of the three psychological needs, they will foster well-being and adjustment. In contrast, when practices are experienced as a threat to these needs, they will undermine development and increase the risk for ill-being. Consistent with these claims, evidence shows that subjectively experienced need-supportive and need-thwarting parenting are related similarly to outcomes across developmental periods (Joussemet et al. 2008a), across cultures (Ahmad et al. 2013; Chirkov and Ryan 2001), and irrespective of children's personality (Mabbe et al. 2016).

We also note that there are limits to the degree to which parental behavior can be interpreted in various ways (Soenens et al. 2015). Although children may differ somewhat in the way they perceive parental practices, there are real and important mean-level differences between parental practices in terms of how need-supportive and motivating they are. For instance, meta-analyses have shown that rewards generally undermine children's intrinsic motivation (Deci et al. 1999), and the provision of choice typically enhances it (Patall et al. 2008). Thus, while children may vary in the degree to which they perceive rewards as controlling, there is a general tendency for them to experience rewards as more controlling than choice. In line with the notion that certain practices are generally more need-supportive than others, Chen et al. (2016) showed that while Chinese adolescents had a more benign interpretation of parental guilt-induction than Belgian adolescents, both Chinese and Belgian adolescents perceived guilt-induction as more controlling and need-thwarting than parental autonomy-support. Thus, autonomy-supportive practices were perceived to be generally more favorable to adolescents' development across cultures.

Clearly, SDT highlights children's agency in the socialization process (Reeve 2013; Soenens et al. 2015). Rather than being passive recipients of environmental influences, children give meaning to parental behaviors and actively develop perceptions and representations of their parents. In addition, children also differ in the way they cope with need-thwarting parental behaviors (Skinner and Edge 2002). While some children respond to controlling parental behavior constructively (e.g., by negotiating and by trying to create a compromise between the parents' goals and their own), other children respond defiantly or in other ways that may contribute to their own need frustration such as simply complying passively. Although these responses appear to be quite different, in both cases children experience frustration of their need for autonomy because they do not stay true to their personal goals and preferences. Future research on these coping responses may reveal why some children are more resilient to need-thwarting parenting than others and why need-thwarting parenting is related to different developmental problems in different children. For instance, while passive compliance may give rise to internalizing difficulties, oppositional defiance may render children more vulnerable to externalizing problems.

Conclusions

Children have a natural tendency to develop towards higher levels of psychosocial maturity as they grow older (Deci and Ryan 2000). Parents can contribute to this psychological-growth process by supporting children's need for relatedness (e.g., by being warm and responsive), need for competence (e.g., by providing clear guidelines and by giving positive feedback and help), and need for autonomy (e.g., by recognizing the children's perspective and by encouraging initiative). When parents thwart these very same needs, they risk forestalling children's development or even increasing vulnerability to psychopathology. Various factors (including age, cultural background, and personality) affect the degree to which potentially need-supportive parental behaviors are actually experienced by children as need-supportive. Regardless, the subjective experience of parental need support is universally related to better psychosocial adjustment, resilience, and well-being.

References

Ahmad, I., Vansteenkiste, M., & Soenens, B. (2013). The relations of Arab Jordanian adolescents' perceived maternal parenting to teacher-rated adjustment and problems: The intervening role of perceived need satisfaction. *Developmental Psychology, 49*, 177–183.

Assor, A., Roth, G., & Deci, E. L. (2004). The emotional costs of parents' conditional regard: A self-determination theory analysis. *Journal of Psychology, 72*, 47–88.

Assor, A., Kanat-Maymon, Y., & Roth, G. (2014). Parental conditional regard: Psychological costs and antecedents. In N. Weinstein (Ed.), *Human motivation and interpersonal relationships* (pp. 215–237). Dordrecht: Springer.

Barber, B. K., Stolz, H. E., & Olsen, J. A. (2005). Parental support, psychological control, and behavioral control: Assessing relevance across time, culture, and method. *Monographs of the Society for Research in Child Development, 70*, 1–137.

Bartholomew, K. J., Ntoumanis, N., Ryan, R. M., Bosch, J. A., & Thogerson-Ntoumani, C. (2011). Self-determination theory and diminished functioning: The role of interpersonal control and psychological need thwarting. *Personality and Social Psychology Bulletin, 37*, 1459–1473.

Baumrind, D. (2012). Differentiating between confrontive and coercive kinds of parental power-assertive disciplinary practices. *Human Development, 55*, 35–51.

Bindman, S. W., Pomerantz, E. M., & Roisman, G. I. (2015). Do children's executive functions account for associations between early autonomy-supportive parenting and achievement through high school? *Journal of Educational Psychology, 107*, 756–770.

Boone, L., Vansteenkiste, M., Soenens, B., Van der kaap-Deeder, J., & Verstuyf, J. (2014). Self critical perfectionism and binge eating symptoms: A longitudinal test of the intervening role of psychological need frustration. *Journal of Counseling Psychology, 61*, 363–373.

Bowlby, J. (1988). *A secure base, clinical applications of attachment theory*. London: Routledge.

Brenning, K., Soenens, B., Van Petegem, S., & Vansteenkiste, M. (2015). Perceived maternal autonomy support and early adolescent emotion regulation: A longitudinal study. *Social Development, 24*, 561–578.

Brummelman, E., Thomaes, S., Nelemans, S. A., De Castro, B. O., Overbeek, G., & Bushman, B. J. (2015). Origins of narcissism in children. *Proceedings of the National Academy of Sciences, 112*, 3659–3662.

Bureau, J. S., & Mageau, G. A. (2014). Parental autonomy support and honesty: The mediating role of identification with the honesty value and perceived costs and benefits of honesty. *Journal of Adolescence, 37*, 225–236.

Chen, B., Vansteenkiste, M., Beyers, W., Boone, L., Deci, E. L., et al. (2015). Basic psychological need satisfaction, need frustration, and need strength across four cultures. *Motivation and Emotion, 39*, 216–236.

Chen, B., Soenens, B., Vansteenkiste, M., Van Petegem, S., & Beyers, W. (2016). Where do the cultural differences in dynamics of controlling parenting lie? Adolescents as active agents in the perception of and coping with parental behavior. *Psychologica Belgica, 56*, 169–192.

Chirkov, V. I., & Ryan, R. M. (2001). Parent and teacher autonomy-support in Russian and U.S. adolescents: Common effects on well-being and academic motivation. *Journal of Cross-Cultural Psychology, 32*, 618–635.

Costa, S., Ntoumanis, N., & Bartholomew, K. J. (2015). Predicting the brighter and darker sides of interpersonal relationships: Does psychological need thwarting matter? *Motivation and Emotion, 39*, 11–24.

Davidov, M., & Grusec, J. E. (2006). Untangling the links of parental responsiveness to distress and warmth to child outcomes. *Child Development, 77*, 44–58.

Deci, E. L., & Ryan, R. M. (1985). The general causality orientations scale: Self-determination in personality. *Journal of Research in Personality, 19*, 109–134.

Deci, E. L., & Ryan, R. M. (2000). The "what" and the "why" of goal pursuits: Human needs and the self-determination of behavior. *Psychological Inquiry, 11*, 227–268.

Deci, E. L., & Ryan, R. M. (2014). Autonomy and need satisfaction in close relationships: Relationships motivation theory. In N. Weinstein (Ed.), *Human motivation and interpersonal relationships* (pp. 53–73). Dordrecht: Springer.

Deci, E. L., Eghrari, H., Patrick, B. C., & Leone, D. (1994). Facilitating internalization: The self-determination theory perspective. *Journal of Personality, 62*, 119–142.

Deci, E. L., Koestner, R., & Ryan, R. M. (1999). A meta-analytic review of experiments examining the effects of extrinsic rewards on intrinsic motivation. *Psychological Bulletin, 125*, 627–668.

Farkas, M. S., & Grolnick, W. S. (2010). Examining the components and concomitants of parental structure in the academic domain. *Motivation and Emotion, 34*, 266–279.

Gagné, M., Ryan, R. M., & Bargmann, K. (2003). Autonomy support and need satisfaction in the motivation and well-being of gymnasts. *Journal of Applied Sport Psychology, 15*, 372–390.

Garn, A. C., & Jolly, J. L. (2015). A model of parental achievement-oriented psychological control in academically gifted students. *High Ability Studies, 26*, 105–116.

Grolnick, W. S. (2003). *The psychology of parental control: How well-meant parenting backfires*. Hillsdale: Erlbaum.

Grolnick, W. S., Kurowski, C. O., & Gurland, S. T. (1999). Family processes and the development of children's selfregulation. *Educational Psychologist, 34*, 3–14.

Grolnick, W. S., & Pomerantz, E. M. (2009). Issues and challenges in studying parental control: Toward a new conceptualization. *Child Development Perspectives, 3*, 165–170.

Grolnick, W. S., Ryan, R. M., & Deci, E. L. (1991). Inner resources for school achievement: Motivational mediators of children's perceptions of their parents. *Journal of Educational Psychology, 83*, 508–517.

Grolnick, W. S., Deci, E. L., & Ryan, R. M. (1997). Internalization within the family: The self-determination theory perspective. In J. E. Grusec & L. Kuczynski (Eds.), *Parenting and children's internalization of values: A handbook of contemporary theory* (pp. 135–161). New York: Wiley.

Grolnick, W. S., Raftery-Helmer, J. N., Marbell, K. N., Flamm, E. S., Cardemil, E. V., & Sanchez, M. (2014). Parental provision of structure: Implementation and correlates in three domains. *Journal of Applied Developmental Psychology, 60*, 355–384.

Grolnick, W. S., Raftery-Helmer, J. N., Flamm, E. S., Marbell, K. N., & Cardemil, E. V. (2015). Parental provision of academic structure and the transition to middle school. *Journal of Research on Adolescence, 25*, 668–684.

Hagger, M. S., & Chatzisarantis, N. L. D. (2011). Causality orientations moderate the undermining effect of rewards on intrinsic motivation. *Journal of Experimental Social Psychology, 47*, 485–489.

Jang, H., Reeve, J., & Deci, E. L. (2010). Engaging students in learning activities: It's not autonomy support or structure, but autonomy support and structure. *Journal of Educational Psychology, 102*, 588–600.

Joussemet, M., Koestner, R., Lekes, N., & Landry, R. (2005). A longitudinal study of the relationship of maternal autonomy support to children's adjustment and achievement in school. *Journal of Personality, 73*, 1215–1235.

Joussemet, M., Landry, R., & Koestner, R. (2008a). A self-determination theory perspective on parenting. *Canadian Psychology, 49*, 194–200.

Joussemet, M., Vitaro, F., Barker, E. D., Côté, S., Nagin, D. S., Zoccolillo, M., & Tremblay, R. E. (2008b). Controlling parenting and physical aggression during elementary school. *Child Development, 79*, 411–425.

Kamins, M. L., & Dweck, C. S. (1999). Person versus process praise and criticism: Implications for contingent self-worth and coping. *Developmental Psychology, 35*, 835–848.

Kanat-Maymon, M., & Assor, A. (2010). Perceived maternal control and responsiveness to distress as predictors of young adults' empathic responses. *Personality and Social Psychology Bulletin, 36*, 33–46.

Koestner, R., Ryan, R. M., Bernieri, F., & Holt, K. (1984). Setting limits on children's behavior: The differential effects of controlling versus informational styles on intrinsic motivation and creativity. *Journal of Personality, 52*, 233–248.

Landry, R., Whipple, N., Mageau, G., Joussemet, M., & Koestner, R. (2008). Trust in organismic development, autonomy-support, and adaptation among mothers and their children. *Motivation and Emotion, 32*, 173–188.

Luyckx, K., Vansteenkiste, M., Goossens, L., & Duriez, B. (2009). Basic need satisfaction and identity exploration and commitment: Bridging self-determination theory and process-oriented identity research. *Journal of Counseling Psychology, 56*, 276–288.

Mabbe, E., Soenens, B., Vansteenkiste, M., & Van Leeuwen, K. (2016). Do personality traits moderate relations between psychologically controlling parenting and problem behavior in adolescents? *Journal of Personality, 84*, 381–392.

Mauras, C. P., Grolnick, W. S., & Friendly, R. W. (2013). Time for "The Talk" … Now what? Autonomy support and structure in mother-daughter conversations about sex. *Journal of Early Adolescence, 33*, 458–481.

Milkie, M. A., Nomaguchi, K. M., & Denny, K. E. (2015). Does the amount of time mothers spend with children or adolescents matter? *Journal of Marriage and Family, 77*, 355–372.

Miller, J. G., Das, R., & Chakravarthy, S. (2011). Culture and the role of choice in agency. *Journal of Personality and Social Psychology, 101*, 46–61.

Mouratidis, A., Vansteenkiste, M., Michou, A., & Lens, W. (2013). Perceived structure and achievement goals as predictors of students' self-regulated learning and affect and the mediating role of competence need satisfaction. *Learning and Individual Differences, 23*, 179–186.

Patall, E. A., Cooper, H., & Robinson, C. (2008). The effects of choice on intrinsic motivation and related outcomes: A meta-analysis of research findings. *Psychological Bulletin, 134*, 270–300.

Pomerantz, E. M., & Eaton, M. M. (2000). Developmental differences in children's conceptions of parental control: "They love me, but they make me feel incompetent". *Merrill-Palmer Quarterly, 46*, 140–167.

Pomerantz, E. M., Moorman, E. A., & Litwack, S. D. (2007). The how, whom, and why of parents' involvement in children's academic lives: More is not always better. *Review of Educational Research, 77*, 373–410.

Putnick, D. L., Bornstein, M. H., Lansford, J. E., Malone, P. S., Pastorelli, C., Skinner, A. T., Sorbring, E., Tapanya, S., Uribe Tirado, L. M., Zelli, A., & Alampay, L. P. (2015). Perceived mother and father acceptance-rejection predict four unique aspects of child adjustment across nine countries. *Journal of Child Psychology and Psychiatry, 56*, 923–932.

Reeve, J. (2006). Extrinsic rewards and inner motivations. In C. Weinstein & T. L. Good (Eds.), *Handbook of classroom management: Research, practice, and contemporary issues* (pp. 645–664). Hillsdale: Erlbaum.

Reeve, J. (2009). Why teachers adopt a controlling motivating style toward students and how they can become more autonomy supportive. *Educational Psychologist, 44*, 159–175.

Reeve, J. (2013). How students create motivationally supportive learning environments for themselves: The concept of agentic engagement. *Journal of Educational Psychology, 105*, 579–595.

Rogers, C. (1961). *On becoming a person*. Boston: Houghton Mifflin.

Roth, G. (2008). Perceived parental conditional regard and autonomy support as predictors of young adults' self- versus other-oriented prosocial tendencies. *Journal of Personality, 76*, 513–533.

Rudy, D., Carlo, G., Lambert, M. C., & Awong, T. (2014). Undergraduates' perceptions of parental relationship-oriented guilt induction versus harsh psychological control: Does cultural group status moderate their associations with self-esteem? *Journal of Cross-Cultural Psychology, 45*, 905–920.

Ryan, R. M., & Deci, E. L. (2000). Self-determination theory and the facilitation of intrinsic motivation, social development and well-being. *American Psychologist, 55*, 68–78.

Ryan, R. M., Deci, E. L., & Vansteenkiste, M. (2016). Autonomy and autonomy disturbances in self-development and psychopathology: Research on motivation, attachment, and clinical process. In D. Cicchetti (Ed.), *Developmental psychopathology* (3rd Ed Vol.1: Theory and Method, pp. 385–438). New York: Wiley.

Sher-Censor, E., Assor, A., & Oppenheim, D. (2015). The interplay between observed maternal perspective taking and clear expectations: Links with male adolescents' externalizing and internalizing problems. *Journal of Child and Family Studies, 24*, 930–936.

Skinner, E. A., & Edge, K. (2002). Parenting, motivation, and the development of children's coping. In L. J. Crockett (Ed.), *Agency, motivation, and the life course: The Nebraska symposium on motivation* (Vol. 48, pp. 77–143). Lincoln: University Of Nebraska Press.

Skinner, E., Johnson, S., & Snyder, T. (2005). Six dimensions of parenting: A motivational model. *Parenting-Science and Practices, 5*, 175–235.

Soenens, B., & Vansteenkiste, M. (2005). Antecedents and outcomes of self-determination in three life domains: The role of parents' and teachers' autonomy support. *Journal of Youth and Adolescence, 34*, 589–604.

Soenens, B., & Vansteenkiste, M. (2010). A theoretical upgrade of the concept of parental psychological control: Proposing new insights on the basis of self-determination theory. *Developmental Review, 30*, 74–99.

Soenens, B., Duriez, B., Vansteenkiste, M., & Goossens, L. (2007a). The intergenerational transmission of empathy-related responding in adolescence: The role of maternal support. *Personality and Social Psychology Bulletin, 33*, 1–13.

Soenens, B., Vansteenkiste, M., Lens, W., Luyckx, K., Goossens, L., Beyers, W., & Ryan, R. M. (2007b). Conceptualizing parental autonomy support: Adolescent perceptions of promotion of independence versus promotion of volitional functioning. *Developmental Psychology, 43*, 633–646.

Soenens, B., Luyckx, K., Vansteenkiste, Duriez, B., & Goossens, L. (2008). Clarifying the link between perceived parental psychological control and adolescents' depressive feelings: A test of reciprocal versus unidirectional models of influence. *Merrill-Palmer Quarterly, 54*, 411–444.

Soenens, B., Vansteenkiste, M., & Van Petegem, S. (2015). Let us not throw out the baby with the bathwater: Applying the principle of universalism without uniformity to autonomy-supportive and controlling parenting. *Child Development Perspectives, 9*, 44–49.

Tilton-Weaver, L., Kerr, M., Pakalniskeine, V., Tokic, A., Salihovic, S., & Stattin, H. (2010). Open up or close down: How do parental reactions affect youth information management? *Journal of Adolescence, 33*, 333–346.

Van IJzendoorn, M. (1995). Adult attachment representations, parental responsiveness, and infant attachment: A meta-analysis on the predictive validity of the adult attachment interview. *Psychological Bulletin, 117*, 387–403.

Vansteenkiste, M., & Ryan, R. M. (2013). On psychological growth and vulnerability: Basic psychological need satisfaction and need frustration as a unifying principle. *Journal of Psychotherapy Integration, 23*, 263–280.

Vansteenkiste, M., & Soenens, B. (2015). *Vitamines voor groei: Ontwikkeling voeden vanuit de zelf-determinatie theorie [Vitamins for psychological growth: A self-determination theory perspective on support for children's development]*. Leuven: Acco.

Vansteenkiste, M., Soenens, B., Van Petegem, S., & Duriez, B. (2014). Longitudinal associations between adolescent perceived degree and style of prohibition and adolescent internalization and defiance. *Developmental Psychology, 50*, 229–236.

Veronneau, M.-H., Koestner, R., & Abela, J. R. Z. (2005). Intrinsic need satisfaction and well-being in children and adolescents: An application of the self-determination theory. *Journal of Social and Clinical Psychology, 24*, 280–292.

Vygotsky, L. S. (1978). *Mind in society: The development of higher psychological processes*. Cambridge, MA: Harvard University Press.

Wuyts, D., Vansteenkiste, M., Soenens, B., & Van Petegem, S. (2015). *The role of observed maternal autonomy support, reciprocity, and psychological need satisfaction in adolescent disclosure*. Manuscript submitted for publication.

Chapter 14
Self Determination Theory, Identity Development, and Adolescence

Luther K. Griffin, Nicole Adams, and Todd D. Little

Abstract This chapter discuss the nature of self-determination in the context of adolescent development and identity development. The chapter reviews definitions of adolescence and the many factors that contribute to the onset and offset of this critical developmental period. Then, two theoretical perspectives for understanding adolescence are introduced: Identity development theory and Self-Determination Theory. The chapter closes with some thoughts on future directions for research on self-determination development during adolescence.

In this chapter, we discuss the nature of self-determination during the period of adolescence. To do so, we first review the varying definitions of adolescence and the many factors that contribution to the onset and offset of this critical developmental period. Then we turn to two theoretical perspectives for understanding adolescence: Identity development and the nature of self-determination development during this epoch. We close with some thoughts on future directions for research on self-determination development during adolescence.

Defining Adolescence

A more detailed discussion of adolescent development is included in Chap. 3, but it is worth revisiting some of the issues in defining adolescence so as to consider identity development during this phase. The adolescent period is generally defined as the developmental time from childhood to adulthood. Traditionally, this developmental time has been classified by age (e.g., the second decade of the life course).

L.K. Griffin (✉)
Texas State University, San Marcos, TX, USA
e-mail: kentgriffin@txstate.edu

N. Adams
Texas Tech University, Lubbock, TX, USA

T.D. Little
Educational Psychology and Leadership, Texas Tech University, Lubbock, TX, USA

M.L. Wehmeyer et al. (eds.), *Development of Self-Determination Through the Life-Course*, DOI 10.1007/978-94-024-1042-6_14

But even age is a controversial way of defining adolescence. Although age is related, it has been difficult for researchers to pinpoint the exact onset and offset of adolescence. This opaque demarcation of adolescence is due primarily to the large number of contributing factors. In an effort to narrowly define the term "adolescent," some researchers have tended toward a biological explanation whereby the human anatomy undergoes accelerated physiological changes resulting in adulthood. These biological changes are often viewed in terms of puberty; however, puberty is a definitive period when the individual is able to reproduce. If puberty defines the end of adolescence, then this period is mostly non-existent given that puberty is commonly achieved by age 15 (Burgeron et al. 2015). Other researchers take a broader perspective and define adolescents in terms of biology as well as from a social science perspective. These researchers investigate adolescent development from a "whole person" idea and include such constructs as culture, gender, race, socioeconomics and others (Bartko and Eccles 2003).

The term adolescent has its earliest foundations in a work by G. Stanley Hall (1904). In his seminal work, Hall coins the term 'adolescence' which has forever changed society's views of the teenager. Prior to the late 1880s the process of adolescent development did not exist. When an individual became a teenager they were considered, by most, to be a full-fledged adult with all of the rights and privileges thereto appertaining. These new adults were expected to conform to the norms of the society and culture of the time. For men this meant they were supposed to get a job, get married, and start a family. For females, they were to get married, have children, and stay home. They were, according to society, to begin their adult life. These cultural norms drastically changed when the industrial revolution began. Central to Hall's work was the concept that adolescence was a time fraught with violence and chaos. Teenagers were viewed not simply as inexperienced adults but as individuals who underwent "storm and stress" during this time. They were incapable of making analytical decisions and were driven by their new found sexual prowess. Hall changed the norm of becoming an adult at age 13 or 14, arguing that teenagers need to weather the adolescent storm before adulthood could be possible.

While most of Hall's work was founded in biological explanations, much of his writing about adolescence has since been redefined, rethought, and redeemed. As society, culture, gender, and so forth have developed over time, so too has our understanding of teenagers. The term adolescent stuck with society, but the ideology of what defines adolescence has not. As mentioned, "teenagerdom" is a period of development that is dependent on many factors and is thus a dynamic process that must undergo continual examination and explanation. Much of the current work on adolescence has centered on education and sport. Since adolescents spend much of their time in one of these two places, school yards and sports fields have become major socializing institutions. Thus, schools and sports provide an avenue for youth development. Within these two bounded systems, two perspectives have come to the forefront in an effort to better understand adolescence: youth identity development and motivation. While these two constructs have been investigated independently, they have a great deal in common.

Identity Development

A major contributor to youth identity development is Marcia (1980). In his original work, Marcia explains youth development via four identity statuses (Achievement, Foreclosure, Diffusion, and Moratorium) (see Table 14.1). When an adolescent is in achievement, they have made a commitment with regard to their decision but yet they may still be searching other possibilities. Foreclosure describes those adolescents who have may have committed to a particular ideology to the point that they are no longer exploring. Diffusion is a progression of Foreclosure and refers to the teenager who may or may not be committed but is also not exploring possibilities. Finally, a teen who is in Moratorium is not committed and is not exploring. An example of the model from a real world perspective may best describe the interactions of these statuses. When an adolescent is hired for a first job, s/he may start out as an identity achiever. This person, especially at the outset, is committed but may also be on the lookout for another job that pays more or provides more satisfaction. If this same individual likes the job, s/he may commit and stop the exploring process. This person has moved into an identity foreclosure. If, after this person gets the first job, they only commit to the point that they do what they must, in order to get the job done, knowing that they will soon be moving to something different, and thereby continually explore s/he is in identity diffusion. The final category, according to Marcia is the most disturbing because it describes a person who is not committed nor exploring. Moratorium is where we would find a teen who may be experiencing depression or behavior issues. This individual could, at the extreme, be psycho-socially disturbed. Marcia went on to describe a moratorium individual as one who is in "identity crisis."

Marcia's work has recently been re-examined and the model has been re-conceptualized to include more descriptor categories (Schwartz 2001; Meeus et al. 2010; Crocetti et al. 2008). Further, much time has been devoted to understanding how adolescents navigate their identity development. In addition, researchers now focus on the category of moratorium as a potential way of understanding adolescents' maladaptive behaviors. While identity development has been a key conceptualization of the adolescent process, one aspect that has not been investigated as a contributing factor is motivation. Several identity development theorists have discussed motivational constructs such as self-esteem and perceived competence, little work has been done to incorporate the two.

Table 14.1 Model depicting Marcia's identity development

Identity decisions	Identity achievement	Foreclosure	Diffusion	Moratorium
Committed	Present	Present	Present or Absent	Absent
Exploring	Present	Absent	Absent	Absent

Self-Determination Theory and Identity Development

Adolescent identity development explanations could benefit greatly when examined through the constructs of autonomy, competence, and relatedness; all, of course, basic psychological needs as postulated by SDT. In addition, the interaction between the individual and the environment is key to the theories application to identity development. Grounded in a framework of organismic integration, SDT views humans as having the innate tendency to organize and integrate internal and external experiences and exchanges in the direction of a unified sense of self (Ryan and Deci 2002) or as identity theorists would say, "identity."

Humans actively seek to experience their environment because of an innate need to develop and express the self, a process energized by intrinsic motivation (Ryan et al. 1995). Self-Determination Theory is concerned with the processes by which individuals develop intrinsic motivation, facilitated by the dialectic between the active, organizing human being and their environment. From this developmental perspective, as discussed in greater detail in Chap. 6, the environment shapes and is shaped by the person (Grolnick et al. 2002). As such, healthy psychological growth involves bi-directional interactions between people and the environment, where organisms actively select and engage with stimuli in order to increase their knowledge of themselves and their external reality (Ryan et al. 1995).

Although identity development and psychological growth occurs as a function of the duality of person and environment, SDT clearly outlines environmental and social conditions where growth is thwarted (Ryan and Deci 2002). According to SDT, optimal development occurs when social environments support satisfaction of three basic psychological needs; those for autonomy, relatedness, and competence.

As discussed in Chap. 4 and other chapters, autonomy from the perspective of SDT is defined as volitional and self-endorsed functioning (Van Petegem et al. 2012) and also considered both a process and outcome of development (Ryan et al. 1995). When individuals engage in intrinsically motivated activities, they experience a sense of vitality and spontaneity, encouraging further engagement and growth through continued experience. Human development therefore is energized by intrinsic motivation and proceeds with the continual interactions between the individual and their environmental and social context (Grolnick et al. 2002). Individuals have an innate tendency to explore their surroundings and act to master increasingly more complex tasks throughout childhood and into adolescence. These behaviors represent autonomous strivings that individuals experience them as originating from themselves and perceive as having an internal locus of causality (Ryan et al. 1995). Environments that support autonomy afford children and adolescents opportunities to engage with their surroundings using choice and autonomous motives.

Adolescence is a particularly important developmental period for self-endorsement and internalization of behavioral regulation (Fousiani et al. 2014). SDT distinguishes the quality of motivation for actions based on a continuum of internal to external regulations, a concept fully elaborated in SDT's sub-theory; organismic integration theory (Deci and Ryan 2008). Organismic integration theory elaborates the process of integrating extrinsically motivated actions and describes the level of autonomy that an individual would feel at various points along this continuum. Because normative physical, cognitive, and social changes occur during adolescence this phase is marked with competing drives and external prompts from significant others (Fousiani et al. 2014; Ryan and Deci 2002). What is most important with respect to autonomy during this phase is the adolescent's integration of extrinsically motivated actions to become internally regulated and therefore performed with a sense of self-endorsement.

Adolescents must successfully integrate motives in a variety of domains in order to function optimally and in increasingly self-responsible ways. These include academics, sport, family responsibilities, and social duties; activities that one would consider instrumental because their outcomes hold certain value (Ryan et al. 1997). An important part of the developmental process is the internalization of these instrumental actions. These actions are not inherently satisfying in their own right but instead lead to ultimate ends that individuals or society holds to be of value. In order to proceed in the direction of positive growth and realization of the self, adolescents must increasingly internally regulate their engagement in the typically externally motivated activities, however, their environment and social milieu must provide adequate supports for this. More internally regulated activities are associated with greater autonomy. It is desirable, therefore, for adolescents to move in the direction of more highly integrated functioning and away from highly externally controlled functioning (Ryan et al. 1997; Ryan and Deci 2002). Increasing levels of internalization are associated with favorable psychosocial functioning, improved well-being, and better quality of relationships (Van Petegem et al. 2012).

Closely related to autonomy, the need for competence reflects the need to feel effective and capable in ones actions (Deci and Ryan 2008). During the adolescent years, the need for competence plays a formidable role in development as teens negotiate the shifting demands of family and academic life (La Guardia and Ryan 2002). Adolescents face a particular challenge with respect to feeling competent in their school-related tasks (Ratelle and Duchesne 2014; Wigfield and Wagner 2005). One possible explanation for this is that adolescents become more familiar with their actual abilities and their comparative abilities because of the evaluative feedback they receive around this phase of schooling (Wigfield and Wagner 2005). Other possible explanations exist for this decline in perceived competence; however, this decline indicates the importance of intrinsic motivation during the adolescent developmental phase. Changes in the school context during the adolescent years typically affect reward structure and increased emphasis on performance. External motivators such a grades and public evaluations of ability such as class ranking can serve to decrease adolescents' perceptions of competence and autonomy, and, therefore, their intrinsic motivation (La Guardia and Ryan 2002).

Adolescents' home, school, social, and sport environments play a key role in supporting or thwarting satisfaction of their needs for autonomy and competence, which impacts the decline in intrinsic motivation (Deci and Ryan 2000; Ratelle and Duchesne 2014). In the school context, environments that support appropriate challenges for adolescents while providing guidance and structure are associated with greater satisfaction of their need for competence and, thereby, their intrinsic motivation (La Guardia and Ryan 2002). Adolescents' perceptions of competence are enhanced when tasks are just challenging enough to stretch their current skill level and when performance feedback is informational as opposed to controlling (Carpentier and Mageau 2013). Finally, environments that emphasize task goals as opposed to performance goals provide adolescents with competency-relevant feedback as opposed to normative feedback; thus enhancing autonomy and intrinsic motivation (Krenn et al. 2013).

Assisting adolescents in adjusting to the many complex demands of their changing social milieu is the sense of belonging and connectedness to others known as *relatedness* in SDT (Deci and Ryan 2000). Although perhaps less central to intrinsic motivation than autonomy and competence, relatedness has been shown to enhance individuals' feelings of engagement and satisfaction in their pursuits (Deci and Ryan 2000, p. 235). Relatedness is particularly important for adolescent functioning because it pertains to the attachment between parents, peers, teachers and other significant others and teens. As teens proceed through the social challenges that adolescence presents, they rely on the secure base provided by their support system. Contrary to some conceptions of adolescent development, SDT views adolescence as a time of movement toward autonomy (as volitional action), internalization of values, and identity development, not a time of separation from adults (La Guardia and Ryan 2002). Relatedness to parents and significant others (teachers, coaches and peers) provides adolescents the secure base from which to pursue their innate tendency toward growth (Deci and Ryan 2000).

Support for the importance of social interactions during adolescent growth is often demonstrated when teens engage in social comparison's. These social comparisons have direct implications concerning autonomy, competence and relatedness. According to Festinger (1956) the social comparison process is an effort to affirm and re-affirm the individuals' actions, decisions and abilities. Many times these comparisons serve to communicate that the teen is acting in an autonomous way, are competent and are accepted by others. Vazou et al. (2005) suggest that there is an interconnectedness between autonomy, competence, relatedness and social comparisons among teens. These same researchers found that youths' perceptions of competence was related to their sense of social support by peers (relatedness). Additionally, competence and relatedness were associated with teens' feeling of autonomy within the social group thereby reinforcing the social comparison process.

Based on the information gathered and interpreted by the individual from the comparison they then adjust behaviors to feel self-determined and motivated. For example, if a teen is with their peer group in a social setting they are likely to communicate both verbally and non-verbally. As their peers respond either negatively or positively the teen is likely to adjust behaviors based on the peer feedback in an effort to feel a sense of autonomy, relatedness and competence. If a negative response is interpreted the adolescent may sense a disturbance in their self-determined beliefs and thus adjust behavior to accommodate. Neighbors and Knee et al. (2003) argue that interpretations in social comparison situations are based on individual differences. What may hold true for one individual may not be true of another. This is not to say that we should not pursue an understanding of these issues. Rather, researchers should focus their attention on the dynamic interactions inherently true of motivation.

Conclusions

Each of the psychological needs described in Self-Determination Theory play an important role in teens' psychological, social, and cognitive development. Situations that enable satisfaction of the basic psychological needs enhance intrinsic motivation and internalization of valued extrinsic pursuits that are of primary importance for identity development and personal growth. Activities and environments that enhance self-determination lead to numerous positive outcomes, including emotional adjustment, well-being, higher academic achievement and identity ratification (Ratelle and Duchesne 2014; Ryan and Deci 2006; Vansteenkiste and Ryan 2013; Marcia 1967).

Much has been accomplished in our understanding of motivation and identity development during adolescence. Currently, what is lacking is a confluence of both concepts. Self-Determination Theory offers an excellent backdrop from which to understand how teenagers develop their sense of being (identity). Likewise, identity development perspectives can shed light on autonomy, competence and relatedness. Thus, a multi-conceptual understanding would be most beneficial in further understanding how adolescents navigate through this important developmental stage.

References

Bartko, W. T., & Eccles, J. S. (2003). Adolescent participation in structured and unstructured activities: A person-oriented analysis. *Journal of Youth and Adolescence, 32*, 233–241.

Burgeron, M. F., Mountjoy, M., Armstrong, N., Chia, M., Cote, J., Emery, C. A., et al. (2015). International Olympic, Committee consensus statement on youth athletic development. *British Journal of Sports Medicine, 49*(13), 843–851.

Carpentier, J., & Mageau, G. A. (2013). When change-oriented feedback enhances motivation, well-being and performance: A look at autonomy-supportive feedback in sport. *Psychology of Sport and Exercise, 14*, 423–435.

Crocetti, E., Rubini, M., & Meeus, W. (2008). Capturing the dynamics of identity formation in various ethnic groups: Development and validation of a three-dimensional model. *Journal of Adolescence, 31*, 207–222.

Deci, E. L., & Ryan, R. M. (2000). The "what" and "why" of goal pursuits: Human needs and the self-determination of behavior. *Psychological Inquiry, 11*, 227–268.

Fousiani, K., Van Petegem, S., Soenens, B., Vansteenkiste, M., & Chen, B. (2014). Does parental autonomy support relate to adolescent autonomy? An in-depth examination of a seemingly simple question. *Journal of Adolescent Research, 29*(3), 299–330.

Grolnick, W. S., Gurland, S. T., Jacob, K. F., & Decourcey, W. (2002). The development of self-determination in middle childhood and adolescence. In A. Wigfield, J. S. Eccles, A. Wigfield, & J. S. Eccles (Eds.), *Development of achievement motivation* (pp. 147–171). San Diego: Academic. doi:10.1016/B978-012750053-9/50008-5.

Hall, G. S. (1904). *Adolescence: Its psychology and its relations to physiology, anthropology, sociology, sex, crime, religion, and education* (Vol. 1). New York: D. Appleton and Company.

Knee, C. R., Patrick, H., & Lonsbary, C. (2003). Implicit theories of relationships: Orientations toward evaluation and cultivation. *Personality and Social Psychology Review, 7*(1), 41–55.

Krenn, B., Wurth, S., & Hergovich, A. (2013). The impact of feedback on goal setting and task performance. *Swiss Journal of Psychology, 72*(2), 79–89.

La Guardia, J. G., & Ryan, R. M. (2002). What adolescents need: A self-determination theory perspective on development within families, school and society. In F. Pajares & T. Urdan (Eds.), *Academic motivation of adolescents*. Greenwich: IAP.

Marcia, J. E. (1980). Adolescent identity. In J. Anderson (Ed.), *Handbook of adolescent psychology* (pp. 100–131). New York: Wiley & Sons.

Meeus, W., van de Schoot, R., Keijsers, L., Schwartz, S. J., & Branje, S. (2010). On the progression and stability of adolescent identity formation. A five-wave longitudinal study in early-to-middle and middle-to-late adolescence. *Child Development, 81*, 1565–1581.

Ratelle, C. C., & Duchesne, S. (2014). Trajectories of psychological need satisfaction from early to late adolescence as a predictor of adjustment in school. *Contemporary Educational Psychology, 39*(4), 388–400. doi:10.1016/j.cedpsych.2014.09.003.

Ryan, R. M., & Deci, E. L. (2002). Overview of self-determination theory: An organismic-dialectical perspective. In E. L. Deci, R. M. Ryan, E. L. Deci, & R. M. Ryan (Eds.), *Handbook of self-determination research* (pp. 3–33). Rochester: University of Rochester Press.

Ryan, R. M., & Deci, E. L. (2006). Self-regulation and the problem of human autonomy: Does psychology need choice, self-determination, and will? *Journal of Personality, 74*, 1557–1585.

Ryan, R. M., Deci, E. L., & Grolnick, W. S. (1995). Autonomy, relatedness, and the self: Their relation to development and psychopathology. In D. Cicchetti & D. J. Cohen (Eds.), *Developmental psychopathology: Theory and methods* (Vol. 1, pp. 618–655). New York: Wiley.

Ryan, R. M., Kuhl, J., & Deci, E. L. (1997). Nature and autonomy: An organizational view of social and neurobiological aspects of self-regulation in behavior and development. *Development and Psychopathology, 9*(04), 701–728.

Schwartz, S. J. (2001). The evolution of Eriksonian and, neo-Eriksonian identity theory and research: A review and integration. *Identity: An International Journal of Theory and Research, 1*, 7–58.

Van Petegem, S., Beyers, W., Vansteenkiste, M., & Soenens, B. (2012). On the association between adolescent autonomy and psychosocial functioning: Examining decisional independence from a self-determination theory perspective. *Developmental Psychology, 48*(1), 76–88. doi:10.1037/a0025307.

Vansteenkiste, M., & Ryan, R. M. (2013). On psychological growth and vulnerability: Basic psychological need satisfaction and need frustration as a unifying principle. *Journal of Psychotherapy Integration, 23*, 263–280. doi:10.1037/a0032359.

Vazou, S., Ntoumanis, N., & Duda, J. L. (2005). Peer motivational climate in youth sport: A qualitative inquiry. *Psychology of Sport and Exercise, 6*, 497–516.

Wigfield, A., & Wagner, A. L. (2005). Competence, motivation, and identity development during adolescence. In A. Elliott & C. Dweck (Eds.), *Handbook of competence and motivation* (pp. 222–239). New York: Guilford Press.

Part IV
The Development of Volitional Action

Synthesis

Essential characteristics of Causal Agency Theory (and, as such, causal action) involve volitional action, agentic action, and action-control beliefs. This part examines the development of skills that are critical to volitional action; that is expressing preferences and initiating action. Chapter 15 reviews the literature in preference and choice making as it pertains to human agentic action and self-determination and provide a description of the development of these skills. Chapter 16 reviews the literature on self-initiation and planning as it pertains to human agentic action and self-determination and provide a description of the development of the ability to self-initiate.

Chapter 15
Preference and Choice-Expression

Karrie A. Shogren and Michael L. Wehmeyer

Abstract Under Causal Agency Theory, volitional action is based on conscious choices that reflect one's preferences. Conscious choices are intentionally conceived, deliberate acts that occur without direct external influence. The expression of preference and choice making are critical components of this process. This chapter reviews the literature in preference and choice making as it pertains to human agentic action and self-determination and provide a description of the development of these skills.

Acting volitionally is at the crux of acting in a self-determined manner. Deci (2003) observed that "self-determination is about the self-initiation and self-regulation of one's own behavior" and "[c]entral to SDT, then, is the idea of encouraging and supporting volition and self-initiation." (Deci 2003, p. 24). As described in Chap. 5, Causal Agency Theory posits three essential characteristics of self-determined action, *Volitional Action*, *Agentic Action*, and *Action-Control Beliefs*. Volitional action involves making conscious choices that reflect one's preferences, interests, values, and goals. Conscious choices are intentionally conceived, deliberate acts that occur without undue external influence. As such, volitional actions are self-initiated and function to enable a person to act autonomously (i.e., engage in self-governed action). Volitional actions involve the initiation and activation of causal capabilities—the capacity to cause something to happen—in one's life.

The purpose of this chapter is to describe key elements associated with volitional action that enable a person to act autonomously, namely the expression of preference and choice making. Specifically, this chapter will review the literature in preference and choice making as it pertains to human agentic action and self-determination, provide a description of the development of these skills, and summarize the role of preference and choice-expression in promoting self-determination.

K.A. Shogren (✉) • M.L. Wehmeyer
Special Education, University of Kansas, Lawrence, KS, USA
e-mail: shogren@ku.edu

M.L. Wehmeyer et al. (eds.), *Development of Self-Determination Through the Life-Course*, DOI 10.1007/978-94-024-1042-6_15

Defining Preference and Choice Making

It may seem unnecessary to define choice making, but it is the case that common parlance often uses choice making and decision making as synonymous, so for our purposes, it is important to clearly distinguish between these two. Making a choice involves, at its simplest, the expression of a preference between two or more alternatives. Having a preference indicates, for example, that one likes one thing or person relatively more than one likes another thing or person. As noted previously, volitional action is action based upon making a conscious choice… expressing a preference. The very nature of human agentic theories, as discussed in detail in Chap. 2, is that organisms act volitionally, using self-regulated and goal-directed action to fulfill basic psychological needs and act as the causal agent in one's life.

It is worth reiterating a point pertaining to the expression of preferences and volitional action that was raised in Chap. 5, that being the distinction between self-determination and the notion of "control." Self-determined action is self-caused—volitional—action, and is not synonymous with the having 'control.' Control "refers to there being a contingency between one's behavior and the outcomes one receives, whereas self-determination refers to the experience of freedom in initiating one's behavior" (Deci and Ryan 1985, p. 31).

Volitional action is, obviously, an important component within SDT in enabling the organism to fulfill the psychological need for autonomy. As noted in Chap. 4, the need for autonomy is satisfied when an individual experiences choice and volition in their action, and perceives themselves to be the origin of their actions. Deci and Ryan (1985) also note that choice, from a motivational standpoint, need not necessarily be deliberate or analytical; that "a person does not need to make a conscious, deliberate decision for there to be a choice" (p. 155).

> Experientially, one way to know whether a behavior was genuinely chosen is whether the other options were (or could have been) fully entertained. We assert that a behavior is truly chosen only if the person could (whether intuitively or deliberately) seriously considered not doing it (Deci and Ryan 1985, p. 155).

So, in defining a choice, one must go beyond just expressing a preference to consider whether someone fully entertained options and that the person could consider not doing whatever is being selected. A choice, as such, indicates some level of preference and the freedom to reject an option. So-called choices in which options are available but not preferred are referred to as dilemmas. A Hobson's choice is a choice in which only one option is available, but the contrasting options are to take the option or not. If there is a preference for the only option, such situations can be true choices, but when the sole option is not preferred, one cannot assert that it is a true choice.

Development of Preference and Choice Making

Developmental aspects of choice making focus on children's capacities to identify and communicate preferences. Once a child develops these capacities, the maturation of choice making ability relies on children's opportunities to make selections and experience the consequences of these choices. Even later, children acquire the capacity for systematic decision making, which includes, as a final step, making a choice of a preferred alternative. The capacity for indicating preferences is present at birth; newborns discriminate between various objects and people in their environment and show evidence of preferences for some of these over others. Other preferences emerge based on infants' interactions with individuals, objects, and the environment (Doll et al. 1996).

Making a selection requires that the child designate a specific option from between two or more choices, an act that requires the emergence of intentional communication. The cry of an infant, the emergence of a social smile, and the use of eye gaze represent forms of communication available to infants by 4–5 months of age, whereas motor skills like reaching, pointing, and moving toward an object are usually in place by 10 months of age. Very young children will select by pointing, reaching, or smiling but initially do so without a fully developed understanding that they can elicit a desired response. Once children learn that these communicative efforts can elicit the outcome they desire, they begin to use communication purposefully and intentionally. Thus, the cry of a 1-year-old when she is hungry becomes not only a notice of an internal state (hunger) but also an attempt to get someone else to meet her need. Independent of how a child communicates, most children develop the necessary skills for indicating preferences and making a selection from options by 12 months of age. When the child's first words emerge, as early as 12 months of age, they are combined with gestures to make the communication of selections and preferences more effective. As children develop more advanced verbal skills at age 3, language typically replaces visual and motor activities as the primary source of information about preferences.

Preference and Choice Making and Disability

One factor that spurred the emphasis on self-determination within the field of special education and that shaped the development of Causal Agency Theory (see Chap. 5), was an emerging recognition of the lack of choice-making opportunities available to people who were educated and living in restrictive (i.e., not inclusive) environments, primarily people with disabilities, and the detrimental effects of these lack of such opportunities on multiple life outcomes (Brotherson et al. 2008; Carr et al. 2002; Dunlap et al. 1994; Neely-Barnes et al. 2008; Stancliffe and Wehmeyer 1995; Wehmeyer 2002; Wehmeyer and Abery 2013; Wehmeyer and Bolding 1999, 2001). A key aspect of the development of the ability to express preferences and make choices is opportunities to engage with the environment and have the opportunity to develop preferences based on exposure to different materials and stimuli. This is critically important in early childhood and remains important throughout lifespan for all people, particularly as adolescents and young adults begin to develop preferences about social relationships (K. W. Fisher and Shogren 2015), employment opportunities (Martin et al. 2005), living arrangements, and so forth. Without opportunities to experience diverse people and environments, people cannot develop preferences and make meaningful choices. As Cullen (1999) noted, with particular emphasis on evaluating choice supports for people with disabilities, the main question in determining the impact of promoting choice supports should be the significance of the choice opportunity for the person. For people with disabilities, as with all people, unless people are exposed to diverse experiences and have opportunities to make real and meaningful choices in their lives, particularly as they enter adolescence and young adulthood, then people cannot become effective choice makers, nor will choices provided be meaningful for the person and their unique life circumstances.

And, the literature clearly shows that people with disabilities, including people with intellectual and developmental disabilities have far fewer opportunities to make choices and express preferences in their lives (Stancliffe et al. 2011; Tichá et al. 2012; Shogren 2011, 2012; Wehmeyer and Abery, 2013). Further, there is a high use of substituted decision making arrangements, for both people with intellectual disability as well as with mental health conditions (Uekert and Van Duizend 2011). These arrangements frequently include legal guardianship that tends to be permanent and often all too encompassing in adulthood that diminishes the capacity of many people with IDD to exercise control over their lives. Wehmeyer and Metzler (1995) found that people with intellectual disability compared to their peers without disabilities experienced significantly fewer choice opportunities pertaining to where they lived, work and leisure activities, who they spent time with, and so forth. For example, in a sample of people without disabilities, 77% indicated that they chose their current job, while Wehmeyer and Metzler found that only 11% of people with intellectual disability made such choices. Similar discrepancies were found in relation to choices about where to live (46–6%), opportunity to control one's own money (91–44%), and choosing who to live with (59–9%). Stancliffe and Wehmeyer (1995) found that choice opportunities varied for people with intellectual disability varied significantly as a function of where a person lived, with people with intellectual disability who lived in their communities having significantly more choice opportunities than did people with intellectual disability living in congregate settings. This body of research highlights the critical role that environments have in shaping choice and preference development (Stancliffe 1995, 1997; Stancliffe et al. 2000, 2011), the same likely holds true for people without disabilities. Further, the attitudes of others play a large role in ensuring choice opportunities. Abery et al. (2013) found that adults with intellectual and developmental disabilities engaged in significantly greater choice and decision making when the staff that were supporting them believed in the importance of choice and self-determination, highlight the role of the context in supporting the development of self-determination.

In addition to promoting the development of environments that facilitate the development of expression of preferences and choice making, a variety of interventions to promote choice-making skills and opportunities has been developed. This is a strong focus on the body of research on choice-making, particularly for students with disabilities (Algozzine et al. 2001). This focus has developed and identified methods to teach people with disabilities the skills needed to make effective choices (Browder et al. 1998; Cobigo et al. 2010; Martin and Marshall 1997; Wehmeyer and Abery 2013), and identified methods to increase choice-making opportunities.

Preference and Choice Making and Its Role in Volitional Action and Causal Agency

As noted throughout the text, self-determined people act volitionally and, as per Fig. 5.1, volitional action involves the initiation and activation of agentic capabilities—the capacity to sustain action toward a goal. Volitional action implies making conscious choices that reflect one's preferences. Conscious choices are intentionally conceived, deliberate acts that occur without direct external influence. As such, volitional actions are self-initiated and function to enable a person to act autonomously (i.e., engage in self-governed action). Volitional actions involve the initiation and activation of causal capabilities—the capacity to cause something to happen—in one's life.

Acting autonomously by expressing preferences and making choices is related to the process of self-identity and the development of agency (Chap. 3). Central to developing a personal identity is having opportunities to develop and express preferences. This process begins early in life, as young children have opportunities to explore their environments and manipulate and play with materials that hold their interest (Odom and Wolery 2003). Through this exploration, young children learn what interests them and develop a personal identity distinct from their caregivers. The level of support in environments for exploration and interactions with of diverse materials and activities shapes the development of one's personal identity, and subsequently the degree to which one can express preferences and make, as interaction with diverse stimuli is necessary to identify preferences and make choices between preferred items (Erikson 1963; Wehmeyer and Palmer 2000).

Adolescents become self-determined—that is, having the dispositional characteristic of self-determination—as they learn, refine, and practice knowledge, skills, beliefs and actions that enable them to respond to contextual and environmental challenges (opportunities, threats) that energize basic psychological needs and resultant autonomous motivation, *manifested by preference expression and choice making*, stimulating a causal action sequence in which volitional and agentic actions are mediated by action-control beliefs, resulting in experiences of causal agency. Repeated experiences of causal agency lead to enhanced self-determination.

Role of Preference and Choice-Expression in Valued Life Outcomes

A wide body of research in special education has suggested an association between enhanced self-determination and choice opportunities and more positive quality of life outcomes (Neely-Barnes et al. 2008; Nota et al. 2007, 2011; Shogren et al. 2006, 2015). For example, Neely-Barnes et al. (2008) found that choice opportunities and living arrangements were significantly associated, and that both predicted higher quality of life. Researchers have also shown when self-determination interventions are systematically implemented in schools, changes in student self-determination result (Wehmeyer et al. 2012, 2013), and that these changes impact environmental factors (i.e. teacher attitudes and perceptions of student potential) (Shogren et al. 2014) as well as valued post-school outcomes, such as employment and community participation (Shogren et al. 2015).

Opportunities to make choices can be infused throughout the lives of all people, and for children and adolescents, multiple opportunities to make choices can be embedded across environments to support preference development, increasingly consequential choices, and a recognition of the relationship between action and outcomes. Research has suggested that simply providing access to basic choice opportunities (i.e., choice in the order of tasks in education contexts) can lead to changes in behavior, namely decreases in disruptive classroom behaviors and increases in on-task classroom behaviors. Research has also suggested the increased choice-making opportunities can promote increased use of adaptive behavior (Heller et al. 2000), work performance, task engagement, accuracy, and social/communicative behavior (Kern et al. 1998; Lancioni et al. 1996). Abery et al. (2013) found the attitudes of others significantly impacted access to choice opportunities, suggesting the role of environmental factors in shaping access to choice opportunities.

Research on the application of SDT to educational settings has also emphasized the importance of autonomy and volition. Reeve (2002) stated that "two decades of empirical work supports the following two conclusions: (1) autonomously-motivated students thrive in educational settings, and (2) students benefit when teachers support their autonomy" (p. 183). Such benefits of autonomy supported teaching include more positive academic achievement, higher levels of creativity, more positive self-esteem and self-worth, and higher rates of retention. Models of instruction, such as the *Self-Determined Learning Model of Instruction* (discussed in Chap. 19), which emphasize student-directed learning through self-regulated problem solving and student active choice in the learning process create autonomy supportive teaching environments.

Thus, there are an array of factors, both external and internal to the person, that impact preference expression and choice making. A key factor, however, is ensuring all people have access to meaningful choice opportunities. Researchers have found that opportunities for choice making is the strongest predictor of self-determination status of adults with disabilities (Wehmeyer and Garner 2003). Developmentally, these skills emerge over time, as children, youth, and adults have opportunities to develop preference and make choices. And, over time, these choices should become more complex and consequential, in relation to the environmental demands related to adolescents and adulthood.

References

Abery, B. H., Ticha, R., Smith, J. G., Welshons, K., & Berlin, S. (2013). Validation of the self-determination and control opportunity and response evaluation scale (SD-CORES). *Manuscript submitted for publication.*

Algozzine, B., Browder, D., Karvonen, M., Test, D. W., & Wood, W. M. (2001). Effects of interventions to promote self-determination for individuals with disabilities. *Review of Educational Research, 71*, 219–277. doi:10.3102/00346543071002219.

Brotherson, M. J., Cook, C. C., Erwin, E. E., & Weigel, C. J. (2008). Understanding self-determination and families of young children with disabilities in home environments. *Journal of Early Intervention, 31*(1), 22–43.

Browder, D. M., Cooper, K. J., & Lim, L. (1998). Teaching adults with severe disabilities to express their choice of settings for leisure activities. *Education and Training in Mental Retardation and Developmental Disabilities, 33*(3), 228–238.

Carr, E. G., Dunlap, G., Horner, R. H., Koegel, R. L., Turnbull, A. P., Sailor, W., et al. (2002). Positive behavior support: Evolution of an applied science. *Journal of Positive Behavior Interventions, 4*(4–16), 20.

Cobigo, V., Lachapelle, Y., & Morin, D. (2010). Choice-making in vocational activities planning: Recommendations from job coaches. *Journal of Policy and Practice in Intellectual Disabilities, 7*(4), 245–249. doi:10.1111/j.1741-1130.2010.00273.x.

Cullen, C. (1999). Contextualism in intellectual disability research: The case of choice behaviour. *Journal of Intellectual Disability Research, 43*(6), 437–444.

Deci, E. L. (2003). Promoting intrinsic motivation and self-determination in people with mental retardation. In H. Switzky, L. Hickson, R. L. Schalock, & M. L. Wehmeyer (Eds.), *Personality and motivational systems in mental retardation* (pp. 1–31). New York: Elsevier.

Deci, E. L., & Ryan, R. M. (1985). *Intrinsic motivation and self-determination in human behavior.* New York: Plenum Press.

Doll, E., Sands, D., Wehmeyer, M. L., & Palmer, S. (1996). Promoting the development and acquisition of self-determined behavior. In D. J. Sands & M. L. Wehmeyer (Eds.), *Self-determination across the life span: Independence and choice for people with disabilities* (pp. 65–90). Baltimore: Paul H. Brookes.

Dunlap, G., Kern-Dunlap, L., Clarke, S., & Robbins, F. R. (1994). Some characteristics of nonaversive intervention for severe behavior problems. In E. Schopler & G. B. Mesibov (Eds.), *Behavioral issues in autism* (pp. 227–245). New York: Plenum.

Erikson, E. H. (1963). *Childhood and society* (2nd ed.). New York: Norton.

Fisher, K. W., & Shogren, K. A. (2015). Does academic tracking impact adolescents' access to social capital? *Manuscript submitted for publication.*

Heller, T., Miller, A. B., Hsieh, K., & Sterns, H. (2000). Later-life planning: Promoting knowledge of options and choice-making. *Mental Retardation, 38*(5), 395–406.

Kern, L., Vorndran, C. M., Hilt, A., Ringdahl, J. E., Adelman, B. E., & Dunlap, G. (1998). Choice as an intervention to improve behavior: A review of the literature. *Journal of Behavioral Education, 8*(2), 151–169.

Lancioni, G. E., O'Reilly, M. F., & Emerson, E. (1996). A review of choice research with people with severe and profound developmental disabilities. *Research in Developmental Disabilities, 17*(5), 391–411.

Martin, J. E., & Marshall, L. H. (1997). Choice making: Description of a model project. In M. Agran (Ed.), *Student-directed learning: Teaching self-determination skills* (pp. 224–248). Pacific Grove: Brooks/Cole Publishing Company.

Martin, J. E., Woods, L. L., Sylvester, L., & Gardner, J. E. (2005). A challenge to self-determination: Disagreement between the vocational choices made by individuals with severe disabilities and their caregivers. *Research and Practice for Persons with Severe Disabilities, 30*, 147–153.

Neely-Barnes, S., Marcenko, M., & Weber, L. (2008). Does choice influence quality of life for people with mild intellectual disabilities? *Intellectual and Developmental Disabilities, 46*(1), 12–26. doi:10.1352/0047-6765(2008)46[12:DCIQOL]2.0.CO;2.

Nota, L., Ferrari, L., Soresi, S., & Wehmeyer, M. (2007). Self-determination, social abilities and the quality of life of people with intellectual disability. *Journal of Intellectual Disability Research, 51*, 850–865. doi:10.1111/j.1365-2788.2006.00939.x.

Nota, L., Soresi, S., Ferrari, L., & Wehmeyer, M. L. (2011). A multivariate analysis of the self-determination of adolescents. *Journal of Happiness Studies, 12*(2), 245–266. doi:10.1007/s10902-010-9191-0.

Odom, S. L., & Wolery, M. (2003). A unified theory of practice in early intervention/early childhood special education: Evidence-based practices. *Journal of Special Education, 37*(3), 164–173.

Reeve, J. (2002). Self-determination theory applied to educational settings. In E. L. Deci & R. M. Ryan (Eds.), *Handbook of self-determination research* (pp. 183–203). Rochester: Rochester University Press.

Shogren, K. A. (2011). Culture and self-determination: A synthesis of the literature and directions for future research and practice. *Career Development for Exceptional Individuals, 34*, 115–127. doi:10.1177/0885728811398271.

Shogren, K. A. (2012). Hispanic mothers' perceptions of self-determination. *Research and Practice for Persons with Severe Disabilities, 37*, 170–184.

Shogren, K. A., Lopez, S. J., Wehmeyer, M. L., Little, T. D., & Pressgrove, C. L. (2006). The role of positive psychology constructs in predicting life satisfaction in adolescents with and without cognitive disabilities: An exploratory study. *The Journal of Positive Psychology, 1*, 37–52.

Shogren, K. A., Plotner, A. J., Palmer, S. B., Wehmeyer, M. L., & Paek, Y. (2014). Impact of the self-determined learning model of instruction on teacher perceptions of student capacity and opportunity for self-determination. *Education and Training in Autism and Developmental Disabilities, 49*, 440–448.

Shogren, K. A., Wehmeyer, M. L., Palmer, S. B., Rifenbark, G. G., & Little, T. D. (2015). Relationships between self-determination and postschool outcomes for youth with disabilities. *Journal of Special Education, 53*, 30–41. doi:10.1177/0022466913489733.

Stancliffe, R. J. (1995). Assessing opportunities for choice-making: A comparison of self- and staff reports. *American Journal on Mental Retardation, 99*(4), 418–429.

Stancliffe, R. J. (1997). Community living-unit size, staff presence, and residents' choice-making. *Mental Retardation, 35*, 1–9. doi:10.1352/0047-6765(1997)035<0001:CLSSPA>2.0.CO;2.

Stancliffe, R. J., & Wehmeyer, M. L. (1995). Variability in the availability of choice to adults with mental retardation. *Journal of Vocational Rehabilitation, 5*, 319–328.

Stancliffe, R. J., Abery, B. H., & Smith, J. (2000). Personal control and the ecology of community living settings: Beyond living-unit size and type. *American Journal on Mental Retardation, 105*(6), 431–454.

Stancliffe, R. J., Lakin, K. C., Larson, S., Engler, J., Taub, S., & Fortune, J. (2011). Choice of living arrangements. *Journal of Intellectual Disability Research, 55*(8), 746–762. doi:10.1111/j.1365-2788.2010.01336.x.

Tichá, R., Lakin, K. C., Larson, S. A., Stancliffe, R. J., Taub, S., Engler, J., et al. (2012). Correlates of everyday choice and support-related choice for 8,892 randomly sampled adults with intellectual and developmental disabilities in 19 states. *Intellectual and Developmental Disabilities, 50*(6), 486–504. doi:10.1352/1934-9556-50.06.486.

Uekert, B. K., & Van Duizend, R. (2011). *Adult guardianships: A "best guess" national estimate and the momentun for reform*. Williamsburg: National Center for State Courts.
Wehmeyer, M. L. (2002). The confluence of person-centered planning and self-determination. In S. Holburn & P. M. Vietze (Eds.), *Person centered planning: Research, practice, and future directions* (pp. 51–69). Baltimore: Paul H. Brookes Publishing Co..
Wehmeyer, M. L., & Abery, B. H. (2013). Self-determination and choice. *Intellectual and Developmental Disabilities, 51*(5), 399–411. doi:10.1352/1934-9556-51.5.399.
Wehmeyer, M. L., & Bolding, N. (1999). Self-determination across living and working environments: A matched-samples study of adults with mental retardation. *Mental Retardation, 37*(5), 353–363.
Wehmeyer, M. L., & Bolding, N. (2001). Enhanced self-determination of adults with intellectual disability as an outcome of moving to community-based work or living environments. *Journal of Intellectual Disability Research, 45*(5), 371–383.
Wehmeyer, M. L., & Garner, N. W. (2003). The impact of personal characteristics of people with intellectual and developmental disability on self-determination and autonomous functioning. *Journal of Applied Research in Intellectual Disabilities, 16*, 255–265.
Wehmeyer, M. L., & Metzler, C. A. (1995). How self-determined are people with mental retardation? The National Consumer Survey. *Mental Retardation, 33*(2), 111–119.
Wehmeyer, M. L., & Palmer, S. B. (2000). Promoting the acquisition and development of self-determination in young children with disabilities. *Early Education and Development, 11*(4), 465–481.
Wehmeyer, M. L., Shogren, K. A., Palmer, S. B., Williams-Diehm, K., Little, T. D., & Boulton, A. (2012). Impact of the self-determined learning model of instruction on student self-determination: A randomized-trial placebo control group study. *Exceptional Children, 78*, 135–153.
Wehmeyer, M. L., Palmer, S. B., Shogren, K. A., Williams-Diehm, K., & Soukup, J. H. (2013). Establishing a causal relationship between interventions to promote self-determination and enhanced student self-determination. *Journal of Special Education, 46*, 195–210. doi:10.1177/0022466910392377.

Chapter 16
Self-Initiation and Planning

Karrie A. Shogren, Michael L. Wehmeyer, and Sheida Khamsi

Abstract Causal Agency Theory describes volitional action as action that is intentionally conceived (planned) and self-initiated. Volitional actions involve the initiation and activation of causal capabilities—the capacity to cause something to happen—in one's life. Acting in an intentionally conceived, self-initiated manner is therefore a critical element of volitional action. This chapter will review the literature on self-initiation and planning as it pertains to human agentic action and self-determination and provide a description of the development of the ability to self-initiate.

The previous chapter described one dimension of volitional action; action based on conscious choices that reflect one's preferences. Self-initiation of action and planning are additional dimensions of volitional action that will be described in this chapter. To act volitionally, actions must not only involve conscious choices that reflect one's preferences, but must also be intentionally conceived (planned) and self-initiated. Essentially, volitional action includes people initiating and activating their causal capabilities to move toward the things they want in their lives.

This chapter will introduce the construct of self-initiation and describe its relationship to planning and causal action, with a particular focus on volitional action and the development of human agentic action, as well as the impact of self-initiation and planning in promoting causal agency and self-determination.

Defining Self-Initiation and Planning

Noted throughout this text, and highlighted in the previous chapter, is that a critical element undergirding theories of human agency is the belief that people are intrinsically motivated to engage with their environment and to act volitionally (Little et al. 2002). As discussed in Chap. 4, Self-Determination Theory (SDT) emphasizes that

K.A. Shogren (✉) • M.L. Wehmeyer
Special Education, University of Kansas, Lawrence, KS, USA
e-mail: shogren@ku.edu

S. Khamsi
University of Kansas, Lawrence, KS, USA

M.L. Wehmeyer et al. (eds.), *Development of Self-Determination Through the Life-Course*, DOI 10.1007/978-94-024-1042-6_16

individuals are intrinsically motivated to address their basic psychological needs for autonomy, competence, and relatedness; that the satisfaction of both autonomy and competence needs are necessary to maintain intrinsic motivation; and that environments can be set up to facilitate such intrinsic motivation by being autonomy-supportive through the promotion of internal (vs. external) control (Niemiec and Ryan 2009). SDT differs from other theories of motivation because of its assumption that both the fulfillment of autonomy and competence needs maintains intrinsic motivation, not just competence related needs, as emphasized in other theories such as self-efficacy theory (Bandura 1997). Essentially, volitional action is driven by an underlying need not only for behavior to be viewed as effective in achieving the intended ends (competence needs), but also for behavior to be perceived as personally meaningful and self-directed (autonomy needs). Research has found, in educational contexts for example, when teachers are autonomy-supportive, rather than focused on directing their student's behavior, that student intrinsic motivation is higher (Deci et al. 2001). Self-Determination Theory focuses on the critical role of creating autonomy-supportive environments to shape intrinsic motivation, enabling autonomy and competence needs to be met.

Although a primary focus of human agentic theories is building intrinsic motivation for learning and behavior because of the strong relationship between intrinsic motivation and outcomes, at times, external factors shape learning and behavior. For example, students may not be internally motivated to study certain topics, however, an external motivator such as getting a certain grade or progressing toward college admittance may shape action. However, such external motivators can be internalized by students if students are supported to develop the ability to recognize how self-initiated action can lead to desired outcomes (i.e., I will study math because it is necessary to get to college, and I want to be able to go to college). When such external contingencies are internalized, this can address the need for autonomy and competence as students are learning to engage in self-initiated actions to achieve their goals (Niemiec and Ryan 2009). In these circumstances, where students are learning to act in service of a goal or an end, even if attainment is delayed, they learn to self-initiate behaviors as a means to act volitionally.

Self-Initiation Self-initiation of action is an important component of causal action beyond just situations of internalizing external contingencies. Causal Agency Theory posits that causal action is in response to environmental or contextual challenges that take the form of opportunities or threats to the organism's self-determination. Opportunities can be found or created. The self-initiation of action is critical in the process of creating opportunities for oneself, as well as for responding to opportunities or threats. In all cases, as discussed more subsequently, there is a direct linkage between self-initiation of action and goal setting and attainment; self-initiated action is in service of a goal.

Positive psychologists also assert that self-initiation as an element of volitional action is linked to the expectations that people hold for the future. Seligman and colleagues discuss teleologic thinking as an alternative to traditional behavioral accounts of how past experiences influence behavior, arguing that past experiences lead to expectations for the future, which leads to people considering future possibilities and selecting and initiating actions based on what they perceive as possibilities in the future, and rationally engaging in actions based on perceived probabilities of certain outcomes occurring in the future (Seligman et al. 2013). This differs from other behavioral accounts that suggest that past outcomes shape future behavior, rather than expectations for the future. When past experiences are viewed as a source of information, rather than circumstances people respond to, self-initiated action can be understood differently. People learn to self-initiate based on their evaluation of past experiences and the perceived likelihood of certain actions leading to desired future outcomes. This situates people as navigators or their future, mentally considering possible futures and actions likely to lead them to desired future states. Further, it suggests that people can learn to conceive and engage in self-initiated acts, based on their vision for the future, using the actions that they perceive as likely to lead them to desired future states.

Of course, self-initiation of action is propelled by the development of intrinsic or internalized extrinsic motivation. This has been well illustrated by research in the field of intellectual disability documenting the phenomenon of *outerdirectdness*. Outerdirectedness is "the term used to describe approaches in which individuals rely on external cues rather than on their internal cognitive abilities to solve a task or problem" (Bybee and Zigler 1998, p. 435). It is, more specifically, a "motivational style of problem solving in which the child uses external cues rather than relying on his own cognitive resources" (MacMillan and Cauffiel 1977, p. 643). Research has established that children with intellectual disability exhibit outerdirectedness at a greater rate than do typically developing children, likely due to multiple factors, including prompt dependency and overreliance, repeated experiences with failure, and task difficulty (Bybee and Zigler 1998). This same body of research documents that outerdirectedness results in the lack of initiation of action, reduced problem solving efficacy, and poorer school performance (Bybee and Zigler 1998).

Self-initiation involves several interrelated actions/processes; when initiating an action, a person chooses when to begin, so there is a temporal aspect to self-initiation. Beginning action also involves considering possibilities and past experiences to make plans, introducing both planning elements and a teleological element of future thinking as well as using past experiences to direct planning and action, as well as using preferences to direct action. We will look at each of these in greater depth subsequently in the chapter, but these elements illustrate the close relationship between self-initiation and planning.

Planning Planning involves "the orchestration of diverse and interdependent cognitive and motivational processes that are influenced by context and that are brought together in the service of reaching a goal" (Friedman and Scholnick 1997a, p. 3). Planning provides a way to "begin" to act (self-initiate) by putting into play the motivational, cognitive, and emotional processes energized by autonomous motivation. That planning serves the goal attainment process is illustrated by research by Masicampo and Baumeister (2011) that examined the role of plan making in eliminating intrusive thoughts brought about by unfulfilled goals. In a series of studies, these researchers showed that unfinished goals cause intrusive thoughts and poorer performance on tasks. However, formulating plans for the unfulfilled goals eliminated the intrusive thoughts.

Most researchers position the planning process within the early stages of the goal setting process, emphasizing (see Fig. 19.1 and Chap.18) the role of planning in what we refer to as solving the goal discrepancy problem: the act of comparing one's current state with one's anticipated goal state, and then generating potential strategies to reduce that gap (Ward and Morris 2005). Further, planning is linked to problem solving as well. In general, research examining the causal relationship between planning and effective problem solving has shown that planning has a positive effect (Ellis and Siegler 1997).

Development of Self-Initiation and Planning

Both self-initiation of action and planning share common developmental antecedents associated with teleologic (future) thinking, the application of past experiences to current circumstances, and using preferences to guide action. We have discussed the developmental sequence of choice and the expression of preference in Chap.15, related to the latter (using preferences to guide action) so will not repeat that information in this context. And, as both self-initiation and planning are in service to goal setting and attainment, developmental descriptions associated with understandings of goal intent, engagement in shared goal pursuits, and the understanding of causality and the identification of causal agents also play a role in the development of self-initiation and planning, and readers are referred to Chap.18 for that information. In fact, the development of planning alone involves consideration of the organism's ability to think about time, place, causes, functions, consequences, evaluation, integration, and decision making (Kreitler and Kreitler 1987) and, thus, we leave for more detailed accounts (e.g., Friedman and Scholnick 1997b) the task of describing such development in full.

With regard to children's development of the conception of time and the capacity to engage in future thinking, Haith (1997) identifies key developmental milestones in the relationship between memory and future thinking. Very young infants, 6 months and older, are able to form expectations with regard to the space and time for the appearance of an object based upon past experience. In general, children as young as nine-months old show expectations for action in the future based upon experiences in the past (Haith, 1997). Temporal sequencing abilities related to planning and self-initiation emerge later in development. Means-end thinking emerges after the child's first year, paralleling the discussion in Chap.18 pertaining to the development of causality thinking. The emergence of language accelerates the development of children's future-oriented processes. Benson (1997) highlights research suggesting that children up to age 18 months focus on the present when talking about what they want, by age 30 months can distinguish and talk about a rough delineation of now or not now references, by 36 months of age can relate two points in time, but not their sequence, and by 52 months of age can coordinate multiple points in time and the sequence in which they occur, and thus can talk about sequences of events that she would do and, thus, engage in planning at a more sophisticated level (Benson 1997). As children get older, they begin to be able to sequence more complex routines (structure of the day) and by early elementary can link past, present, and future events. By ages 10–11 years, children have acquired the basic skills needed to engage in planning (Nurmi, 1991).

In adolescence, research has shown that, not surprisingly, parents and family members strongly influence the future orientation of their son or daughter (Nurmi, 1991). Adolescents goals, values, and beliefs tend to mirror those of their parents, as do adolescents' planning skills. By adolescence, most young people can formulate hypotheses that are contrary to fact, and explore multiple courses of actions so as to facilitate planning and goal setting. As was discussed in Chap.3, the process of identify development and agency beliefs, including adolescents establishing individual goals and interests, are primary developmental tasks during late adolescence and early adulthood (Nurmi, 1991).

The Role of Self-Initiation and Planning in Volitional Action and Causal Agency

We have discussed the importance of self-initiation and planning in the volitional action process, and specifically, the important role these play in enabling people to begin actions associated with goals and/or in response to threats and opportunities in the environment. Self-initiation and planning spur volitional action in service of a goal, leading to agentic action and experiences of causal agency, which, over time, enhance self-determination.

For some populations of adolescents, and particularly, perhaps, young people with disabilities, these issues of self-initiation and planning are of particular importance in interventions to promote causal agency and self-determination. In discussing issues of outerdirectedness or prompt dependence, Bybee and Zigler (1998) identify people with intellectual disability as particularly prone, for various reasons, to develop outerdirectedness and prompt dependence. It is, as such important to consider the need for instruction and supports leading to self-initiation and planning. One important aspect of supporting self-initiation is simply creating opportunities for self-initiation, often associated with opportunities to express preferences and make choices. Interveners often need to consider response ranges beyond typical verbal or behavioral actions as indicators of self-initiation, interest, preferences, and so forth. For example, researchers have highlighted the importance of initiation and responses to self-initiations for adolescents with severe disabilities, emphasizing how self-initiation can take many forms, including showing alertness, looking at something that is desired, and other behavioral indicators that can be detected by people supporting the initiation (Munde and Vlaskamp 2015). Similarly for people without disabilities, educators and family and community members can be sensitive to actions begin taken by others to initiate steps toward achieving an end.

Researchers have also identified the criticality of initiation, particularly for youth with autism (Koegel et al. 2001), and suggest the importance of five elements when teaching and supporting youth to begin to engage in self-initiation: planning, processing of information, attention to relevant stimuli, motivation, and expectations (Hume et al. 2009). This line of work suggests that people need to learn how to plan to initiate action (e.g., what are the first steps to begin action toward an intended outcome), process information that enables them to recognize the need to self-initiate, attend to relevant cues in the environment that provide information on when and how to initiate, be motivated to engage in action based on a belief that the action will be supported in the environment, and have clearly laid out expectations for what is expected and how the environment will respond. As further discussed in Chap.17, for example, people can learn how to engage in self-regulated problem solving in service of goals enabling them to develop an understanding of the link between their actions and outcomes, enhancing motivation to self-initiate actions. Part of the instruction and support, however, must be enabling students to develop the capacity to identify future possibilities, and evaluate the actions that are most likely (based on past experiences) to lead them to these outcomes. Then, students can self-initiate behavior that enables them to act based on their preferences, interests, and vision for the future.

Self-Initiation, Planning, and Valued Outcomes

As mentioned previously, researchers have identified self-initiation as a critical skill for people with and without disabilities and found that structuring the environment to be supportive of self-initiation can lead to increases in self-initiation and valued outcomes. For example, researchers have found that when teachers and other authority figures in youth's lives are autonomy-supportive, meaning they encourage choice, self-initiation, and self-regulation in the youth they support, that youth tend to feel more competent, autonomous, and related or connected to others (Amorose and Anderson-Butcher 2007; Deci et al. 2001; Deci and Ryan 1994). Researchers have also found that people that are driven by autonomous motivation tend to have better coping skills and put forward more effort in preferred athletic activities (Mouratidis and Michou 2011) and in after school activities (Beiswenger and Grolnick 2010). College students who demonstrate greater self-initiation and autonomous motivation tend to show greater motivation for learning, and students chose their own major they tend to be more motivated to learn (Pan and Gauvain 2012). In adulthood, people with higher autonomous motivation, have also been found to have higher work related motivation and greater satisfaction with their jobs (Gillet et al. 2013) as well as report greater overall well-being (Hortop et al. 2013).

With regard to youth with disabilities, researchers have found that when youth with disabilities learn to self-initiate in specific domains, such as conversing with peers and building social relationships, and that increases in self-initiation support the development of relationships and the reciprocity of interactions (Reilly et al. 2014). For youth with physical disabilities, higher levels of autonomous motivation contribute to higher levels of physical activity during rehabilitation (Saebu et al. 2013). Researchers have also found that when environments for adults with disabilities are highly directive, people with disabilities tend to engage in fewer self-initiations and have higher levels of problematic behavior (Shukla et al. 1995). Researchers have found that youth and adults with disabilities can learn and implement strategies for self-initiating behavior. For example, a strategy "Did-Next-Now" was developed to teach students with severe disabilities to being (and complete) work routines without external prompting and direction, and multiple studies have shown the utility on self-initiation strategies in promoting increased performance and self-initiation (Browder and Minarovic 2000; Smith et al. 2015).

Self-initiation, in combination with making conscious choices based on one's preference, defines volitional action. The construct of self-initiation provides an important way of understanding how internal motivation is expressed, and provides a framework for understanding how our expectations for the future can shape our current behavior. The environment can play a key role in enabling and supporting self-initiation, and engaging in self-initiated action has been shown to impact outcomes in multiple domains. Strategies for people, including people with disabilities, who may need more support to engage in self-initiation have been developed, and developing there may be differing demands for initiation as children and youth develop. Overall, creating environments that are autonomy-supportive and creating opportunities for self-determination will be critical to enabling children and youth to initiate and activate their causal capabilities, a critical element of going after what they want and need in life to achieve desired goals and future states.

References

Amorose, A. J., & Anderson-Butcher, D. (2007). Autonomy-supportive coaching and self-determined motivation in high school and college athletes: A test of self-determination theory. *Psychology of Sport and Exercise, 8*(5), 654–670. doi: http://dx.doi.org/10.1016/j.psychsport.2006.11.003

Bandura, A. (1997). *Self-efficacy: The exercise of control*. New York: W.H. Freeman and Co..

Beiswenger, K. L., & Grolnick, W. S. (2010). Interpersonal and intrapersonal factors associated with autonomous motivation in adolescents' after-school activities. *The Journal of Early Adolescence, 30*(3), 369–394. doi: http://dx.doi.org/10.1177/0272431609333298

Benson, J. B. (1997). The development of planning: It's about time. In S. L. Friedman & E. K. Scholnick (Eds.), *The developmental psychology of planning: Why, how, and when do we plan?* (pp. 43–75). Mahweh: Lawrence Erlbaum Associates.

Browder, D. M., & Minarovic, T. J. (2000). Utilizing sight words in self-instruction training for employees with moderate mental retardation in competitive jobs. *Education and Training in Mental Retardation and Developmental Disabilities, 35*(1), 78–89.

Bybee, J., & Zigler, E. (1998). Outerdirectedness in individuals with and without mental retardation: A review. In J. A. Burack, R. M. Hodapp, & E. Zigler (Eds.), *Handbook of mental retardation and development* (pp. 434–461). Cambridge/UK: Cambridge University Press.

Deci, E. L., & Ryan, R. M. (1994). Promoting self-determined education. *Scandinavian Journal of Educational Research, 38*(1), 3–14.

Deci, E. L., Koestner, R., & Ryan, R. M. (2001). Extrinsic rewards and intrinsic motivation in education: Reconsidered once again. *Review of Educational Research, 71*, 1–27.

Ellis, S., & Siegler, R. S. (1997). Planning as a strategy choice, or why don't children plan when they should? In S. L. Friedman & E. K. Scholnick (Eds.), *The developmental psychology of planning: Why, how, and when do we plan?* (pp. 183–208). Mahweh: Lawrence Erlbaum Associates.

Friedman, S. L., & Scholnick, E. K. (1997a). An evolving "blueprint" for planning: Psychological resquirements, task characteristics, and social-cultural inlfuences. In S. L. Friedman & E. K. Scholnick (Eds.), *The developmental psychology of planning: Why, how, and when do we plan?* (pp. 3–22). Mahweh: Lawrence Erlbaum Associates.

Friedman, S. L., & Scholnick, E. K. (1997b). *The developmental psychology of planning: Why, how, and when do we plan?* Mahweh: Lawrence Erlbaum Associates.

Gillet, N., Gagné, M., Sauvagère, S., & Fouquereau, E. (2013). The role of supervisor autonomy support, organizational support, and autonomous and controlled motivation in predicting employees' satisfaction and turnover intentions. *European Journal of Work and Organizational Psychology, 22*(4), 450–460. doi: http://dx.doi.org/10.1080/1359432X.2012.665228

Hortop, E. G., Wrosch, C., & Gagné, M. (2013). The why and how of goal pursuits: Effects of global autonomous motivation and perceived control on emotional well-being. *Motivation and Emotion, 37*(4), 675–687. doi: http://dx.doi.org/10.1007/s11031-013-9349-2

Hume, K., Loftin, R., & Lantz, J. (2009). Increasing independence in autism spectrum disorders: A review of three focused interventions. *Journal of Autism and Developmental Disorders, 39*(9), 1329–1338.

Koegel, R. L., Koegel, L. K., & McNerney, E. K. (2001). Pivotal areas in intervention for autism. *Journal of Clinical Child Psychology, 30*(1), 19–32.

Kreitler, S., & Kreitler, H. (1987). Conceptions and processes of planning: The developmental perspective. In S. L. Friedman, E. K. Scholnick, & R. R. Cocking (Eds.), *Blueprints for thinking; The role of planning in cognitive development* (pp. 205–272). Cambridge: Cambridge University Press.

Little, T. D., Hawley, P. H., Henrich, C. C., & Marsland, K. (2002). Three views of the agentic self: A developmental synthesis. In E. L. Deci & R. M. Ryan (Eds.), *Handbook of self-determination research* (pp. 389–404). Rochester/NY: University of Rochester Press.

MacMillan, D. L., & Cauffiel, S. R. (1977). Outerdirectedness as a function of success and failure in educationally handicapped boys. *Journal of Learning Disabilities, 10*(10), 643–654.

Masicampo, E. J., & Baumeister, R. F. (2011). Consider it done! Plan making can eliminate the cognitive effects of unfulfilled goals. *Journal of Personality and Social Psychology, 101*(4), 667–683.

Mouratidis, A., & Michou, A. (2011). Perfectionism, self-determined motivation, and coping among adolescent athletes. *Psychology of Sport and Exercise, 12*(4), 355–367. doi: http://dx.doi.org/10.1016/j.psychsport.2011.03.006

Munde, V., & Vlaskamp, C. (2015). Initiation of activities and alertness in individuals with profound intellectual and multiple disabilities. *Journal of Intellectual Disability Research, 59*(3), 284–292.

Niemiec, C. P., & Ryan, R. M. (2009). Autonomy, competence, and relatedness in the classroom: Applying self-determination theory to educational practice. *Theory and Research in Education, 7*(2), 133–144. doi:10.1177/1477878509104318.

Pan, Y., & Gauvain, M. (2012). The continuity of college students' autonomous learning motivation and its predictors: A three-year longitudinal study. *Learning and Individual Differences, 22*(1), 92–99. doi: http://dx.doi.org/10.1016/j.lindif.2011.11.010

Reilly, C., Hughes, C., Harvey, M., Brigham, N., Cosgriff, J., Kaplan, L., & Bernstein, R. (2014). "Let's Talk": Increasing novel peer-directed questions by high school students with autism to their general education peers. *Education and Training in Autism and Developmental Disabilities, 49*, 214–231.

Saebu, M., Sørensen, M., & Halvari, H. (2013). Motivation for physical activity in young adults with physical disabilities during a rehabilitation stay: A longitudinal test of self-determination theory. *Journal of Applied Social Psychology, 43*(3), 612–625. doi: http://dx.doi.org/10.1111/j.1559-1816.2013.01042.x

Seligman, M. E. P., Railton, P., Baumeister, R. F., & Sripada, C. (2013). Navigating into the future or driven by the past. *Perspectives on Psychological Science, 8*(2), 119–141. doi:10.1177/1745691612474317.

Shukla, S., Surratt, A. V., Horner, R. H., & Albin, R. W. (1995). Examining the relationship between self-initiations of an individual with disabilities and directive behavior of staff persons in a residential setting. *Behavioral Interventions, 10*(2), 101–110. doi: http://dx.doi.org/10.1002/bin.2360100206

Smith, K. A., Shepley, S. B., Alexander, J. L., & Ayres, K. M. (2015). The independent use of self-instructions for the acquisition of untrained multi-step tasks for individuals with an intellectual disability: A review of the literature. *Research in Developmental Disabilities, 40*, 19–30. doi:10.1901/jaba.1980.13-119.

Ward, G., & Morris, R. (2005). Introduction to the psychology of planning. In R. Morris & G. Ward (Eds.), *The cognitive psychology of planning* (pp. 1–35). New York: Taylor & Francis.

Part V
The Development of Agentic Action

Synthesis

Essential characteristics of causal agency theory (and, as such, causal action) involve volitional action, agentic action, and action-control beliefs. This part examines the development of skills that are critical to agentic action; that is, the skills needed to sustain action toward and to achieve a goal. Chapter 17 examines the role of self-regulation in self-determination, explores the uses of the self-regulation construct in psychology, and examines how theories of self-regulation relate to and differ from self-determination and, specifically, Self-Determination Theory. The chapter also examines a continuum of regulation 'types' that range from extrinsically-motivated to intrinsically and autonomously motivated, then concludes with a discussion of the development of self-regulation across multiple age spans. Chapter 18 describes the role of goal setting and attainment in agentic action and Causal Agency Theory, as well as research on the development of goal setting and attainment. The role of self-regulated problem-solving skills in the development of agentic capacities is discussed, as is the relationship of goal setting and attainment to valued outcomes. Chapter 19 reviews the role of problem solving in agentic action and Causal Agency Theory. It also describes the role of autonomous motivation, as defined by Self-Determination Theory in problem solving. The literature on the development of problem solving, interventions to promote problem solving skills, and the linkages between problem solving and valued outcomes is reviewed. Another process critical to agentic action and, thus, causal agency, involves making a decision. Developmentally, the emergence of decision-making capacity occurs in early adolescence, on the heels of the development of problem-solving skills. Like problem solving, decision making is undertaken by agentic people in service of a goal. Chapter 20 explores in greater depth what is meant by the term decision (and by a decision-making process), how decision making is situated within SDT and Causal Agency Theory, and the relationship (again within SDT and Causal Agency Theory) between decision making and autonomy. The development of decision-making skills is discussed. The chapter concludes by discussing the decision-making process and autonomy-supportive interventions to promote more effective decision making. Pathways thinking and agency thinking are critical elements of Hope Theory, and Chap. 21 concludes the section on the development of agentic action by examining the role of hope, and Hope Theory, in the development of self-determination. The chapter begins with an overview of Hope Theory, followed by an examination of the development of hopeful thought and hope. Next, the chapter discusses measurement and the Hope Scale. The chapter concludes with a review of the literature in hope and by exploring interventions to promote hope and linkages between hope and Causal Agency Theory.

Chapter 17
A Self-Determination Perspective on Self-Regulation across the Life Span

G. John Geldhof, Meghann L. Fenn, and Jennifer K. Finders

Abstract As a core component of human functioning, self-regulation has persisted as a focus of psychological inquiry since the field's inception. The study of self-regulation plays a central role in understanding the development of self-determination, particularly within the context of initiating and sustaining agentic action. This chapter examines the role of self-regulation in self-determination, explores uses of the self-regulation construct in psychology, and examines how theories of self-regulation relate to and differ from self-determination and, specifically, Self-Determination Theory. The chapter examines a continuum of regulation 'types' that range from extrinsically motivated to intrinsically and autonomously motivated, then concludes with a discussion of the development of self-regulation across multiple age spans.

As a core component of human functioning, self-regulation has persisted as a focus of psychological inquiry since the field's inception. Aspects of self-regulation can be found in some of psychology's earliest writings (e.g., Freud 1923/1961; James 1890). These issues motivated research during the neo-positivist era (e.g., Skinner 1953), were critical during the cognitive revolution (see also Freund 2001), and lie at the heart of contemporary theories of human development (e.g., Gestsdottir and Lerner 2008; McClelland et al. 2015). So too does the study of self-regulation play a central role in understanding the development of self-determination, particularly within the context of initiating and sustaining agentic action. As noted in previous chapters, when acting agentically, action is self-regulated, self-directed, and enables progress toward freely chosen goals. Goal setting and attainment are discussed in the following chapter.

G.J. Geldhof (✉) • M.L. Fenn • J.K. Finders
Oregon State University, Corvallis, OR, USA
e-mail: John.Geldhof@oregonstate.edu

M.L. Wehmeyer et al. (eds.), *Development of Self-Determination Through the Life-Course*, DOI 10.1007/978-94-024-1042-6_17

Defining Self-Regulation

Despite its long history in psychological research, the study of self-regulation remains disorganized at best. Scholars from diverse sub-disciplines use the same terms to refer to different processes, use different terms to describe the same processes, and even conceptualize self-regulation as comprising completely different components. Only a few threads unite the field, meaning most theorists would only agree to broad generalizations when describing self-regulated actions. For instance, a majority of psychologists would acknowledge that self-regulation promotes goal attainment (regardless of whether the goals are consciously selected, see Bargh et al. 2001).

Viewing self-regulation through the lens of self-determination therefore requires a broad definition of self-regulated action within which one can frame self-determined action. For instance, Gestsdottir and Lerner (2008) define self-regulation from a developmental systems perspective. They assert that development occurs through bidirectional causal interactions between individuals and their contexts (represented as person ←→ context relations). These interactions form the rules (regulations) of development and are accordingly called developmental regulations (Brandtstädter 1998). Self-regulation is then defined as the individual's impact on developmental regulations (Gestsdottir and Lerner 2008).

Defining self-regulation as the person → context component of person ←→context processes leaves considerable room for both agentic and non-agentic behaviors. Indeed, Gestsdottir and Lerner (2008) further parse self-regulation into organismic and intentional components. Organismic self-regulation includes, "broad, consistent attributes of a person that involve biologically based, physiological structures," (p. 204), whereas intentional self-regulation represents, "contextualized actions that are actively aimed towards harmonizing demands and resources in the context with personal goals" (p. 204). Intentional self-regulation thus comprises a wide swath of an individual's actions, ranging from fully conscious actions to automized behaviors.

Despite the breadth of self-regulation as a concept, Little et al. (2006, p. 67) noted that, "self-determination is a function of self-regulated agentic action." Unsurprisingly, theories of self-determination therefore share many similarities with contemporary theories of self-regulation. The complementarity between the literatures surrounding self-regulation and self-determination indicates that understanding how these concepts promote adaptive development also requires an understanding of their synthesis. In the present chapter we frame a discussion of this synthesis by asking two questions. We first ask, "How do theories of self-regulation relate to self-determination (and, specifically, Self-Determination Theory)?" Using the parallels between self-regulation and SDT as a starting point, we then ask, "What can the development of self-regulation tell us about self-determination?"

Self-Regulation and Self-Determination Theory

The organismic roots of Self-Determination Theory (SDT; Deci and Ryan 1991) strongly reflect the importance of person ←→ context interactions. Rather than viewing self-determined action as a direct and additive function of associative bonds (e.g., operant conditioning, strictly additive gene x environment interactions), self-determined actions must be truly agentic. They reflect the "inherent tendency of organisms to originate behavior, to relate to and assimilate events, and to gain a sense of effectance," (Deci and Ryan 1991, p. 251). Agency therefore develops through repeated person ←→ context interactions and mirrors the definition of intentional self-regulation presented above. Agentic actions require, "conscious or preconscious formulation[s] about some future behavior or outcome the person will attempt to perform or achieve," (Deci and Ryan 1991, p. 247).

The literature on intentional self-regulation typically focuses on processes that facilitate goal attainment (e.g., goal selection, goal pursuit strategies, strategies for accommodating unexpected events or failures) (see Chap. 18), whereas SDT describes the role of internal vs. external factors in motivating regulation. This elaboration, called Organismic Integration Theory (Deci and Ryan 1985), results in the continuum of regulation 'types' presented in Fig. 17.1. At the far left of this continuum we see non-regulated actions—actions that the self has little or no role in. Non-regulated actions are not motivated by internal or external factors and therefore represent actions done without a specific purpose (e.g., learned helplessness) or an event that has happened *to* an individual. For instance, Deci and Ryan (1991) use the example of a person being pushed from behind. Non-regulated actions thus fall outside the definition of self-regulation presented above. These actions are neither intentional, nor are they driven by organismic, biological factors. By definition, such actions are also not self-determined.

The next type of regulation in Fig. 17.1, external regulation, represents actions driven by factors entirely outside the self. Externally regulated actions are extrinsically motivated (i.e., are directly contingent on rewards or punishments offered by others) and have a strictly external perceived locus of causality. That is, individuals

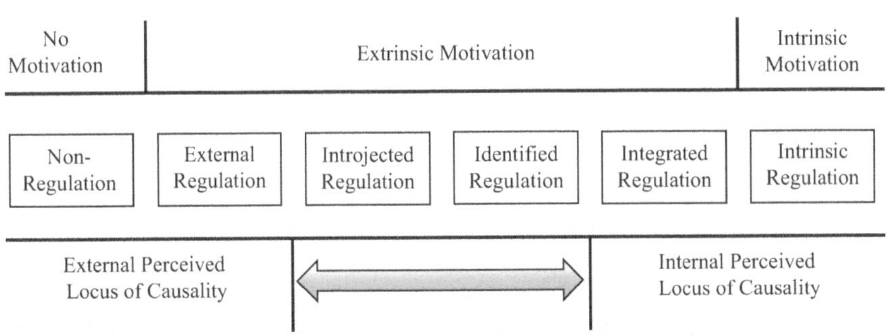

Fig. 17.1 Levels of self-regulation arranged according to their degrees of self-determination (Adapted from Figure 1 in Ryan and Deci 2000)

see the direct cause of externally regulated actions as being outside of themselves. External regulation qualifies as a form of intentional self-regulation, although the externally regulated actions are decidedly non-agentic.

The next level of self-regulation is introjected regulation. Introjected regulation represents actions that individuals perform strictly due to self-administered rewards or punishments (e.g., allowing oneself to go fishing after writing a certain number of pages, feelings of pride or shame). Although still extrinsically motivated, individuals perceive a slightly internal locus of causality when performing introjectedly regulated actions. Introjected regulation requires that the individual has at least partially internalized relevant motivations (e.g., individuals who follow a norm, but only because they are 'supposed to'). Introjected regulation therefore also qualifies as a kind of intentional self-regulation, as do all forms of regulation discussed in the remainder of this section.

Introjected regulation only requires an individual to internalize an action or motivation. Identified regulation, the next level of self-regulation presented in Fig. 17.1, instead requires that an action aligns with personally-valued goals. As indicated by the arrow in Fig. 17.1, identified regulation encompasses a more internal perceived locus of causality than introjected regulation, although both types of behavior are motivated by reward or punishment.

The next form of regulation, integrated regulation, occurs when an individual integrates the importance of an action with other valued aspects of his or her self. Integrated regulation remains motivated by goals, but such actions reflect and are wholly consistent with one's core beliefs. As such, individuals perceive integrated regulation as arising from a fully internal locus of causality. Individuals believe that integrated regulation is motivated by their own wishes and desires. Integrated regulation therefore closely resembles stereotypical definitions of self-regulation (e.g., selecting a goal and seeing it through to completion).

Intrinsic regulation is the last form of regulation specified by Deci and Ryan's (1985) Organismic Integration Theory. Intrinsically regulated behaviors are both intrinsically motivated (i.e., self-rewarding) and have an internal locus of causality. Thus, intrinsic regulation presents something of a conundrum for theories of self-regulation. Although intrinsic regulation fits nicely under the umbrella of intentional self-regulation, it does not require the degree of effort often associated with self-regulated actions. For instance, Baumeister and colleagues (e.g., Baumeister and Heatherton 1996) describe self-regulation as a limited resource. Self-regulation requires effort, and engaging in self-regulation therefore depletes one's energy. Intrinsic regulation may actually increase vitality, however (see Deci and Ryan 2008 for a discussion).

Intrinsic regulation has been associated with adaptive outcomes (Ng et al. 2012; Van Petegem et al. 2012). By providing additional elaboration to the concept of intentional self-regulation, the self-determination perspective may therefore be especially useful for understanding the associations between self-regulation and adaptive functioning across the life span—a unifying thread across many self-regulation theories. Optimally leveraging the links between self-determination and self-regulation requires an understanding of their joint development, however, and we turn to this topic next.

Development of Self-Regulation

Previous chapters provided an overview of developmental aspects of self-determination more globally from childhood through late adulthood. This chapter looks more closely at the developmental perspectives of self-regulation in each of these periods. From a developmental perspective, aspects of organismic regulation are especially relevant during infancy and early childhood. Intentional self-regulation becomes increasingly important from middle childhood through adolescence and maintains its importance throughout adulthood. For example, studies of children's self-regulation often emphasize emotion regulation (Eisenberg et al. 1996) or executive functioning (McClelland et al. 2007). By adolescence, self-regulation researchers focus instead on the increasing relevance of distal goals (Moilanen 2007; Nurmi 1991; Salmela-Aro et al. 2007) and begin to describe intentional self-regulation in the terms used to discuss adult-like functioning (e.g., Baltes and colleagues' Selection, Optimization, and Compensation model; see Baltes et al. 1999; Gestsdottir and Lerner 2008).

A similar transition during adolescence is reflected in the self-determination literature. Heller et al. (2011) note that "children are not seen as 'self-determined'—they are not yet developmentally or emotionally capable of acting autonomously and regulating behavior." (p. 32). Simultaneously, intrinsic motivations may be less common as children mature and become increasingly swayed by their peers during adolescence. Thus, the development of both self-regulation and self-determination are related but not fully yoked. The remainder of this chapter describes the development of self-regulation across the life course and explicates congruencies between self-regulation and self-determination during key developmental periods.

Childhood: Emergence of Self-Related Processes

From birth onward, human beings are active, inquisitive, curious, and playful. They even exhibit these characteristics in the absence of specific rewards (e.g., Harter 1978). Despite these seemingly in-born tendencies, however, decades of research suggests that the environment must support such behaviors in order for individuals to thrive. Infants and young children are not equipped to exhibit truly self-determined behaviors (Heller et al. 2011), meaning the context plays an especially important role in determining self-regulation during these periods. In particular, one can consider the conditions that elicit and sustain self-regulation in early childhood, and how early experiences act as precursors to goal-directed actions in middle childhood. In this section we therefore describe processes of organismic self-regulation in infancy, the progression from extrinsic to intrinsic motivation during early childhood, and how self-regulated behaviors become internalized throughout middle childhood. This progression allows older children to exhibit increasing autonomy and, eventually, supports the emergence of self-determined actions.

Infancy researchers often examine self-regulation in terms of temperament, which represents a unification of the cognitive and emotional aspects of development (Wolfe and Bell 2007). Individual differences in temperament are understood as differences in biologically based tendencies, such as emotional reactivity (e.g. arousal), as well as the regulation of this reactivity through behavioral strategies (e.g. executive attention; Posner and Rothbart 2000). As newborns transition from simple arousal to greater attentional control during the first few years of life, they develop an increased capacity for emotion regulation (Sheese et al. 2008), or the ability to appropriately regulate emotions and behaviors influenced by emotional reactions (Bridges et al. 2004).

Children's actions tend to become more internalized, or self-regulated, over time (e.g., Chandler and Connell 1987). Although still exogenously driven, the actions of infants between 12 and 18 months reflect increasing awareness of social demands, and the ability to initiate, maintain, and cease behavior to comply with caregivers' requests. By 24 months, children acquire endogenous (i.e., intrinsically motivated) self-control, even in the absence of external monitors (Kochanska et al. 2001). In other words, the development of executive attention supports the transition from primarily extrinsic toward primarily intrinsic sources of control, where the locus of causality becomes increasingly internal.

Attention and emotion regulation continue to develop throughout infancy and are highly related to the emergence of the executive functions in early childhood (Cuevas and Bell 2014), allowing self-regulation to emerge by around 36 months. Specifically, executive functions such as inhibitory control (the ability to stop an automatic response in favor of a more adaptive behavior), working memory (holding multiple rules in mind), and attentional/cognitive flexibility (focusing on a task while simultaneously ignoring distractions), likely underlie self-regulated behaviors during this period. These cognitive processes enable rudimentary forms of the future oriented, goal directed behaviors that allow children to become active producers of their own development (e.g., planning, organization, and regulation). Together, top-down (executive functions) and bottom-up (temperamental and socioemotional) processes become integral aspects children's self-regulated functioning (Ursache et al. 2012).

The integration of top-down and bottom-up processes lays the foundation for autonomy and adaptive development. For instance, Mischel and colleagues (e.g., Mischel et al. 1989) have shown that children capable of distracting their attention away from visually salient rewards, and therefore capable of delaying gratification longer than their peers, displayed greater academic achievement 10 years later. In a more recent study, researchers found that children rated as having strong attention and persistence at age 4 had nearly 50% greater odds of completing college by age 25 (McClelland et al. 2013). Thus, evidence from a variety of perspectives, including

SDT, converges on the conclusion that intrinsic motivation and self-regulation are associated with adaptive outcomes.

The development of self-regulation during childhood equips children to better differentiate self from other, thus facilitating the ability to differentiate between internal versus external loci of causality (see also Geldhof and Little 2011). In terms of self-determination, the developmental processes that support autonomous functioning facilitate self-determined, rather than extrinsically controlled, actions. Children who fail to develop self-regulation skills may remain controlled by external contingencies, which can in turn foster the development of an external perceived locus of causality. When individuals perceive that their actions are controlled by extrinsic processes, regulatory process becomes more aligned with compliance (Deci and Ryan 1991) than with self-regulation.

Furthermore, children's motivation, performance, and development can be maximized by contexts that provide opportunities to satisfy their innate needs for competence, relatedness, and autonomy. In particular, opportunities to satisfy the need for autonomy serve a fundamental role in ensuring that individuals develop endogenous, rather than exogenous, control (Deci et al. 1991), which they can then carry forward into later stages of development. For example, children will have difficulty developing greater levels of self-determination during adolescence unless their early socialization and educational experiences lay a solid foundation upon which to build more sophisticated skills and capacities. An emphasis on intrinsic goals during childhood may therefore serve an important role in supporting adaptive development across the life span.

Adolescence and Early Adulthood: Establishing Autonomy

The self-regulatory skills forged during childhood must be honed and refined during the second decade. Adolescents face novel contexts that both challenge the skills they developed as children and also prepare them for autonomous functioning during adulthood. Thus, the development of self-regulation during adolescence requires a diverse array of internal skills as well as myriad contextual supports that facilitate the autonomous application of those skills.

Through increasingly complex person ←→ context interactions, adolescents develop a nuanced repertoire of self-regulation skills that facilitate their own self-development. For instance, Gestsdottir and colleagues (e.g., Gestsdottir and Lerner 2008) note that adolescents develop the processes of adult-like self-regulation specified by the Selection, Optimization, Compensation (SOC) model (Freund and Baltes 2000). According to this model, self-regulated actions can be parsimoniously clustered into three categories. *Selection* occurs when an individual chooses an attainable goal to pursue, either as a result of increased capacity (elective selection) or in reaction to the loss of a previously held capacity (loss-based selection). *Optimization* occurs when individuals perform actions that move them iteratively closer to a selected goal (e.g., practice, actual goal-directed actions). *Compensation* occurs when one approach to goal attainment is blocked and an alternative means must be implemented.

The processes of selection, optimization, and compensation align closely with the concept of Intentional Self-Regulation (Gestsdottir and Lerner 2008), and therefore share many features associated with self-determination. For instance, implementation of the SOC processes assumes a degree of agency and allows for an increased ability to direct one's own developmental trajectory. Often called developmental regulation (Hekhausen et al. 2010), the ability to be an active and intentional producer of one's own development lies at the heart of Intentional Self-Regulation. In this respect, successful self-regulation during adolescence requires increasing awareness of one's long-term self and an explicit orientation toward distal goals. Future orientation (Moilanen 2007; Nurmi 1991; Salmela-Aro et al. 2007) and hope for one's future (Schmid et al. 2011) play especially important roles during adolescence and also likely motivate self-determined actions during this period.

Although adolescents as a whole are capable of substantially more complex self-regulation than children, this complexity does not translate directly into capabilities for self-determination. The development of self-determination during adolescence requires appropriate scaffolding from important parental and non-parental adults. For instance, adolescents with positive adult role models and supportive parental attachments exhibit more positive developmental trajectories (Bowers et al. 2011, 2014). Furthermore, we cannot expect adolescents to display uniformly self-determined actions, nor would it be adaptive for them to do so. In one study, youth who were allowed to exercise autonomy at too early an age showed setbacks in later adolescence and early adulthood (Haase et al. 2008). Too much autonomy at too young an age can stunt the development of self-determination and prevent a successful transition into adult life.

Society instead allots certain freedoms that help young people solidify their identities as independent and autonomous agents. External controls, such as the structure provided by families and schools, are slowly removed and individuals must increasingly rely on intrinsically motivated self-regulation in order to thrive. As such, individuals are given greater leverage to control their behaviors and emotions during the transition into adulthood.

From the perspective of self-regulation, the transition into adulthood therefore necessitates further refinement and application of self-regulatory processes established during adolescence. For instance, the skills learned during adolescence, in conjunction with the autonomy allotted by adult independence, allow individuals to begin planning for long-term accomplishments. Young adults often select and pursue goals related to obtaining a higher education, establishing themselves in a career, and starting a family. Selecting and pursuing these goals over extended periods requires the continued refinement and application of advanced self-regulatory skills, such as those described by the SOC model, and also has implications for the types of behaviors that become self-determined during the transition to adulthood.

Adulthood and Aging: Skill Refinement and Performance Maintenance

Adaptive functioning during adulthood, especially during the third and fourth decades, provides a benchmark for research on self-regulation and its development across the life span. The development of self-regulation from birth through early adulthood unfolds as a nearly teleological journey beginning with a purely reactive biological system and culminating in the complex biopsychosocial processes we call 'adult-like functioning.' The adult-like system is not only self-aware and self-regulating, but it is also capable of selecting and striving for distal goals that can extend even beyond the individual's own lifetime (e.g., generativity). The development of self-regulation from midlife through old age is then typically treated in one of two respects. Research on self-regulation in later life often examines why older adults regulate their behavior toward different goals than their younger counterparts (e.g., Carstensen et al. 1999) or emphasizes the processes that older adults use to maintain their 'adult-like' functioning. For instance, Baltes and colleagues (e.g., Baltes et al. 2006) discuss how the development of crystallized, pragmatic skills support adaptive functioning despite declines in fluid, mechanic abilities.

The importance of self-regulation throughout the life span, coupled with the perception that its development apexes during adulthood, has resulted in myriad theoretical perspectives of adult-like self-regulation. For instance, action theories comprise just one segment of the self-regulation literature, and the diversity of action-theoretical perspectives alone has justified models meant to assist their organization (Brandtstädter 2006; see also Geldhof et al. 2010).

Perhaps as a result of their diversity, theories of adult-like self-regulation are not uniformly aligned with theories of self-determination. As noted above, for instance, self-determined actions may increase vitality, whereas limited resource models of self-regulation hypothesize that self-regulated actions should instead deplete one's energy stores (see Deci and Ryan 2008). One can only rectify these opposing hypotheses (and the empirical support for each) by emphasizing the non-equivalence of self-regulation and self-determination at any stage of the life span.

Despite these differences, models of self-determination and self-regulation during adulthood converge to acknowledge the importance of autonomous action across all periods of the life span. For instance, now-classic research highlights the importance of aligning older adults' level of self-determination motivation with their opportunities for self-determined action (O'Connor and Vallerand 1994). It is therefore not surprising that developmental theories of self-regulation that focus most explicitly on autonomous self-development also tend to align with the self-determination literature. We have already described one such model of adult-like self-regulation (Baltes and colleagues' SOC model), and briefly summarize two additional models below. These models explicitly highlight the two general approaches to self-regulation and its development during late life described earlier in this section.

Carstensen and colleagues' Socioemotional Selectivity Theory (e.g., 1999) describes how an individual's time perspective can moderate the target of self-regulated actions. In short, Socioemotional Selectivity Theory emphasizes that individuals focused on their own distal futures will select social goals that emphasize knowledge acquisition. Individuals with a truncated time orientation will instead select social goals that emphasize emotion regulation. For instance, an individual who expects to live long into the future may be motivated to meet a diverse set of acquaintances who introduce the individual to novel experiences. An older individual (who accordingly has a shorter life expectancy) is more likely to focus his or her efforts on nurturing relationships with close friends and relatives. In this way, we can anticipate that self-determined actions will typically favor skill attainment and knowledge acquisition during early adulthood and midlife (see also Morgan and Robinson 2013). Such goals will facilitate the individual's long-term self-development. Toward the end of the life span, however, we can anticipate that self-determined actions will emphasize emotion-related goals, such as deepening close social ties.

Aside from suggesting how self-determination may manifest across adulthood, it is worth noting that the theoretical foundations of Socioemotional Selectivity Theory parallel many assumptions of SDT. For instance, Carstensen et al. (1999) note three assumptions that underlie their theory. The first two of these assumptions center on the fact that humans are intrinsically driven to establish social relationships and to establish agency. These assumptions reflect the relatedness and autonomy needs described in the self-determination literature and the importance of agency as discussed above. Carstensen et al. (1999) also assume that goal selection is a precursor to action. This assumption parallels the above discussion of how goal preferences can influence which actions are most likely to be self-determined during which age period while also mirroring the fact that goal selection serves an important function in models of intentional self-development (e.g., SOC).

The second model of adult-like self-regulation we will discuss in this section, the Motivational Theory of Life-Span Development (Heckhausen et al. 2010), provides an exemplary model that simultaneously emphasizes intentional self-development and the maintenance of functioning during the decline in self-regulatory skills that occurs during late life. Although space limitations prohibit a complete description of this model, the concepts of primary and secondary control (see also Brandtstädter and Renner 1990) form key components of this model and are especially relevant for self-determination. Primary control represents an individual's ability to actively shape the context in ways that promote goal attainment. Secondary control represents an individual's thoughts or actions that change internal perceptions and/or motivations.

Each type of control can be further decomposed into selective and compensatory components. Selective primary control involves persistent goal pursuit, whereas compensatory primary control requires that an individual finds alternative means to reach a selected goal (e.g., eliciting help from a friend). Selective secondary control involves cognitive and motivational processes that facilitate goal pursuit (e.g., enhancing one's motivation), whereas compensatory secondary control may manifest as the disengagement of difficult-to-attain goals (see also Wrosch et al. 2003).

According to this model, individuals intrinsically strive for primary control throughout the life span. One's actual capacity for primary control waxes from childhood until adulthood and wanes into late life, however. Secondary control may therefore become especially important for supporting primary control and for maintaining a sense of autonomous efficacy in old age. From a self-determination perspective, the emphasis on primary control aligns with the need for autonomy while also reflecting the importance of agency for self-determination.

Combined, theories such as Socioemotional Selectivity Theory and the Motivational Theory of Life-Span Development highlight the possible degree of correspondence between theories of self-regulation during adulthood and concepts central to self-determination perspectives. This alignment is especially strong for self-regulation models that emphasize intentional self-development, which has been a running theme throughout this chapter. Although self-regulation has established a substantially firmer foothold in the child development literature when compared to the adult development literature, this alignment suggests that further attempts to align self-determination perspectives with theories of intentional self-development during adulthood may prove especially useful.

Self-Regulation, Causal Capability, and Causal Action

Figure 5.2 (Chap. 5) highlighted the causal action sequence involving the implementation of causal and agentic capabilities. Agentic individuals possess various capabilities that enable them to respond to challenges and opportunities in the environment. Two types of capabilities are important to causal action: causal capability and agentic capability. These capabilities differentiate between two aspects of goal-focused actions: (a) initiating goal pursuit (causal capability) and (b) directing actions toward a preferred end (agentic capability). Causal capability includes the knowledge, skills, self-perceptions, and beliefs about one's environment that enable the expression of causal action. Agentic capabilities involve the mental or physical capacities to direct behavior toward an end. Such capacities include the skills and knowledge associated with self-management, goal attainment, problem solving, and self-advocacy; the skills and behaviors that enable self-regulation, self-direction, pathways thinking and, as such, agentic action. Agentic capability enables one to identify pathways and manage the steps toward goal attainment. As discussed in Chap. 5 (and depicted in Fig. 5.2), the outcome of the capacity-challenge discrepancy analysis in which causal capacity to solve the goal discrepancy problem is evaluated, and appropriate agentic actions utilizing agentic capabilities that maximize the relationship between capacities and challenges by creating a "just-right match" between capacity and challenge to optimize the probability of solving the goal discrepancy problem, is a discrepancy reduction plan, in which self-regulation plays a significant role.

As the person implements this discrepancy reduction plan and after time has passed, uses information derived from self-monitoring to self-evaluate progress toward reducing the discrepancy between current and goal status. If progress is satisfactory, the person will continue implementing the discrepancy reduction plan. If not, the person either reconsiders the discrepancy reduction plan and modifies that or returns to the goal generation process to re-examine the goal and its priority and, possibly, cycle through the process with a revised or new goal.

Conclusions

Contemporary research suggests that thriving during any period of the life span is associated with both self-regulation and self-determination. The self-regulation and self-determination literatures emphasize slightly different aspects of human functioning, however. These literatures are therefore well-poised to provide complementary insights into successful human development. To this end, the present chapter attempted to address two broad questions.

First, we asked "How do theories of self-regulation relate to self-determination?" In response, we highlighted the meta-theoretical similarities between contemporary theories related to each concept and paid especially close attention to Gestsdottir and Lerner's (2008) definition of self-regulation. According to this definition, self-regulation represents the person → context component of mutually influential person ← → context relations. We then emphasized the parallels between agency and the process that Gestsdottir and Lerner (2008) called Intentional Self-Regulation. This discussion highlighted differences between definitions of self-determination and self-regulation. We described how theories of self-regulation typically focus on goal-directed actions, whereas theories of self-determination are more strongly concerned with (perceived) internal vs. external loci of causality.

We next asked "What can the development of self-regulation tell us about self-determination?" In response, we presented a bird's eye summary of self-regulation and its development, highlighting areas where the development of self-regulation is especially relevant to understanding self-determination. We described the transition from extrinsic to intrinsic control during childhood, the resulting importance of executive functioning for children's self-regulation, and the increasing reliance on diverse, future-oriented self-regulation skills during adolescence and adulthood. We then noted a particular alignment between theories of self-determination and theories self-regulation that center on intentional self-development. Finally, we described how self-regulation plays a critical role in agentic capacity and goal attainment, contributing to experiences of causal action and, ultimately, self-determination.

References

Baltes, P. B., Staudinger, U. M., & Lindenberger, U. (1999). Lifespan psychology: Theory and application to intellectual functioning. *Annual Review of Psychology, 50*, 471–507.

Baltes, P. B., Lindenberger, U., & Staudinger, U. M. (2006). Life-span theory in developmental psychology. In W. Damon & R. M. Lerner (Eds.), *Handbook of child psychology: Theoretical models of human development* (6th ed., pp. 569–664). New York: Wiley.

Bargh, J. A., Lee-Chai, A., Barndollar, K., Gollwitzer, P. M., & Trötschel, R. (2001). The automated will: Nonconscious activation and pursuit of behavioral goals. *Journal of Personality and Social Psychology, 81*, 1014–1027.

Baumeister, R. F., & Heatherton, T. F. (1996). Self-regulation failure: An overview. *Psychological Inquiry, 7*, 1–15.

Bowers, E. P., Gestsdottir, S., Geldhof, G. J., Nikitin, J., von Eye, A., & Lerner, R. M. (2011). Developmental trajectories of intentional self regulation in adolescence: The role of parenting and implications for positive and problematic outcomes among diverse youth. *Journal of Adolescence, 34*, 1193–1206.

Bowers, E. P., Johnson, S. K., Buckingham, M. H., Gasca, S., Warren, D. J., Lerner, J. V., & Lerner, R. M. (2014). Important non-parental adults and positive youth development across mid-to late-adolescence: The moderating effect of parenting profiles. *Journal of Youth and Adolescence, 43*, 897–918.

Brandstädter, J. (1998). Action perspectives on human development. In W. Damon (Series Ed.), & R. Lerner (Vol. Ed.), *Handbook of child psychology: Vol. 1. Theoretical models of human development* (pp. 1029–1144). New York: Wiley.

Brandtstädter, J. (2006). Action perspectives on human development. In W. Damon (Editor-in-Chief) & R. Lerner (Vol. Ed.), *Handbook of child psychology: Vol. 1. Theoretical models of human development* (5th edn., pp. 516–568). Hoboken: Wiley.

Brandtstädter, J., & Renner, G. (1990). Tenacious goal pursuit and flexible goal adjustment: Explication and age-related analysis of assimilative and accommodative strategies of coping. *Psychology and Aging, 5*, 58–67.

Bridges, L. J., Denham, S. A., & Ganiban, J. M. (2004). Definitional issues in emotion regulation research. *Child Development, 75*, 340–345.

Carstensen, L. L., Isaacowitz, D. M., & Charles, S. T. (1999). Taking time seriously: A theory of socioemotional selectivity. *American Psychologist, 54*, 165–181.

Chandler, C. L., & Connell, J. P. (1987). Children's intrinsic, extrinsic and internalized motivation: A developmental study of children's reasons for liked and disliked behaviours. *British Journal of Developmental Psychology, 5*, 357–365.

Cuevas, K., & Bell, M. A. (2014). Infant attention and early childhood executive function. *Child Development, 85*, 397–404.

Deci, E. L., & Ryan, R. M. (1985). The general causality orientations scale: Self-determination in personality. *Journal of Research in Personality, 19*, 109–134.

Deci, E. L., & Ryan, R. M. (1991). A motivational approach to self: Integration in personality. In R. Dienstbier (Ed.), *Nebraska symposium on motivation: Vol. 38. Perspectives on motivation* (pp. 237–288). Lincoln: University of Nebraska Press.

Deci, E. L., & Ryan, R. M. (2008). Self-determination theory: A macrotheory of human motivation, development, and health. *Canadian Psychology/Psychologie Canadienne, 49*, 182–185.

Deci, E. L., Vallerand, R. J., Pelletier, L. G., & Ryan, R. M. (1991). Motivation and education: The self determination perspective. *Educational Psychologist, 26*, 325–346.

Eisenberg, N., Fabes, R. A., Guthrie, I. K., Murphy, B. C., Maszk, P., Holmgren, R., & Suh, K. (1996). The relations of regulation and emotionality to problem behavior in elementary school children. *Development and Psychopathology, 8*, 141–162.

Freud, S. (1923/1961). *The ego and the id*. New York: Norton.

Freund, A. M. (2001). Developmental psychology of life-management. In N. J. Smelser & P. B. Baltes (Eds.), *International encyclopedia of the social & behavioral sciences* (Vol. 13, pp. 8827–8832). Oxford: Elsevier Science.

Freund, A. M., & Baltes, P. B. (2000). The orchestration of selection, optimization, and compensation: An action-theoretical conceptualization of a theory of developmental regulation. In W. J. Perrig & A. Grob (Eds.), *Control of human behavior, mental processes and consciousness: Essays in honor of the 60th birthday of August Flammer* (pp. 35–58). New York: Erlbaum.

Geldhof, G. J., & Little, T. D. (2011). Influences of children's and adolescents' action-control processes on school achievement, peer relationships, and coping with challenging life events. *New Directions for Child and Adolescent Development, 2011*(133), 45–59.

Geldhof, G. J., Little, T. D., & Colombo, J. (2010). Self-regulation across the lifespan. In R. M. Lerner (Editor-in-Chief), and M. E. Lamb, & A. M. Freund (Vol. Eds.). *Social and emotional development. Volume 2 of the handbook of lifespan development* (pp. 116–157). Hoboken: Wiley.

Gestsdottir, S., & Lerner, R. M. (2008). Positive development in adolescence: The development and role of intentional self-regulation. *Human Development, 51*, 202–224.

Haase, C. M., Tomasik, M. J., & Silbereisen, R. K. (2008). Premature behavioral autonomy: Correlates in late adolescence and young adulthood. *European Psychologist, 13*, 255–266.

Harter, S. (1978). Effectance motivation reconsidered: Toward a developmental model. *Human Development, 21*, 34–64.

Hekhausen, J., Wrosch, C., & Schulz, R. (2010). A motivational theory of life-span development. *Psychological Review, 117*, 32–60.

Heller, T., Schindler, A., Palmer, S. B., Wehmeyer, M. L., Parent, W., Jenson, R., et al. (2011). Self-determination across the life span: Issues and gaps. *Exceptionality, 19*, 31–45.

James, W. (1890). *The principles of psychology*. New York: Henry Holt and Company.

Kochanska, G., Coy, K. C., & Murray, K. T. (2001). The development of self-regulation in the first four years of life. *Child Development, 72*, 1091–1111.

Little, T. D., Snyder, C. R., & Wehmeyer, M. (2006). The agentic self: On the nature and origins of personal agency across the lifespan. In D. Mroczek & T. D. Little (Eds.), *The handbook of personality development* (pp. 61–79). Mahwah: Lawrence Erlbaum and Associates.

McClelland, M. M., Cameron, C. E., Wanless, S. B., & Murray, A. (2007). Executive function, behavioral self-regulation, and social-emotional competence. *Contemporary Perspectives on Social Learning in Early Childhood Education, 1*, 113–137.

McClelland, M. M., Acock, A. C., Piccinin, A., Rhea, S. A., & Stallings, M. C. (2013). Relations between preschool attention span-persistence and age 25 educational outcomes. *Early Childhood Research Quarterly, 28*, 314–324.

McClelland, M. M., Geldhof, J. G., Cameron, C. E., & Wanless, S. B. (2015). Development and self-regulation. In R. M. Lerner, W. F. Overton, & P. C. M. Molenaar (Eds.), *Handbook of child psychology and developmental science, theory and method* (pp. 523–565). Hoboken: Wiley.

Mischel, W., Shoda, Y., & Rodriguez, M. I. (1989). Delay of gratification in children. *Science, 244*, 933–938.

Moilanen, K. L. (2007). The adolescent self-regulatory inventory: The development and validation of a questionnaire of short-term and long-term self-regulation. *Journal of Youth and Adolescence, 36*, 835–848.

Morgan, J., & Robinson, O. (2013). Intrinsic aspirations and personal meaning across adulthood: Conceptual interrelations and age/sex differences. *Developmental Psychology, 49*, 999–1010.

Ng, J. Y., Ntoumanis, N., Thøgersen-Ntoumani, C., Deci, E. L., Ryan, R. M., Duda, J. L., & Williams, G. C. (2012). Self-determination theory applied to health contexts a meta-analysis. *Perspectives on Psychological Science, 7*, 325–340.

Nurmi, J. E. (1991). How do adolescents see their future? A review of the development of future orientation and planning. *Developmental Review, 11*, 1–59.

O'Connor, B. P., & Vallerand, R. J. (1994). Motivation, self-determination, and person-environment fit as predictors of psychological adjustment among nursing home residents. *Psychology and Aging, 9*, 189–194.

Posner, M. I., & Rothbart, M. K. (2000). Developing mechanisms of self-regulation. *Development and Psychopathology, 12*, 427–441.
Ryan, R. M., & Deci, E. L. (2000). Self-determination theory and the facilitation of intrinsic motivation, social development, and well-being. *American Psychologist, 55*, 68–78.
Salmela-Aro, K., Aunola, K., & Nurmi, J. E. (2007). Personal goals during emerging adulthood: A 10-year follow-up. *Journal of Adolescent Research, 22*, 690–715.
Schmid, K. L., Phelps, E., Kiely, M. K., Napolitano, C. M., Boyd, M. J., & Lerner, R. M. (2011). The role of adolescents' hopeful futures in predicting positive and negative developmental trajectories: Findings from the 4-H Study of Positive Youth Development. *The Journal of Positive Psychology, 6*, 45–56.
Sheese, B. E., Rothbart, M. K., Posner, M. I., White, L. K., & Fraundorf, S. H. (2008). Executive attention and self-regulation in infancy. *Infant Behavior & Development, 31*, 501–510.
Skinner, B. F. (1953). *Science and Human Behavior*. New York: Simon and Schuster.
Ursache, A., Blair, C., & Raver, C. C. (2012). The promotion of self-regulation as a means of enhancing school readiness and early achievement in children at risk for school failure. *Child Development Perspectives, 6*, 122–128.
Van Petegem, S., Beyers, W., Vansteenkiste, M., & Soenens, B. (2012). On the association between adolescent autonomy and psychosocial functioning: Examining decisional independence from a self-determination theory perspective. *Developmental Psychology, 48*(1), 76–88.
Wolfe, C. D., & Bell, M. A. (2007). The integration of cognition and emotion during infancy and early childhood: Regulatory processes associated with the development of working memory. *Brain and Cognition, 65*, 3–13.
Wrosch, C., Scheier, M. F., Miller, G. E., Schulz, R., & Carver, C. S. (2003). Adaptive self-regulation of unattainable goals: Goal disengagement, goal reengagement, and subjective well-being. *Personality and Social Psychology Bulletin, 29*, 1494–1508.

Chapter 18
Goal Setting and Attainment

Karrie A. Shogren and Michael L. Wehmeyer

Abstract Goal setting and attainment skills are a critical component of the development of agentic capacities that lead to agentic action. This chapter describes the role of goal setting and attainment in agentic action and Causal Agency Theory, as well as research on the development of goal setting and attainment. The role of self-regulated problem solving skills in the development of agentic capacities is discussed, as is the relationship of goal setting and attainment to valued outcomes.

Chapter 17 provided an overview of the development of self-regulation. A second component element in the development of agentic capacities that lead to agentic action is goal setting and attainment skills. As noted in Chap. 5, self-determined people identify pathways that lead to a specific ends to cause or create change. The identification of pathways, or pathways thinking, is a proactive, purposive process. When acting agentically, action is self-regulated, self-directed, and enables progress toward freely chosen goals. As noted briefly in Chap. 15 (Choice and Preferences), the goal setting process is part of volitional action, which involves causal capacities leading to the initiation and activation of action. Goal attainment is also a large part of agentic action, involving the agentic capacities to sustain action toward a goal. We have opted to address goal setting and attainment in a single chapter, and position it within the section on Agentic Action, acknowledging, though, that goal setting is critical to Causal Action. As such, this chapter will describe current research on goal setting and attainment, with a specific focus on how goal-directed action can be supported through self-regulated problem-solving skills. We will also review what research suggests about the relationship between goal-directed behavior and outcomes.

K.A. Shogren (✉) • M.L. Wehmeyer
Special Education, University of Kansas, Lawrence, KS, USA
e-mail: shogren@ku.edu

M.L. Wehmeyer et al. (eds.), *Development of Self-Determination Through the Life-Course*, DOI 10.1007/978-94-024-1042-6_18

Defining Goal Setting and Attainment

Agentic actions are purposeful; that is people use agentic actions to achieve an end. Agentic actions can be responses to planned circumstances (e.g., a goal that a person has set for themselves), or can be responses to circumstances that emerge in the environment (e.g., an opportunity that emerges in the environment that a person decides to capitalize upon). Thus, the end or goal that people are working toward can be shaped by a variety of factors, but agentic action and goal-directed behavior enables people to act as a causal agent and, over time, such action leads to enhanced causal agency and self-determination. Identifying and responding to opportunities requires pathways thinking in the process of setting goals, developing action plans to achieve goals, implementing and following action plans, evaluating the outcomes of the action plan, and changing action plans if the goal was not achieved or if sufficient progress is not being made (Mithaug et al. 2003). The skills associated with self-regulation (Chap. 17) enable people to examine their environments, evaluate their repertoire of possible responses, and implement and evaluate a response (Whitman 1990).

Goal setting and attainment skills, therefore, are critical to agentic action and the development of self-determination. Goals specify what a person wishes to achieve and act as regulators of human behavior. If a person sets a goal, it increases the probability that he or she will perform behaviors related to that goal (Latham and Locke 1991; Locke and Latham 2006). The process of goal-setting and attainment involves: (1) identifying and defining a goal clearly and concretely, (2) identifying pathways to achieve the goal, and (3) specifying and implementing the pathways most likely to achieve the desired outcome. At each step, choices and decisions must be made about what goals to pursue and what actions are will lead to goal attainment.

Research has suggested that the most effective goals are those that are challenging, but not so challenging that they are unattainable. If goals are too easy, there is no motivation to engage in the work necessary to attain them, nor is there a feeling of accomplishment after achieving them. Further, goals (even when shaped by environmental opportunities) should be shaped by the preferences and interests of the individual as this will influence motivation to pursue the goal (Hortop et al. 2013). Goals that have personal meaning are more likely to be attained (Locke and Latham 2002, 2006).

Goals and Motivation

Goals play multiple roles within Self-Determination Theory (SDT) and motivation, in general. As described in Chap. 4 and elsewhere in this text, satisfaction of three basic needs—competence, autonomy, and relatedness—are foundational within SDT for maintaining intrinsic motivation and the self-regulation of extrinsic motivations. Deci and Ryan (2000) observed that SDT has "maintained that a full understanding not only of goal-directed behavior, but also of psychological development and well-being, cannot be achieved without addressing the needs that give goals their psychological potency and that influence which regulatory processes direct people's goal pursuits" (p. 228).

So, one function for goals within SDT, as articulated in one SDT mini-theory, *goal content theory* (GCT), is to explain the role of goal orientation on fulfillment of basic psychological needs; extrinsic goals are less likely to satisfy these psychological needs than are intrinsic goals (e.g., personal growth, etc.), and pursuit of the latter leads to greater well-being. Koestner and Hope (2014) suggested that the "central issue for an SDT perspective on goal setting is whether the way in which individuals select and pursue their goals reflects processes related to autonomy" (p. 402). On the other hand, goal-oriented action is particularly important to the fulfillment of the need for competence. In discussing the benefits of a broader conceptualization of the need for competence, Elliot et al. (2002) described the difference between needs, motives, and goals. As noted in Chap. 4, the *need for competence* reflects humans' desire to effectively master their environment and experience a sense of competence in it. As per Elliot and colleagues:

> Our view is that goals may be distinguished from needs and motives in that the latter are affectively-based dispositions that energize behavior and orient the individual in a general way, whereas the former are cognitive representations that serve a directional function for behavior by focusing the individual on more specific possibilities. Goals are related to needs and motives in the self-regulatory process, in that individuals sometimes adopt goals that help serve their dispositional desires by channeling them in a more concrete direction. Needs or motives can and often do lead directly to behavior, but these general dispositional desires sometimes need to be strategically channeled in a specific direction to be satisfied in an effective and efficient manner. Thus the need for competence can influence behavior in two ways: it can impel competence-based behavior directly, or it can lead to competence-based behavior indirectly by prompting the adoption of competence goals that proximally regulate behavior (p. 373).

SDT "differentiates the content of goals or outcomes and the regulatory process through with the outcomes are pursued…" and "uses the concept of innate psychological needs as the basis for integrating the differentiation of goal contents and regulatory processes." (Deci and Ryan 2000, p. 227). Deci and Ryan summarized the issues pertaining to goal pursuit and attainment as:

> Specifically, according to SDT, a critical issue in the effects of goal pursuit and attainment concerns the degree to which people are able to satisfy their basic psychological needs as they pursue and attain their valued outcomes (p. 227).

Thus, goal pursuit, and the outcomes of goal attainment, differ according to the degree to which they (goals-directed activities) are autonomous or self-determined versus controlled.

Development of Goal Setting and Attainment

The intent of this chapter is not to describe in detail all aspects of the development of goal-oriented action, but instead to describe and define the role of goal setting and attainment in the development of causal agency and self-determination. That said, understanding the developmental trajectory for goal-oriented action can provide information to practitioners interested in promoting some of the early foundational skills leading to later self-determination, as discussed in Chap. 6. Autonomy-focused goal-oriented action is, in many ways, at the heart of causal agency and the development of self-determination; goals energize action to satisfy psychological needs, motivate organisms to use resources and energy in one direction rather than another direction, and, in essence, enable someone to act as a causal agent in one's life. As such, part of the developmental trajectory of goal-directed behavior lies in the development of instrumental and communicative agency; the understanding of intent and intentionality, causality, and means-end action (Gergely 2011).

By at least the second year of life, infants can attribute goal intent to others, predict novel means-ends actions, and learn new goals and means-ends action by observing and imitating adults (Gergely 2011, p. 81). Meltzoff (2011) has shown that 18-month old infants imitate an action they observe in the same way whether the actor was successful or not. That is, 18-month old infants infer the intent or goal of the action of an actor, and don't just imitate the failed attempt. Once children develop an understanding of goal intention, the next step, developmentally, involves engagement in shared goal pursuit activities. Carpenter (2011) describes a series of studies that showed, essentially, that children as young as 2 years of age are able to coordinate with adults in goal-focused tasks.

The understanding of causality, and the identification of causal agents, unfolds during early elementary years. In children's earliest understandings of causality (ages 5–6), they attribute excessive importance to effort for producing success and preventing failure, ignoring the contributions of ability and chance. Research in causal reasoning shows that children as early as third of fourth-grade begin to understand the rudiments of hypothesis testing, understanding that there is a need to perform some sort of contrast to determine what caused something to happen. A subsequent, more mature understanding is that something needs to remain constant (e.g., a control) so as to successfully test the hypothesis (Koslowski & Masnick 2011). Even at 8 and 9 years of age, children fail to differentiate between successes they could control and those that they could not, believing that practice could improve their chances of winning a game of chance. Not surprisingly, children's internal perceptions of control at this age appear unrelated to their achievement. By the age of 10 years, children begin to distinguish between effort and luck, understanding that a game of chance is non-contingent and uncontrollable, whereas effort can improve one's performance only on tasks one can control. An understanding of the contribution of ability to task success is late to develop; until the age of 11, children believe that if they try hard they will succeed and view other children as smart when they devote extensive effort or practice to a task as well as when they have exceptional ability (Doll et al. 1996).

Goal Setting and Attainment Processes in the Development of Self-Determination

As people are pursuing goals, a number of factors impact the process of goal setting and attainment, including the (a) the capability to perform causal actions, which can subdivided into causal capacity and agentic capacity, and (b) the threats to and opportunities for self-determination that emerge in the environment and promote causal action. Figure 2.1 (Chap. 2) depicted the Causal Action schema leading to enhanced causal agency. Figure 5.2 (Chap. 5) highlighted the causal action sequence involving the implementation of causal and agentic capabilities. Figure 18.1 provides this goal generation sequence to illustrate the process by which goal setting and attainment occurs.

As noted in Chap. 2, capability refers to having the requisite ability to execute chosen actions to accomplish a particular task. Agentic individuals possess various capabilities that enable them to respond to challenges and opportunities in the environment. Two types of capabilities are important to causal action: *causal capability* and *agentic capability*. These capabilities differentiate between two aspects of goal-focused actions: (a) initiating goal pursuit (causal capability) and (b) directing actions toward a preferred end (agentic capability). Causal capability includes the knowledge, skills, self-perceptions, and beliefs about one's environment that enable the expression of causal action. Having the capacity to engage in goal pursuit enables a person to prioritize goals, identifying what is in line with personal preferences and interests, and initiating actions that enable one to choose and pursue a goal. Agentic capabilities involve the mental or physical capacities to direct behavior toward an end. Such capacities include the skills and knowledge associated with self-management, goal attainment, problem solving, and self-advocacy; the skills and behaviors that enable self-regulation, self-direction, pathways thinking and, as such, agentic action. Agentic capability enables one to identify pathways and manage the steps toward goal attainment. A critical element of agentic capability is the act of comparing one's current state with one's anticipated goal state, self-regulating and evaluating if the chosen pathway is leading to progress toward the outcome.

Both causal and agentic capability work together in complex ways to achieve or maintain a desired goal (i.e., a schema for self-determined action; see Fig. 18.1). When opportunities or challenges emerge in the environment, a person begins a *goal generation process*, consisting of self-analysis and exploration concerning one's strengths, limitations, preferences, values, and wants with regard to the environmental circumstances. After prioritizing actions, the goal state is defined in terms of the most important action. Knowledge of oneself and one's vision for the future is central to this prioritization process. With a goal state in mind, the person

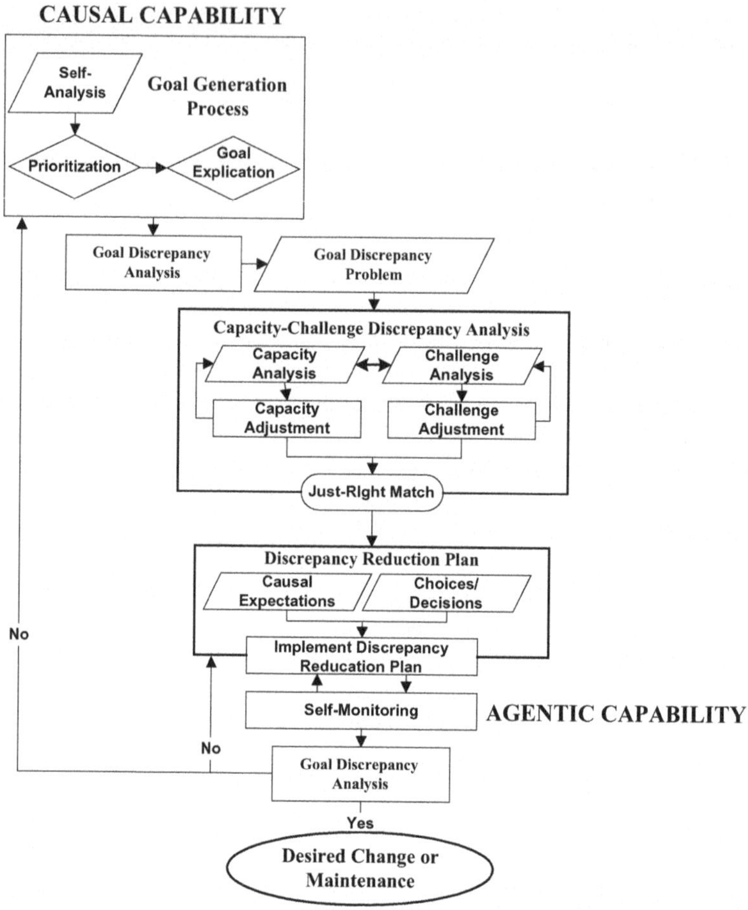

Fig. 18.1 Overview of goal action schema

engages in a *goal-discrepancy analysis* wherein the current status and the goal status are reconciled and pathways and action steps are identified. This is the *goal-discrepancy problem*, essentially the person needs to identify the pathways they need to take to reduce the discrepancy and achieve their goal by conducting a *capacity-challenge discrepancy* analysis. The person evaluates his or her capacity to solve the problem and examines the degree to which the challenge will support goal attainment. In this process, the person maximizes adjustment in capacity (e.g., acquires new or refines existing action skills) or adjusts the challenge presented to create a "just-right match" between capacity and challenge so as to optimize his or her probability of solving the goal-discrepancy problem (Mithaug 1996; Wehmeyer et al. 2003).

Next, a person creates a *discrepancy-reduction plan* that is regulated by the person's action-control beliefs (see Chap. 22). As discussed in Chaps. 2 and 22, such beliefs influence the expectations and choices a person makes in service of their goal. The person then monitors their progress to reducing the discrepancy between their current status and goal status, determining if their actions led to goal attainment, or they encountered barriers and must reevaluate their goal or the action plan. If the goal is achieved, an agentic person will return to the goal-generation process, identifying the next goal in the sequence. If progress is satisfactory but the goal is not yet achieved, the person will continue implementing the discrepancy reduction plan. If progress is not satisfactory, the person either reconsiders the discrepancy reduction plan and modifies that component, or returns to the goal-generation process to re-examine the overall goal, its priority, and, possibly, cycling through the process with a revised or new goal.

Enhancing Goal Setting and Attainment Skills

To enable children, youth and adults to go through the actions described in Fig. 18.1, researchers have developed models of teaching self-regulated problem solving skills in service of a goal. One such model, *The Self-Determined Learning Model of Instruction*, is rooted in Causal Agency Theory, and has significant evidence for its efficacy, particularly when applied with in educational contexts, although it also has relevance in other contexts such as the home environment or in work or community environments.

Self-Determined Learning Model of Instruction

The Self-Determined Learning Model of Instruction (SDLMI) was developed to capitalize on opportunities to support the development of self-determination, enabling children, youth and young adults to learn the skills associated with self-determined action based on research on the process of self-regulated problem solving and student-directed learning. It was developed to be used across goal domains, with adolescents with and without disabilities. The SLDMI is increasingly being conceptualized within systems of support that teach all young people critical problem solving and goal setting skills, and providing additional supports to address the unique needs of students with disabilities or other life circumstances that necessitate more intensive supports to learn to take action toward goals (Shogren et al. in press).

The SDLMI is a model of teaching. Models of teaching can be defined as "a plan or pattern that can be used to shape curriculums (long term courses of study), to design instructional materials, and to guide instruction in the classroom and other settings" (Joyce and Weil 1980, p. 1). Many teachers use multiple models in their instruction based on the specific content and the characteristics of learners. However, many models that are adopted in educational contexts are characterized by other-direction, not self-direction. The SDLMI changes this, by specifically emphasizing self-direction of learning, changing the role of educators and others that are supporting learning to one of a facilitator or a coach, enabling student self-direction.

Implementation of the SDLMI consists of a three-phase instructional process. Each instructional phase presents a problem to be solved by the student. To solve the problem, the student works through a series of four *Student Questions* per phase. The students learn the questions, make them their own, and apply them to reach self-selected goals. Each student question is also linked to a set of *Teacher Objectives* that provides teachers with guidance on what they are trying to support each student to achieve in answering the questions. Each instructional phase also includes a list of *Educational Supports* that teachers can use to enable students to self-direct learning. This process, across the three phases of the model, is depicted in Figs. 18.2, 18.3, and 18.4 (Wehmeyer et al. 1999).

The *Student Questions* in the model can be used in any goal domain – academic, social, community, postsecondary education. In generating a solution to the problem posed in each phase, students learn to lead themselves through the phases of the SDLMI (set a goal, take action, adjust goal or plan). Facilitators focus on teaching students to solve the sequence of problems to construct a means-ends chain – a causal sequence – that moves them from where they are (an actual state of not having their needs and interests satisfied) to where they want to be (a goal state of having those needs and interests satisfied). Students are learning how to self-regulate their actions to reduce or eliminate the discrepancy between what they want or need and what they currently have or know. Essentially, these steps teach students to engage in the action schema depicted in Figs. 18.2, 18.3, and 18.4 in a self-directed agentic way.

Each of the three phases (set a goal, take action, adjust goal or plan) has four questions that students work through, and the four questions differ from phase to phase, but represent identical steps in the problem-solving sequence. That is, students answering the questions must: (1) identify the problem, (2) identify potential solutions to the problem, (3) identify barriers to solving the problem, and (4) identify consequences of each solution. These steps are the fundamental steps in any problem-solving process and they form the means-end problem-solving sequence represented by the *Student Questions* in each phase.

Because the model itself is designed for teachers or facilitators to implement, the language of the *Student Questions* are, intentionally, not written to be understandable by every student nor does the model assume that students have life experiences that enable them to fully answer each question. Again, however, the facilitator acts as a supporter of student self-direction. The goal is for the facilitator to provide support for the student to act agentically, not to do things for the student. For this reason, the *Student Questions* are written in first-person voice in a relatively simple format with the intention that they are the starting point for discussion and can be modified based on the specific needs of each student and the goal they are working to attain. Some students will learn and use all 12 questions as they are written. Other students will need to have the questions rephrased to be more understandable. Still other students, due to the intensity of their instructional needs, may have the facilitator paraphrase the questions for them.

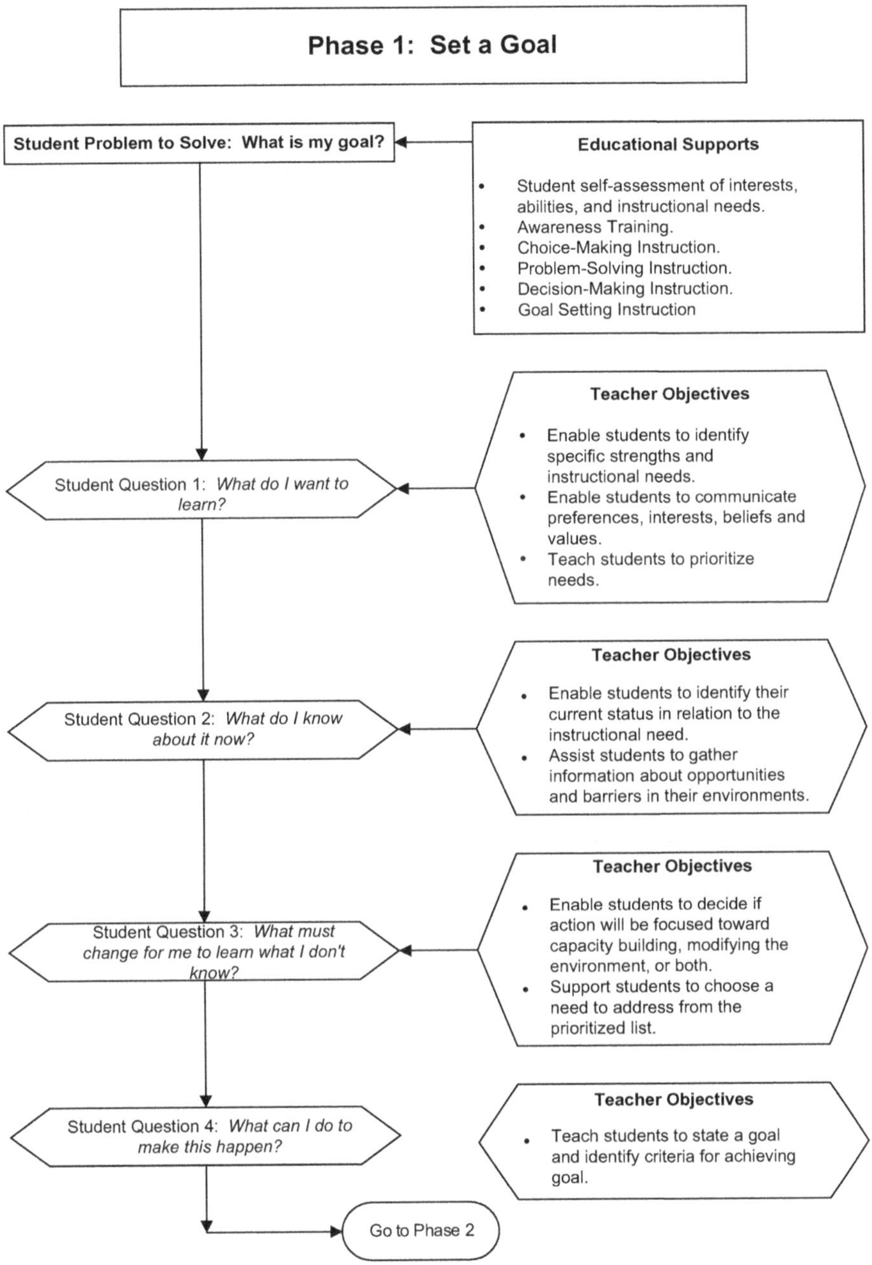

Fig. 18.2 Self-determined learning model of instruction, phase 1

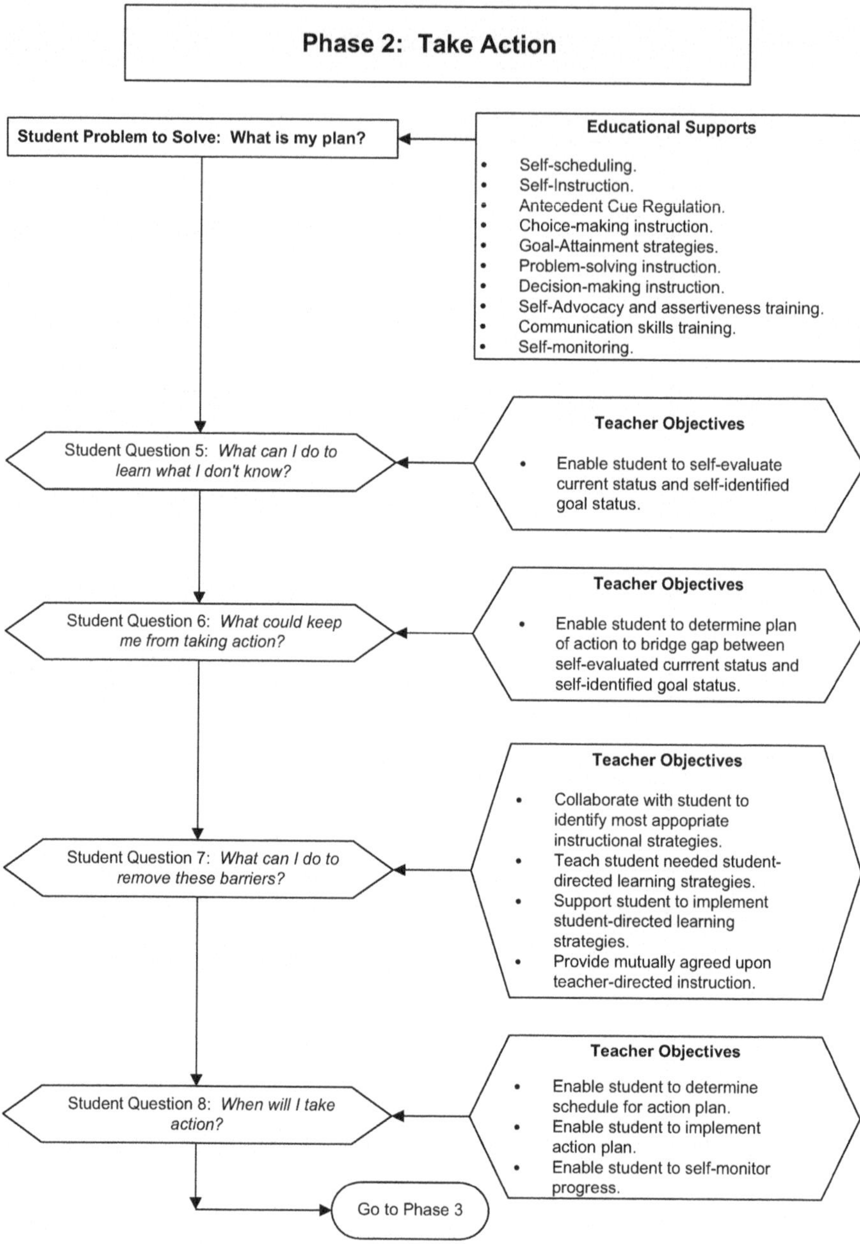

Fig. 18.3 Self-determined learning model of instruction, phase 2

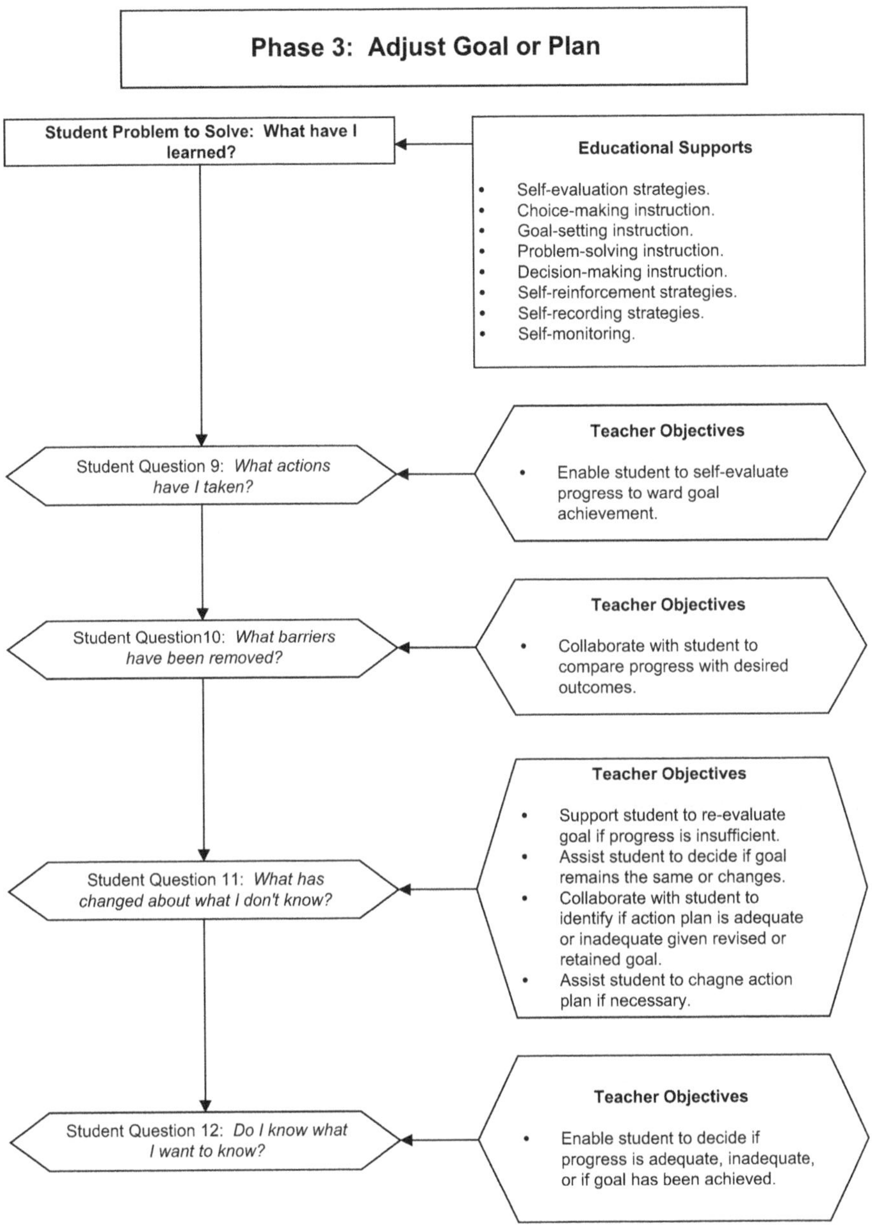

Fig. 18.4 Self-determined learning model of instruction, phase 3

The first time a teacher uses the model with a student or a group of students, the initial step in the implementation process is to read the question with or to the student, discuss what the question means and then, if necessary, change the wording to enable that student to better understand the intent of the question. Such wording changes must, however, be made such that the problem-solving intent of the question remains intact. For example, changing *Student Question 1* from "What do I want to learn?" to "What is my goal?" changes the nature of the question. The *Teacher's Objectives* associated with each student question provide direction for teachers regarding the intent of the questions.

The *Teacher Objectives* provide the objectives a teacher will be trying to accomplish by implementing the model. In each instructional phase, the objectives are linked directly to the *Student Questions*. These objectives can be met by utilizing strategies provided in the *Educational Supports* section of the model, which include instructional and support strategies that can enable students to learn how to perform the actions necessary to answer each question. The *Teacher Objectives* provide teachers with a road map to assist the teacher in enabling students to o solve the problem stated in the student question. For example, regarding the first *Student Question*: What do I want to learn? *Teacher Objectives* clarify that the goal of the facilitator is to enable students to identify their specific strengths and instructional needs, to identify and communicate preferences, interests, beliefs and values, and to prioritize their instructional needs.

Linkages Between Goal Setting and Attainment Skills and Valued Outcomes

The previous sections have described goal setting and attainment, the role of these skills in agentic action, and a model that can be implemented by educators or others that are supporting adolescents to become more self-determining to teach and create opportunities for the development of skills associated with agentic action. And, research has suggested that interventions to promote skills associated with agentic action, such as intervention with the SDLMI substantially benefit students. For example, Wehmeyer et al. (2012) conducted a group randomized control trial study of over 300 adolescents with intellectual and learning disabilities and found that when students were exposed to instruction with the SDLMI they showed significantly greater growth in their self-determination scores after two years of exposure compared to students that did not receive such instruction. Shogren et al. (2012) found in another group randomized control trial study that students with disabilities exposed to the SDLMI had greater academic and transition-related goal attainment and greater access to the general education curriculum, critical outcomes to promote access to challenging curricular content for students with disabilities. Further, teachers felt that students had significantly higher capacity and that access to more opportunities or self-determination when they were in the treatment group, compared to being in a control group (Shogren et al. 2014). And, when following students exposed to self-determination interventions post school, Shogren et al. (2015) found that students with disabilities not only left high school with higher levels of self-determination after exposure to interventions to promote self-determination, but also had better employment and community access outcomes one and two years post school.

Overall, the results of this body of research suggest the power of interventions to promote agentic action in service of goals on the outcomes of adolescents with disabilities, and those that support them. Further work is needed to expand this body of research to all adolescents, supporting the development of skills related to goal setting and attainment in all students, as descriptive work has suggested that goal setting and self-regulation skills can be important factors that impact school performance in adolescents without disabilities (Bird and Markle 2012), but few interventions have been developed that can be flexibly applied across content areas to enable students to learn to use and apply these skills in their lives, creating multiple opportunities to go through the goal generation process, engaging in *goal-discrepancy analysis* and implementing and evaluating *discrepancy-reduction plans.* Researchers have found, however, that when students as young as elementary age are supported to set their own goals for learning they are able they were able to take steps to achieve their goals, show changes in their behavior directed toward achieving their goals, and express pride in their behavior changes (Hallenbeck and Fleming 2011). Only with these repeated opportunities will adolescents and young people build the skills that enable them to act agentically, benefiting from the positive outcomes of directing their actions in service of a goal.

References

Bird, J. M., & Markle, R. S. (2012). Subjective well-being in school environments: Promoting positive youth development through evidence-based assessment and intervention. *American Journal of Orthopsychiatry, 82*, 61–66. doi:10.1111/j.1939-0025.2011.01127.x.

Carpenter, M. (2011). Social cognition and social motivations in infancy. In U. Guswami (Ed.), *The Wiley-Blackwell handbook of childhood cognitive development* (2nd ed., pp. 106–128). London: Wiley-Blackwell.

Deci, E. L., & Ryan, R. M. (2000). The "what" and "why" of goal pursuits: Human needs and the self-determination of behavior. *Psychological Inquiry, 11*(4), 227–268.

Doll, E., Sands, D., Wehmeyer, M. L., & Palmer, S. (1996). Promoting the development and acquisition of self-determined behavior. In D. J. Sands & M. L. Wehmeyer (Eds.), *Self-determination across the life span: Independence and choice for people with disabilities* (pp. 65–90). Baltimore: Paul H. Brookes.

Elliot, A. J., McGregor, H. A., & Thrash, T. M. (2002). The need for competence. In E. L. Deci & R. M. Ryan (Eds.), *Handbook of self-determination research* (pp. 360–387). Rochester: University of Rochester Press.

Gergely, G. (2011). Kinds of agents: The origins of understanding instrumental and communicative agency. In U. Guswami (Ed.), *The Wiley-Blackwell handbook of childhood cognitive development* (2nd ed., pp. 76–105). London: Wiley-Blackwell.

Hallenbeck, A., & Fleming, D. (2011). Don't you want to do better? Implementing a goal-setting intervention in an afterschool program. *Afterschool Matters, 13*, 38–28.

Hortop, E. G., Wrosch, C., & Gagné, M. (2013). The why and how of goal pursuits: Effects of global autonomous motivation and perceived control on emotional well-being. *Motivation and Emotion, 37*(4), 675–687. doi:10.1007/s11031-013-9349-2.

Joyce, B., & Weil, M. (1980). *Models of teaching* (2nd ed.). Englewood Cliffs: Prentice Hall.

Koestner, R., & Hope, N. (2014). A self-detemination theory approach to goals. In M. Gagne (Ed.), *The Oxford handbook of work engagement, motivation, and self-determination theory* (pp. 400–413). Oxford: Oxford University Press.

Koslowski, B., & Masnick, A. (2011). Social cognition and social motivations in infancy. In U. Guswami (Ed.), *The Wiley-Blackwell handbook of childhood cognitive development* (2nd ed., pp. 377–398). London: Wiley-Blackwell.

Latham, G. P., & Locke, E. A. (1991). Self-regulation through goal setting. *Organizational Behavior and Human Decision Processes, 50*(2), 212–247.

Locke, E. A., & Latham, G. P. (2002). Building a practically useful theory of goal setting and task motivation: A 35-year odyssey. *American Psychologist, 57*(9), 705–717.

Locke, E. A., & Latham, G. P. (2006). New directions in goal-setting theory. *Current Directions in Psychological Science, 15*, 265–268. doi:10.1111/j.1467-8721.2006.00449.x.

Meltzoff, A. N. (2011). Social cognition and the origins of imitation, empathy, and theory of mind. In U. Guswami (Ed.), *The Wiley-Blackwell handbook of childhood cognitive development* (2nd ed., pp. 49–75). London: Wiley-Blackwell.

Mithaug, D. E. (1996). *Equal opportunity theory*. Thousand Oaks: Sage.

Mithaug, D. E., Mithaug, D. K., Agran, M., Martin, J. E., & Wehmeyer, M. L. (2003). The credibility and worth of self-determined learning theory. In D. E. Mithaug, D. K. Mithaug, M. Agran, J. E. Martin, & M. L. Wehmeyer (Eds.), *Self determined learning theory: Construction, verification, and evaluation* (pp. 223–245). Mahwah: Lawrence Erlbaum Associates, Publishers.

Shogren, K. A., Palmer, S. B., Wehmeyer, M. L., Williams-Diehm, K., & Little, T. D. (2012). Effect of intervention with the self-determined learning model of instruction on access and goal attainment. *Remedial and Special Education, 33*, 320–330. doi:10.1177/0741932511410072.

Shogren, K. A., Plotner, A. J., Palmer, S. B., Wehmeyer, M. L., & Paek, Y. (2014). Impact of the self-determined learning model of instruction on teacher perceptions of student capacity and opportunity for self-determination. *Education and Training in Autism and Developmental Disabilities, 49*, 440–448.

Shogren, K. A., Wehmeyer, M. L., Palmer, S. B., Rifenbark, G. G., & Little, T. D. (2015). Relationships between self-determination and postschool outcomes for youth with disabilities. *Journal of Special Education, 53*, 30–41. doi:10.1177/0022466913489733.

Shogren, K. A., Wehmeyer, M. L., & Lane, K. L. (in press). Embedding interventions to promote self-determination within multi-tiered systems of supports. *Exceptionality*.

Wehmeyer, M. L., Agran, M., Palmer, S. B., & Mithaug, D. (1999). *A teacher's guide to implementing the self-determined learning model of instruction: Adolescent version*. Lawrence: Beach Center on Disability, University of Kansas.

Wehmeyer, M. L., Abery, B., Mithaug, D. E., & Stancliffe, R. (2003). *Theory in self-determination: Foundations for educational practice*. Springfield: Charles C. Thomas Publishing Company.

Wehmeyer, M. L., Shogren, K. A., Palmer, S. B., Williams-Diehm, K., Little, T. D., & Boulton, A. (2012). Impact of the self-determined learning model of instruction on student self-determination: A randomized-trial placebo control group study. *Exceptional Children, 78*, 135–153.

Whitman, T. L. (1990). Self-regulation and mental retardation. *American Journal on Mental Retardation, 94*, 347–362.

Chapter 19
Problem Solving

Karrie A. Shogren and Michael L. Wehmeyer

Abstract Problem solving is another element of agentic action. This chapter reviews the role of problem solving in agentic action and Causal Agency Theory. It also describes the role of autonomous motivation, as defined by Self-Determination Theory in problem solving. The literature on the development of problem solving, interventions to promote problem solving skills, and the linkages between problem solving and valued outcomes is reviewed.

To act agentically, one must regulate one's actions in service of goals, responding to opportunities and challenges that emerge in the environment. Previous chapters have discussed the critical role of self-regulation of action (Chap. 17) and goal setting and attainment skills (Chap. 18) in enabling people to act agentically (e.g., engage in agentic action). This chapter will discuss another skill that enables people to act agentically, problem solving. Specifically, the chapter will define problem solving, review the literature on the development of problem solving and the role of problem solving in human agentic action, and summarize what is known about the linkages between problem solving and the attainment of valued psychological outcomes.

Defining Problem Solving

To engage in agentic action, one must respond to opportunities or threats encountered. When working toward goals and self-regulating one's actions in service of goals, situations will be encountered where the best solution or pathway to goal attainment is unknown, not clear, or not available. This can occur when responding to a planned circumstances (e.g., a goal that a person has set for themselves) or when responding to circumstances that emerge in the environment (e.g., an opportunity that emerges in the environment that a person decides to capitalize upon).

K.A. Shogren (✉) • M.L. Wehmeyer
Special Education, University of Kansas, Lawrence, KS, USA
e-mail: shogren@ku.edu

M.L. Wehmeyer et al. (eds.), *Development of Self-Determination Through the Life-Course*, DOI 10.1007/978-94-024-1042-6_19

When a solution is not known or readily encountered, this presents a problem. Problems can be defined as "existing or anticipated life situations or tasks that require responses for adaptive functioning, but for which no effective coping responses are immediately identifiable or available to the individual" (Nezu 2004, p. 3). The demands of problem solving can emerge from the person (e.g., unsure the best steps to act agentically to reach a goal), from the environment (e.g., lack of opportunities for agentic action), or from both.

The ability to solve problems is critical to enabling people to engage with their environment and act agentically (Little et al. 2002), and addresses the psychological need for competence through the act of solving problems, described in Self-Determination Theory (see Chap. 4). The process of navigating problems and engaging in self-regulated, goal-directed actions gives rise to a sense of personal empowerment and action-control beliefs, or the sense that one knows and has what it takes to achieve goals, which contributes to the development of a sense of causal agency. The process of solving a problem is generally assumed to involve five steps: (a) identifying and defining the problem, (b) listing possible solutions, (c) identifying the impact of each solution, (d) making a judgment about a preferred solution, and (e) evaluating the efficacy of the judgment (D'Zurilla and Goldfried 1971).

While early work focused on the application of these steps to solving problems with finite solutions, more recent research has focused on applications of problem solving in more complex situations, where there is not a finite solution, and when environments are highly dynamic. Some researchers have described this as *complex problem solving*. Complex problem solving requires the use of cognitive skills related to acquiring information in dynamic situations, generating novel solutions, and representing complex information. Buchner (1995) defines complex problem solving as "the successful interaction with task environments that are dynamic (i.e., change as a function of user's intervention and/or as a function of time) and in which some, if not all, of the environment's regularities can only be revealed by successful exploration and integration of the information gained in that process" (p. 14). Within these dynamic environmental situations, problem-solving skills are critical to acting agentically and making progress toward one's goals, as it is necessary to integrate information and make a judgement about a preferred solution to continue to make progress toward one's goals even as the environment changes. Researchers have focused on specific applications of complex problem solving situations or tasks such as social problem solving, which addresses the application of problem solving skills within social and interpersonal situations that tend to be highly dynamic and require nuanced understandings to identify, generate, and evaluate possible solutions (Chang et al. 2004; Elias and Tobias 1996) as well as every day or practical problem solving skills, which also emphasize dynamic situations or tasks, but focus more on the complexity inherent in everyday environments and tasks across environments (Berg et al. 2009; Sinnott 1989). Researchers that focus on everyday problem solving emphasize the importance of being able to generate more than one potential solution, particularly when dealing with a dynamic or complex situation, and the role of evaluating alternate solutions using logical thinking skills and defining or redefining of the problem to enable the generation of alternative solutions (Pezzuti et al. 2014).

In addition to the specific skills needed to solve complex problems, researchers have also emphasized the role of self-appraisal in solving problems. This body of research suggests that how a person perceives their ability to solve problems directly influences their application of their problem solving skills across situations, with one's self-appraisal affecting "how (and whether) they will solve problems" (Butler and Meichenbaum 1981, p. 219). Essentially, consistent with Causal Agency Theory, as people develop a sense of personal empowerment and action-control beliefs, their perceptions or appraisals about their ability to navigate the complex problem solving process change. If these changes lead to more adaptive appraisals, people are more able to effectively apply their problem solving skills to acting agentically.

Development of Problem Solving Skills

Problem solving skills develop over the lifespan, and researchers have linked the development of complex problem solving skills with the development of cognitive skills, such as fluid reasoning, in childhood and adolescence (Funke 2010). In adolescence between the ages of 12 and 17, for example, children develop an increasing ability to cognitively understand and process complex situations. Their evolving executive functioning skills and increased processing speed allow for increased fluid reasoning when generating and evaluating alternate solutions to complex problems (Frischkorn et al. 2014). Opportunities for the development of these skills occur across environments, and more and more complex problems are encountered both socially and academically as adolescents participate in educational and social contexts particularly as they move to high school and early adult life. Much attention has been directed to the development of complex problem solving skills as well as social problem solving skills in the context of the general education curriculum throughout the schools years, particularly in the context of teaching math and science skills, as well as in developing "soft skills" related to working with peers and navigating complex social situations. Researchers have found that as students age, they show more flexibility in their problem solving strategies (i.e., more ability to address complex problems) and that there are strong correlations between problem solving strategies used across content areas, such as math and literacy, but differences in the specific strategies that are most effective in solving problems in the differing content areas, suggesting the need for developmentally appropriate activities for teaching both content-specific and generalized problem solving strategies (Farrington-Flint et al. 2009).

In early childhood, the precursors of the skills associated with complex problem solving emerge. In infancy, young children encounter problems on a routine basis, such as needing to find a way to get attention or objects from caregivers. Infants frequently use trial and error approaches to navigate these problems, identifying the pathways that enable them to solve their problem and achieve their intended goal state. Over time, children become more and more able to engage in means-ends analysis, recognizing that their actions impact their environment and developing an understanding of the linkage between problems, solutions, and their implementation of those solutions. As this understanding develops, young children begin to act with intentionality, and use specific means to solve problems, although the ability use strategies is largely restricted to problems with finite solutions in younger children. Young children also struggle to generalize what they learn in solving problem to another problem. Toddlers and young children frequently need hints or models of strategies to solve simple problems; it is not until the age of 7–9 that most children are able to begin to solve more complex problems without extensive supports from adults (Chen et al. 2000; Ellis and Siegler 1994; Willatts 1990).

During early childhood modeling problem solving strategies and creating opportunities to children to participate in identifying solutions can promote the development of the precursors to agentic action (Shogren and Turnbull 2006). Researchers have found that when families model effective problem, this predicts adolescents' mastery of problem solving skills and their effectiveness in solving problems, suggesting a social influence on learning and using problem solving skills during adolescence (Conger et al. 2009).

The Role of Problem Solving in the Development of Self-Determination

As discussed in Chap. 5, Causal Agency Theory holds that as people use their causal and agentic capabilities, they engage in a *goal generation process*, and that the process of analyzing the discrepancy between the one's current goal status with one's intended goal state leads to the identification of a *goal-discrepancy problem.* Solving this problem, is central to acting agentically. Problem solving is, therefore, central both to identifying a goal and developing pathways to achieve that goal, as well as navigating the obstacles encountered in progressing toward goal attainment. Researchers have found that individuals with high levels of personal agency tend to be better problem solvers, using more effective problem solving strategies. This suggests a reciprocal relationship between the development of causal agency and problem solving abilities.

Researchers have also found that when autonomously motivated, as defined by SDT (Chap. 4) people tend to show more persistence and motivation in completing problem solving tasks, both when solutions are known and unknown. Interestingly, when solutions are unknown, researchers have found people tend to report lower levels of perceived competence; however, people still persist if they were autonomously motivated, even if they did not feel competence, enabling them to make more progress toward their goal and show greater persistence in generating solutions to the problem (Keatley et al. 2013).

Enhancing Problem-Solving Skills

Most of the research in enhancing problem solving skills has derived from the work of D'Zurilla and colleagues (D'Zurilla 1986; D'Zurilla and Goldfried 1971) and Spivack, Shure, and colleagues (Shure et al. 1972; Spivack and Shure 1974). D'Zurilla and Goldfried (1971) suggested a five-step training model: (a) problem orientation, (b) problem definition and formulation, (c) generation of alternative solutions, (d) decision making, and (e) solution implementation. It is worth noting, though, that an important prerequisite to engaging in problem solving is to recognize that there is a problem. Young children are not, developmentally, aware of problem situations, and as such, instruction to promote problem-solving skills typically begins in late elementary school.

Instruction focuses first on problem perception—the recognition and labeling of problems. As part of this step, children should address the following questions: (a) Is the problem caused by myself or someone else?, and (b) How important is the problem? Children should also learn how to estimate the time they will need to solve a problem during this step.

Second, children learn to gather as much information about the problem as possible, set problem-solving goals, and reexamine the importance of the problem's resolution to their well-being. This will allow them to better understand how to identify effective solutions.

Third, children learn to generate alternative solutions to the problem. This may involve expanding the experience base from which the child can draw when generating alternatives; "instruction" may be as simple as expanding a student's experiences in social interactions. You also might provide instructional opportunities that would enable students to generate at least one solution for a frequently encountered social dilemma. After generating one solution, they should learn to generate a small list of alternatives, and finally to brainstorm alternatives. Many programs have been developed that follow this basic problem-solving model. The following is an example of one such program.

Benjamin (1996a, b) developed programs to get students thinking about problems they encounter at school and work. Students are taught the following four-step process:

1. Understand: Students are taught, through role playing and simulated activities, to observe and analyze the situation, to identify the problem in the situation, and to name that problem.
2. Plan and Solve: Students are taught to think about possible options that might be a solution to the problem. If they cannot identify any existing solutions, they are taught how to access resources, such as libraries and talking to others, to generate possible solutions.
3. Check: Once a student has identified specific solutions and selected one, the student is encouraged to see if there is still a problem. If so, what can he or she do to change the plan?

4. Review: Students explore how they can use strategies to solve similar problems in other circumstances.

Linkages Between Problem Solving and Valued Outcomes

A wide array of research has suggested a strong and positive relationship between problem solving, well-being and other positive psychological outcomes (Smith 2003). For example, social problem solving has been defined as a key contributor to quality relationships and enhanced quality of life (Chang et al. 2004). Specifically, the ability to bond with others, work cooperatively, and handle differences and conflicts all require social problem solving skills, and the effective application of these social problem solving skills is linked with more positive social relationships. Social problem solving skills have been identified as key elements of child development, correlated with lower stress and greater well-being as well as lower levels of anxiety and depression (Siu and Shek 2010). Social problem solving interventions have been implemented to support people with autism (Bernard-Opitz et al. 2001), intellectual disability (Ailey et al. 2012; Crites and Dunn 2004), traumatic brain injury (Wade et al. 2015) as well as personality disorders (McMurran et al. 2008) with positive results.

With regard to problem-solving skills, generally, researchers have found that teaching problem-solving skills to children and youth can lead to enhanced literacy and mathematics skills (Goodwin in press; Muis et al. in press), and that such instruction benefits students who are struggling with learning specific skills (Swanson et al. 2015), including students with learning disabilities, intellectual disability, and autism (Hua et al. 2015; Jitendra and Xin 1997; Montague et al. 2011; Whitby 2013). For example, Montague et al. (2014) found that teaching mathematical problem-solving skills to students with and without learning disabilities in an inclusive classroom, the problem-solving instruction was effective across all ability groups and led to a significantly greater growth rate on the curriculum-based measures for students in the problem-solving intervention compared to students in a control group who received the standard district curriculum.

Teaching problem-solving skills has also been linked to enhanced health outcomes and well-being in diabetes self-management (Hill-Briggs 2003; Hill-Briggs and Gemmell 2007) as well as in individual and family management of cancer diagnoses and treatment (Cameron et al. 2004; Meyers et al. 2011; Nezu et al. 1998; Sahler et al. 2002). Enhanced problem-solving skills have been linked to better outcomes in treatment for depression and anxiety (Kleiboer et al. 2015).

Those that develop positive perceptions of their problem-solving ability also tend to show more positive outcomes generally, and specific to problem-solving. For example, researchers have found that both problem-solving skills and appraisals are linked with general psychological adjustment as well as positive perceptions of social competence, lower levels of depression and hopefulness, and enhanced vocational decision making. Inversely, diminished perceptions of one's problem-solving effectiveness, is a consistent predictor of hopelessness and suicidal ideation across multiple populations, including college students, those in correctional facilities, and with psychiatric diagnoses (M. J. Heppner et al. 2004; P. P. Heppner and Lee 2009).

Conclusions

Problem solving is a key element of acting agentically, and is central to identifying and selecting pathways to achieve self-selected goals, reducing the *goal-discrepancy problem*. The problems that people face in acting agentically tend to be highly complex and cut across social, learning, and everyday activities. To solve these problems people must use cognitive skills to generate alternative solutions, recognizing the dynamic and changing nature of the problems as solutions are generated and implemented, and evaluate the best solutions. Repeatedly engaging in these activities over the lifespan will lead to enhanced appraisals of one's problem-solving skills, and enhanced action-control beliefs, another critical element of causal agency.

References

Ailey, S. H., Friese, T. R., & Nezu, A. M. (2012). Modifying a social problem-solving program with the input of individuals with intellectual disabilities and their staff. *Research in Nursing & Health, 35*, 610–623.

Benjamin, C. (1996a). *Problem solving in school*. Upper Saddle River: Globe Fearon Educational Publisher.

Benjamin, C. (1996b). *Problem solving on the job*. Upper Saddle River: Globe Fearon Educational Publisher.

Berg, C. A., Skinner, M., & Ko, K. (2009). An integrative model of everyday problem solving across the adult life span. In *Handbook of research on adult learning and development* (pp. 524–552). New York: Routledge/Taylor & Francis Group.

Bernard-Opitz, V., Sriram, N., & Nakhoda-Sapuan, S. (2001). Enhancing social problem solving in children with autism and normal children through computer-assisted instruction. *Journal of Autism and Developmental Disorders, 31*, 377–398.

Buchner, A. (1995). Basic topics and approaches to the study of complex problem solving. In *Complex problem solving: The European perspective* (pp. 27–63). Hillsdale: Lawrence Erlbaum Associates.

Butler, L., & Meichenbaum, D. (1981). The assessment of interpersonal problem-solving skills. In P. Kendall & S. D. Hollon (Eds.), *Assessment strategies for cognitive-behavioral interventions* (pp. 197–225). New York: Academic.

Cameron, J. I., Shin, J. L., Williams, D., & Stewart, D. E. (2004). A brief problem-solving intervention for family caregivers to individuals with advanced cancer. *Journal of Psychosomatic Research, 57*, 137–143. doi:http://dx.doi.org/10.1016/S0022-3999(03)00609-3.

Chang, E., D'Zurilla, T. J., & Sanna, L.J, J (Eds.). (2004). Social problem solving: Theory, research, and training. Washington, DC: American Psychological Association.

Chen, Z., Siegler, R. S., & Daehler, M. W. (2000). Across the great divide: Bridging the gap between understanding of toddlers' and older children's thinking. *Monographs of the Society for Research in Child Development, 65*, 1–105. doi:10.2307/3181574.

Conger, K. J., Williams, S. T., Little, W. M., Masyn, K. E., & Shebloski, B. (2009). Development of mastery during adolescence: The role of family problem-solving. *Journal of Health and Social Behavior, 50*, 99–114.

Crites, S. A., & Dunn, C. (2004). Teaching social problem solving to individuals with mental retardation. *Education and Training in Developmental Disabilities, 39*, 301–309.

D'Zurilla, T. J. (1986). *Problem solving therapy*. New York: Springer.

D'Zurilla, T. J., & Goldfried, M. R. (1971). Problem solving and behavior modification. *Journal of Abnormal Psychology, 78*, 107–126.

Elias, M. J., & Tobias, S. E. (1996). *Social problem solving: Interventions in the schools*. New York: Guilford Press.

Ellis, S., & Siegler, R. S. (1994). Development of problem solving. In *Thinking and problem solving* (pp. 333–367). San Diego: Academic.

Farrington-Flint, L., Vanuxem-Cotterill, S., & Stiller, J. (2009). Patterns of problem-solving in children's literacy and arithmetic. *British Journal of Developmental Psychology, 27*, 815–834. doi:10.1348/026151008X383148.

Frischkorn, G. T., Greiff, S., & Wüstenberg, S. (2014). The development of complex problem solving in adolescence: A latent growth curve analysis. *Journal of Educational Psychology, 106*, 1007–1020. doi:http://dx.doi.org/10.1037/a0037114.

Funke, J. (2010). Complex problem solving: A case for complex cognition? *Cognitive Processing, 11*, 133–142. doi:10.1007/s10339-009-0345-0.

Goodwin, A. P. (in press). Effectiveness of word solving: Integrating morphological problem-solving within comprehension instruction for middle school students. *Reading and Writing*. doi:http://dx.doi.org/10.1007/s11145-015-9581-0.

Heppner, P. P., & Lee, D.-G. (2009). Problem-solving appraisal and psychological adjustment. In *Oxford handbook of positive psychology* (2nd ed., pp. 345–355). New York: Oxford University Press.

Heppner, M. J., Lee, D.-G., Heppner, P. P., McKinnon, L. C., Multon, K. D., & Gysbers, N. C. (2004). The role of problem-solving appraisal in the process and outcome of career counseling. *Journal of Vocational Behavior, 65*, 217–238. doi:http://dx.doi.org/10.1016/S0001-8791(03)00100-3.

Hill-Briggs, F. (2003). Problem solving in diabetes self-management: A model of chronic illness self-management behavior. *Annals of Behavioral Medicine, 25*, 182–193. doi:http://dx.doi.org/10.1207/S15324796ABM2503_04.

Hill-Briggs, F., & Gemmell, L. (2007). Problem solving in diabetes self-management and control: A systematic review of the literature. *The Diabetes Educator, 33*, 1032–1050. doi:10.1177/1049732304273888.

Hua, Y., Woods-Groves, S., Kaldenberg, E. R., Lucas, K. G., & Therrien, W. J. (2015). Effects of the TIP strategy on problem solving skills of young adults with intellectual disability. *Education and Training in Autism and Developmental Disabilities, 50*, 31–42.

Jitendra, A., & Xin, Y. P. (1997). Mathematical word-problem-solving instruction for students with mild disabilities and students at risk for math failure: A research synthesis. *The Journal of Special Education, 30*, 412–438. doi:http://dx.doi.org/10.1177/002246699703000404.

Keatley, D., Clarke, D. D., & Hagger, M. S. (2013). Investigating the predictive validity of implicit and explicit measures of motivation in problem-solving behavioural tasks. *British Journal of Social Psychology, 52*, 510–524. doi:10.1111/j.2044-8309.2012.02107.x.

Kleiboer, A., Donker, T., Seekles, W., van Straten, A., Riper, H., & Cuijpers, P. (2015). A randomized controlled trial on the role of support in internet-based problem solving therapy for depression and anxiety. *Behaviour Research and Therapy, 72*, 63–71. doi:http://dx.doi.org/10.1016/j.brat.2015.06.013.

Little, T. D., Hawley, P. H., Henrich, C. C., & Marsland, K. (2002). Three views of the agentic self: A developmental synthesis. In E. L. Deci & R. M. Ryan (Eds.), *Handbook of self-determination research* (pp. 389–404). Rochester: University of Rochester Press.

McMurran, M., Huband, N., & Duggan, C. (2008). The role of social problem solving in improving social functioning in therapy for adults with personality disorder. *Personality and Mental Health, 2*, 1–6. doi:http://dx.doi.org/10.1002/pmh.19.

Meyers, F. J., Carducci, M., Loscalzo, M. J., Linder, J., Greasby, T., & Beckett, L. A. (2011). Effects of a problem-solving intervention (COPE) on quality of life for patients with advanced cancer on clinical trials and their caregivers: Simultaneous care educational intervention (SCEI): Linking palliation and clinical trials. *Journal of Palliative Medicine, 14*, 465–473. doi:http://dx.doi.org/10.1089/jpm.2010.0416.

Montague, M., Enders, C., & Dietz, S. (2011). Effects of cognitive strategy instruction on math problem solving of middle school students with learning disabilities. *Learning Disability Quarterly, 34*, 262–272.

Montague, M., Krawec, J., Enders, C., & Dietz, S. (2014). The effects of cognitive strategy instruction on math problem solving of middle-school students of varying ability. *Journal of Educational Psychology, 106*(2), 469–481. doi:http://dx.doi.org/10.1037/a0035176.

Muis, K. R., Psaradellis, C., Chevrier, M., Leo, I. D., & Lajoie, S. P. (in press). Learning by preparing to teach: Fostering Self-regulatory processes and achievement during complex mathematics problem solving. *Journal of Educational Psychology*. doi:http://dx.doi.org/10.1037/edu0000071.

Nezu, A. M. (2004). Problem solving and behavior therpay revisited. *Behavior Therapy, 35*, 1–33.

Nezu, A. M., Nezu, C. M., Friedman, S. H., Faddis, S., & Houts, P. S. (1998). *Helping cancer patients cope: A problem-solving approach*. Washington, DC: American Psychological Association.

Pezzuti, L., Artistico, D., Chirumbolo, A., Picone, L., & Dowd, S. M. (2014). The relevance of logical thinking and cognitive style to everyday problem solving among older adults. *Learning and Individual Differences, 36*, 218–223. doi:http://dx.doi.org/10.1016/j.lindif.2014.07.011.

Sahler, O. J. Z., Varni, J. W., Fairclough, D. L., Butler, R. W., Noll, R. B., Dolgin, M. J., … Mulhern, R. K. (2002). Problem-solving skills training for mothers of children with newly diagnosed cancer: A randomized trial. *Journal of Developmental and Behavioral Pediatrics, 23*, 77–86. doi:http://dx.doi.org/10.1097/00004703-200204000-00003.

Shogren, K. A., & Turnbull, A. P. (2006). Promoting self-determination in young children with disabilities: The critical role of families. *Infants and Young Children, 19*, 338–352.

Shure, M. B., Spivack, G., & Jaeger, M. (1972). Problem-solving thinking and adjustment among disadvantaged preschool children. *Child Development, 42*, 1791–1803.

Sinnott, J. D. (Ed.). (1989). *Everyday problem solving: Theory and applications*. New York: Praeger Publishers.

Siu, A. M. H., & Shek, D. T. L. (2010). Social problem solving as a predictor of well-being in adolescents and young adults. *Social Indicators Research, 95*, 393–406. doi:http://dx.doi.org/10.1007/s11205-009-9527-5.

Smith, D. C. (2003). Problem solving as an element of development well-being. In *Well-being: Positive development across the life course* (pp. 321–330). Mahwah: Lawrence Erlbaum Associates Publishers.

Spivack, G., & Shure, M. (1974). *Social adjustment of young children*. San Francisco: Jossey-Bass Publishers.

Swanson, H. L., Lussier, C. M., & Orosco, M. J. (2015). Cognitive strategies, working memory, and growth in word problem solving in children with math difficulties. *Journal of Learning Disabilities, 48*, 339–358. doi:10.1177/0022219413498771.

Wade, S. L., Kurowski, B. G., Kirkwood, M. W., Zhang, N., Cassedy, A., Brown, T. M., … Taylor, H. G. (2015). Online problem-solving therapy after traumatic brain injury: A randomized controlled trial. *Pediatrics, 135*, 487–495. doi:http://dx.doi.org/10.1542/peds.2014-1386.

Whitby, P. J. S. (2013). The effects of Solve it! on the mathematical word problem solving ability of adolescents with autism spectrum disorders. *Focus on Autism and Other Developmental Disabilities, 28*(2), 78–88. doi:http://dx.doi.org/10.1177/1088357612468764.

Willatts, P. (1990). Development of problem-solving strategies in infancy. In *Children's strategies: Contemporary views of cognitive development* (pp. 23–66). Hillsdale: Lawrence Erlbaum Associates.

Chapter 20
Decision Making

Michael L. Wehmeyer and Karrie A. Shogren

Abstract Another process critical to agentic action and, thus, causal agency, involves making a decision. Developmentally, the emergence of decision-making capacity occurs in early adolescence, on the heels of the development of problem-solving skills. Like problem solving, decision making is undertaken by agentic people in service of a goal. In this chapter, we explore in greater depth what is meant by the term decision (and by a decision-making process), how decision making is situated within SDT and Causal Agency Theory, and the relationship (again within SDT and Causal Agency Theory) between decision making and autonomy. The development of decision-making skills is discussed. The chapter concludes by discussing the decision-making process and autonomy-supportive interventions to promote more effective decision making.

Another process critical to agentic action and, thus, causal agency, involves making a decision. Developmentally, the emergence of decision-making capacity occurs in early adolescence, on the heels of the development of problem-solving skills (Chap. 19). As was emphasized in Chap. 2, theories of human agentic behavior suggest that actions are volitional and that an agentic person uses self-regulated and goal-directed agentic actions to "plot and navigate a chosen course through the uncertainties and challenges of the social and ecological environments… continuously interpreting and evaluating actions and their consequences" (Little, Hawley, Henrich and Marsland 2002, p. 390). Like problem solving, decision making is undertaken by agentic people in service of a goal. In the next section, we explore in greater depth what is meant by the term decision (and by a decision-making process), but we begin by situating decision making within SDT and Causal Agency Theory.

A decision is "goal-directed behavior made by the individual in response to a certain need, with the intention of satisfying the motive that the need occasions" (Jabes 1978, p. 86). As we have articulated throughout this text, our model of the development of self-determination (Fig. 2.1) proposes that the organism's desire to satisfy the basic needs postulated by SDT (autonomy, competence, relatedness) in

M.L. Wehmeyer (✉) • K.A. Shogren
Special Education, University of Kansas, Lawrence, KS, USA
e-mail: wehmeyer@ku.edu

M.L. Wehmeyer et al. (eds.), *Development of Self-Determination Through the Life-Course*, DOI 10.1007/978-94-024-1042-6_20

response to environmental challenges (opportunities, threats) facilitates autonomous motivation, which initiates a causal action sequence in which volitional and agentic actions are mediated by action-control beliefs, resulting in experiences of causal agency. Thus, we contextualize the decision-making process as part of the causal action sequence, and, specifically, the agentic action process, enabling the person to satisfy the need for autonomy, competence, and relatedness, stimulated by environmental challenges through goal-directed volitional and agentic action.

Perhaps more than any other component element of causal action, decision-making is closely associated with autonomous functioning, and it is worth a brief discussion about autonomy and adolescence before defining the construct. Autonomy, or literally self-rule, is often used to refer to behavioral independence. The adolescent years are often described by theorists as "a period characterized by a normative increase in autonomous functioning" (Van Petegem et al. 2012, p. 76). This is roughly equivalent to saying that adolescence is characterized by greater independent functioning. Decision making is a critical skill in attaining greater levels of independence and functional autonomy. This sense of autonomy as self-reliance, however, contrasts with SDT's use (and our use within this text) of autonomy as reflecting self-endorsement of functioning. Within SDT, "autonomy is defined as volitional or self-endorsed, functioning and is contrasted with pressured or controlled functioning" (Van Petegem et al. 2012, p. 76). A litmus test for contrasting these two uses of the term autonomy is the degree to which autonomous or independent decision making by adolescents contributes to more positive psychosocial development and well-being. Van Petegem and colleagues determined, in fact, that whether a decision was independent or whether it was controlled, if the decisions are fully endorsed by the adolescent, the result is more positive psychosocial development, including well-being.

Defining Decisions and Decision Making

Even in psychological literature, the terms decision, problem, and choice are often used interchangeably. In fact, however, they comprise unique processes serving different, albeit closely related, purposes within the causal action sequence. We have explained, in Chap. 15, that a choice, at its simplest, is the expression of a preference between two or more alternatives and, more complexly, implies that the organism had the freedom to reject options. A problem, as discussed in Chap. 19, is a circumstance, activity, or task for which a solution is not known or readily apparent. A decision is "the end state of a … series of linked stages of activity," an important element of which is uncertainty (McGrew and Wilson 1982, p. 4); it is a judgement about which solution is best at a given time. Thus, the decision-making process begins with a problem-solving process (identifying the action alternatives from which a decision is to be made) and ends with making a choice; selecting the alternative that best meets the individual's goal. A decision is "goal-directed behavior

Table 20.1 Decision-making process

1. Recognition of the circumstances that are creating the threat or opportunity that leads to a decision needing to be made
2. Awareness of the need to make a decision
3. Identification of the goal in which the decision is in service of
4. Identification of action alternatives
(a) Recognition of known action alternatives
(b) Generation of unknown action alternatives
(c) Determination of the relevancy of the action alternatives
(i) Determination if action alternatives are feasible and actionable
(ii) Determination if the action alternatives serve the goal
(iii) Determination of the relevance of action alternatives to the circumstances that are creating the threat or opportunity
(d) Determination if there is a sufficient pool of relevant action alternatives
5. Determination of consequences of each action alternative
(a) Recognition of known consequences of each action alternative
(b) Generation of not previously known consequences of each action alternative
(c) Recognition of known risks associated with each action alternative
(d) Generation of unknown risks associated with each relevant action alternative
(e) Recognition of known benefits associated with each action alternative
(f) Generation of unknown benefits associated with each relevant action alternative
6. Determination of probability of each consequence occurring if the action were undertaken
7. Establishment of the relative importance (value or utility) of each relative action alternative and consequence
(a) Ranking preference for each of the relevant action alternatives
(b) Ranking preference for each of the consequences
(c) Determining preference for self-directed vs. other-directed action alternatives
(d) Determination of just-right match for an action alternative and associated consequence
(e) Determination of the efficacy of each action alternative and its associated consequence for achieving the goal
8. Integration of the probability and importance determinations to identify the most attractive course of action

made by the individual in response to a certain need, with the intention of satisfying the motive that the need occasions" (Jabes 1978, p. 86).

The decision-making process is, simply, a taxonomy of how decisions are typically made. Table 20.1 provides our synthesis of steps typically discussed in the literature. We return to our prior discussion of the differences between autonomy as self-reliant action and autonomy as self-endorsed action at this juncture, however, to point out that "how" one makes a decision is not at the core of self-determined behavior. Because of its conflation with autonomous functioning, critics of self-psychology often point out that the model of decision-making reflected in Table 20.1 reflects one way of making decisions typically associated with Western cultures.

Wehmeyer et al. (2011) discussed the role of culture as a moderating variable pertaining to self-determination and Chap. 12 in this volume extends that discussion. Hall (1981) identified low and high context cultures, in which low context cultures emphasize independence, the importance of the individual, and a future-time orientation. These cultures highly value individual rights and choice. High context cultures value interdependence and relationships with others having a present-time orientation. In many cultures though, as Hall suggested, a sense of self is understood in relationship(s) with and to others; individuals often set their goals considering both their own needs and family needs (e.g., bringing honor to the family). Turnbull and Turnbull (2001) listed contrasting beliefs, values, and practices between Anglo-European culture and other cultures, including personal control over the environment, individualism, self-help, competition, future orientation, and goal orientation (Turnbull and Turnbull 2001; Zhang 2006). Non-Western cultures may encourage values and behaviors that differ from those associated with the Western emphasis on individualism (Zhang et al. 2005). The critical point to be made here is that efforts to promote self-determination must be culturally relevant and address efforts that promote self- (versus other-) determination in ways that emphasize the values, beliefs, and practices associated with the developmental process. Again, Chap. 12 provides a broader discussion of these issues.

So, given the caveats mentioned in the above discussion, most research on decision-making processes follow steps similar to those depicted in Table 20.1. As discussed in Chap. 2, the interaction between the organism's efforts to meet basic psychological needs and the resultant autonomous motivation and the environmental conditions of opportunity or threat stimulates causal action. Thus, a de facto first step in the decision-making process involves the person's recognition of the environmental or contextual challenges that create the opportunity or threat that is leading to the need to make a decision and, consequently, the recognition of the need that a decision must be made. Causal action, and thus decision making, is in service of a goal, so the person must identify the goal of which the decision is in service.

These lead to the more traditional steps in the decision-making process, the first being the identification of relevant action alternatives. Some such alternatives are probably already known to the decision maker, others will not be known and the person will need to engage in actions (talking to others, searching, etc.) that enable him or her to identify those additional action alternatives. As the person generates alternatives, he or she must evaluate the relevancy of alternatives in terms of feasibility and actionability, the relevancy of alternatives to the goal, and the relevancy to the circumstances creating the treat or opportunity. As is frequently noted, this first action step is, essentially, a problem-solving process.

Next, decision-makers must determine the consequences if each relevant action alternative is undertaken. Again, some consequences will already be known to the person, while he or she will need to generate other, unknown consequences. As consequences are identified, the person must identify (or generate if not known) information about the relative risks associated with each consequence and the potential benefits associated with each consequence. Once consequences are known, and relative risks and benefits associated with each consequence considered, the person must determine the probability that a give consequence would occur if the action was undertaken, taking into about likely frequency information, knowledge, and past experience.

After this, decision-makers consider the relative importance (e.g., value, utility) of each action alternative and related consequence as a function of the person's preferences, his or her preferences pertaining to self- versus other-directed action, and the just-right match between the action and consequence, particularly as a function of its efficacy for achieving the desired goal. Based upon all of this information, the person then integrates the probability and importance information to identify the most attractive course of action to them at that time.

The Development of Decision Making

The development of decision-making skills occurs, primarily, during early adolescence. As noted, the decision-making process begins with solving a problem (what are my action alternatives?) and ends with making a choice, so it is necessary for those skills to have been developed and available to adolescents as part of the development of decision making. Byrne (2002) posed a series of questions pertaining to what is known about the development of decision-making in adolescence, and they serve as a useful rubric to consider developmental issues. We pose them not as questions, but as topics in the following discussion.

The Role of Knowledge and Experience in Decision Making It stands to reason that greater knowledge about alternatives, consequences, risks, benefits, and so forth, as well as more life experiences pertaining to such, would be a factor in the development of decision-making skills. The evidence to support his is, however, mixed. As Byrne pointed out, for example, multiple studies show that for adolescents, knowledge about risky behaviors such as smoking, alcohol use, and so forth, is unrelated to the engagement in such behaviors. Not only is knowledge disregarded (often because of faulty consequential thinking) by adolescents, but research has shown that "experienced individuals are not necessarily experts" (Byrne 2002, p. 210). That is, supposed knowledge retained from past experience is, often as not, incorrect, inaccurate, or misremembered and, as such, of no more use than no knowledge in coming to competent decisions. That said, adults with greater experience are less likely to repeat options that have not been successful in the past than are children or adolescents who may have only tried an option once or twice and still not concluded that it is an ineffective option, and, as Byrne noted, values and preferences change over time, so the type of decision made will change as a function of those shifts in values and preferences. These changes in preference and values are, likely a function of maturity and experience.

Access to Knowledgeable Sources or Individuals The development of social networks and the accumulation of social capital benefits decision makers by expanding the network to which a person can turn to identify alternatives, consequences, risks, and benefits. Adolescence is a period of time in which young people are taking greater and greater responsibility for their lives. One strategy used by mature decision makers to make competent decisions is to seek the advice of knowledgeable sources or people with expertise or experience in the domain in which the decision must be made. Research suggests that adolescents are less likely to seek assistance from knowledgeable sources or experts and to rely, instead, on friends. Newman (2002) has looked at adaptive help seeking by adolescents in the context of academic performance. Newman notes that "[w]hen students monitor their academic performance, show awareness of difficulty they cannot overcome on their own, and exhibit the wherewithal and self-determination to remedy that difficulty by requesting assistance from a more knowledgeable individual, they are exhibiting mature, strategic behavior" (p. 132). Students who are successful at seeking help when needed evidence a set of competencies and motivations that facilitate such action, including:

- knowing when help is necessary;
- knowing that others can help;
- knowing how to ask a question that yields the needed information;
- knowing who is the best person to approach for help;
- knowing how to carry out a request for help in a socially appropriate manner;
- having motivational resources (goal knowledge, action-control beliefs) associated with tolerance for difficult tasks;
- willingness to express a need for help to others;
- a sense of personal agency (Newman 2002, pp. 132–133).

Using the need for competence, relatedness, and autonomy underlying SDT, Newman (2002) identified ways in which teachers can facilitate the development of adaptive help seeking. These begin with teacher-student intersubjectivity, defined by Newman (2002) as "attunement of teacher's and student's purposes, focus, and affect" (p. 133). Teachers who promote relatedness listen, ask questions, and inquire about student need for support, creating a learning environment in which students feel free to seek help. Newman notes that very young children seek help based upon global traits of niceness and kindness, but that as students enter adolescence such help seeking is weighted in more complex interactions pertaining to cost/benefit analyses comparing the benefits of obtaining information to the costs (might result in embarrassment, might look "dumb"). As the costs of seeking help from a teacher or an adult begin to include perceptions that doing so (e.g., seeking help from an adult) might jeopardize the increasingly important goals of friendships, social acceptance, and social affiliation for adolescents, they turn increasingly to their peers for such support. Asking for help in the classroom comes in conflict, according to the adolescent's perceptions, with fitting in or being socially accepted. Teachers can structure environments in which these important aspects of development don't clash and support students and peers to seek assistance as a group and not just individually. Focusing on the intrinsic value of learning, as opposed, for example, to just getting good grades, responds to students' needs for competence. Finally, autonomy supportive classrooms emphasize both the normality of help-seeking and minimize social comparisons.

Ability to Weight Multiple Pros and Cons Evaluations are at the heart of the decision-making process. The ability to evaluate the relative benefits and disadvantages among and between options is a critical developmental skill. Research shows that students develop the capacity to remember information that is relevant to evaluating an option over time, and that adolescents become increasingly skilled at both retaining relevant and important information, but also to being able to search for new information. Another aspect of the evaluation process—awareness of the number of consequences associated with any given option—is yoked to age. Adolescents are more aware of a greater number of consequences than younger children. As Byrne (2002) noted, however, it is unclear as to whether this is a true age difference in knowledge or an age difference in reporting information. Either way, a focus on providing experiences leading to greater knowledge about consequences is important in the development of evaluative thinking.

Differences in Goal Setting Strategies and Abilities We have discussed developmental aspects of the goal setting process in Chap. 18 and readers are referred to that chapter for more detail. With regard to decision making, the developmental issue that arises pertaining to goal-setting strategies involves the issue of coordinating multiple goals that arise in the course of the decision-making process, and there are age differences in this, with adolescents better able to coordinate multiple subgoals in service of a decision toward a larger goal.

Other Developmental Issues in Decision Making

In addition to the issues highlighted by Byrne (2002) described in the prior section, there are a number of other developmental issues that warrant mention. The first, decision control or willingness to choose, is related to the previous discussion pertaining to social affiliation and seeking help. That is, younger adolescents (13–15 year olds) are more prone to seek conformity and be influenced by peers in making a decision than older adolescents (Mann et al. 1989b). Further, the development of problem-solving abilities (discussed in Chap. 19) influence decision-making development for the simple fact that the decision-making process begins with a problem-solving sequence.

The Role of Decision Making in the Development of Self-Determination

Like problem solving, we have opted to situate the development of decision-making capacity within the context of agentic action. As discussed in Chap. 5, agentic action is a means by which something is done or achieved; agentic actions are self-directed toward a goal. When acting agentically, action is self-regulated, self-directed and enables progress toward freely chosen goals. Volitional actions involve the initiation and activation of agentic capabilities—the capacity to sustain action toward a goal. As shown in Fig. 5.2, there are multiple points within both the causal and agentic capability processes in which decisions serve the interest of goal attainment. From decisions about which goal to select in the goal generation process, to decisions about which outcomes of the goal discrepancy process to act upon, to decisions about what options are best to implement to reduce the discrepancy between a person's current state compared to her desired state, to decisions about what strategies to implement in the discrepancy reduction plan: decision-making opportunities are scattered throughout and making decisions becomes a critical aspect to be a causal agent in one's life.

Enhancing Decision-Making Skills

Beyth-Marom et al. (1991) pointed out that uncertainty is a basic element in many decisions. Research indicates that adults and children alike tend to underestimate the uncertainty in most decisions, often leading to less than optimal outcomes from decisions. There are a number of sources of uncertainty in any decision. Identifying the consequences of any given alternative is usually a "best guess" situation. This may result either from a lack of information about a particular option, or may just be a factor of the type of alternative. It is also often the case that there is uncertainty as to whether a particular alternative is actually available or will be available after a decision is made. The degree of uncertainty in each of these steps should be treated as a factor in reaching a decision, and the fact that such uncertainty typically exists should be a topic of instruction for students with disabilities.

Beyth-Marom et al. (1991) suggested that instruction which focuses on teaching adolescents about uncertainty should address questions like:

1. What is uncertainty?
2. What are the different kinds of uncertainty?
3. What is the relationship between uncertainty and amount of information?

Another factor which will impact the decision-making process is the amount of risk involved in making a particular decision. Schloss, Alper and Jayne (1994) detailed four levels of risk-taking associated with making a choice, and these dimensions are equally relevant when considering alternatives in the decision-making process. These levels are:

1. *The alternative involves limited potential for immediate risk, but little possibility of long-term harm to the individual or others.* Examples include choosing what to eat or wear. This first step also emphasizes that almost no choice is risk-free. For example, choosing to wear one's hair in a non-traditional manner may result in others making judgments and holding expectations that are limiting or unfair.

2. *The alternative involves mild risk with minimal possibility of long-lasting harm to the individual or others.* An example is choosing to spend one's lunch money on a video game and, as a result, having to go without lunch (Schloss et al. p. 218).
3. *The alternative results in a moderate probability for long-lasting harm to the individual or others.* Examples include becoming sexually active without adequate birth control (moderate risk of becoming pregnant) or choosing to smoke cigarettes (moderate risk of cancer or other illness).
4. *The alternative involves an almost certain outcome that includes personal injury.* Schloss and colleagues (1994) identify daily use of addictive substances as an example of this level. Another example might be unprotected sexual contact with multiple partners over a long period of time (risk of HIV infection).

Again, instruction can be targeted to assisting students to understand and discriminate amongst these levels of risk.

There is generally a dearth of research-based interventions to promote decision-making skills, and most instruction simply teaches, through role playing and modeling, the skills depicted in Table 20.1. Byrne (1998) and Beyth-Marom et al. (1991) identified several intervention programs addressing adolescent decision making, grouping them into two general types: programs geared toward improving general decision making skills (not content specific) and those geared toward decisions with specific (and often high risk) decision categories (e.g., drug/alcohol awareness and education). In the former (general decision making skills), work by Mann et al. (1989a) on the GOFER program has applicability. GOFER is an acronym for steps to sound decision making:

- Goals clarification
- Option generation
- Fact finding
- Consideration of Effects
- Review

Unfortunately, Byrne (1998) and Beyth-Marom et al. (1991) both commented on the limited data to support the utility of any of the general decision-making programs and were critical of the theoretical underpinnings for each program as well. To illustrate that there have been few efforts to create more systematic approaches to teaching decision-making skills to adolescents, a 2009 monograph from the American Academy of Arts and Sciences titled *Education and a Civil Society: Teaching Evidence-based Decision Making* (Callan et al. 2009) simply repeated the information provided by Byrne (1998) and Beyth-Marom et al. (1991). In essence, efforts to promote more effective decision making by adolescents and to promote the development of these skills should focus on the skills identified in Table 20.1 and teach these in a learning environment that offers autonomy supports and in the context of actually engaging in decision-making activities.

References

Beyth-Marom, R., Fischhoff, B., Jacobs Quadrel, M., & Furby, L. (1991). Teaching decision-making to adolescents: A critical review. In J. Baron & R. V. Brown (Eds.), *Teaching decision making to adolescents*. Hillsdale: Lawrence Erlbaum Associates.

Byrne, J. P. (1998). *The nature and development of decision making*. Mahwah: Lawrence Erlbaum Associates.

Byrne, J. P. (2002). The development of decision-making. *Journal of Adolescent Health, 31*, 208–215.

Callan, E., Grotzer, T., Kagan, J., Nisbett, R. E., Perkins, D. N., & Shulman, L. (2009). *Education and a civil society: Teaching evidence-based decision making*. Washington, DC: American Academy of Arts and Sciences.

Hall, E. (1981). *Beyond culture*. New York: Doubleday.

Jabes, J. (1978). *Individual processes in organizational behavior*. Arlington Heights: Harlam Davidson, Inc..

Mann, L., Harmoni, R., Power, C., Beswick, G., & Ormand, C. (1989a). Effectiveness of the GOFER course in decision making for high school students. *Journal of Behavioral Decision Making, 1*, 159–168.

Little, T. D., Hawley, P. H., Henrich, C. C., & Marsland, K. (2002). Three views of the agentic self: A developmental synthesis. In E. L. Deci & R. M. Ryan (Eds.), *Handbook of self-determination research* (pp. 389–404). Rochester/NY: University of Rochester Press.

Mann, L., Harmoni, R., & Power, C. (1989b). Adolescent decision-making: The development of competence. *Journal of adolescence, 12*, 265–278.

McGrew, A. G., & Wilson, M. J. (1982). Introduction. In A. G. McGrew & M. J. Wilson (Eds.), *Decision making: Approaches and analysis* (pp. 1–11). Manchester: Manchester University Press.

Newman, R. S. (2002). How self-regulated learners cope with academic difficulty: The role of adaptive help seeking. *Theory into Practice, 41*(2), 132–138.

Turnbull, A. P., & Turnbull, H. R. (2001). Self-determination for individuals with significant cognitive disabilities and their families. *Journal of the Association for Persons with Severe Handicaps, 26*(1), 56–62.

Schloss, P. J., Alper, S., & Jayne, D. (1994). Self-determination for persons with disabilities: Choice, risk, and dignity. *Exceptional Children, 60*, 215–225.

Van Petegem, S., Beyers, W., Vansteenkiste, M., & Soenens, B. (2012). On the association between adolescent autonomy and psychosocial functioning: Determining decisional independence from the Self-Determination Theory perspective. *Developmental Psychology, 48*(1), 76–88.

Wehmeyer, M. L., Abery, B., Zhang, D., Ward, K., Willis, D., Amin, W. H., et al. (2011). Personal self-determination and moderating variables that impact efforts to promote self-determination. *Exceptionality, 19*, 19–30.

Zhang, D. (2006). Parent practices in facilitating self-determination skills: The influences of context, socioeconomic status, and children's special education status. *Research and Practice for Persons with Severe Disabilities, 30*, 154–162.

Zhang, D., Wehmeyer, M., & Chen, L. J. (2005). Parent and teacher engagement in fostering the self-determination of students with disabilities: A comparison between the U.S. and the Republic of China. *Remedial and Special Education, 26*, 55–64.

Chapter 21
The Development of Hope

Susana C. Marques and Shane J. Lopez

Abstract Agentic action refers to the process of identifying pathways that lead to specific ends and engaging in self-directing and self-regulating action to navigate environmental opportunities and threats. Pathways thinking and agency thinking are critical elements of Hope Theory, and this this chapter concludes the section of this text on the development of agentic action by examining the role of hope, and Hope Theory, in the development of self-determination. The chapter begins with an overview of Hope Theory, followed by an examination of the development of hopeful thought and hope. Next, the chapter discusses measurement and the Hope Scale. The chapter concludes with a review of the literature in hope and by exploring interventions to promote hope and linkages between hope and Causal Agency Theory.

As noted in Chap. 2, agentic action refers to the process of identifying pathways that lead to specific ends and engaging in self-directing and self-regulating action to navigate environmental opportunities and threats. Pathways thinking and agency thinking are critical elements of Hope Theory, and this this chapter concludes the section of this text on the development of agentic action.

In the late-twentieth century, social scientists turned their attention to hope. Previous reviews (e.g., Lopez et al. 2003) have located more than two dozen scholarly theories or definitions of hope (and a handful of validated measures) and discussed some of their common characteristics. Generally conceptualizations of hope emphasize a person's thoughts and feelings about the future and thoughts and feelings about personal capacity to make the future better.

S.C. Marques (✉)
University of Porto, Porto, Portugal
e-mail: smarques@fpce.up.pt

S.J. Lopez
Gallup and The Clifton Strengths School, Omaha, NE, USA

M.L. Wehmeyer et al. (eds.), *Development of Self-Determination Through the Life-Course*, DOI 10.1007/978-94-024-1042-6_21

Hope Theory

Snyder and his colleagues (Snyder 1994; Snyder et al. 1991) developed a psychological theory and cognitive motivational model of hope based in goal-directed thinking that has received much attention both within and outside the field of psychology (Marques et al. 2014). According to hope theory (Snyder et al. 1991), hope reflects peoples' perceptions regarding their capacities to: (1) clearly conceptualize goals; (2) develop the specific strategies to reach those goals (pathways thinking); and (3) initiate and sustain the motivation for using those strategies (agency thinking). Goals, whether short-term or long-term, provide the targets of mental action sequences and vary in the degree to which they are specified, but all goals must be of sufficient value to warrant sustained conscious thought about them (Snyder 2002). Pathways thinking refers to a person's perceived ability to generate workable routes to desired goals (Snyder et al. 2002a) and the production of several pathways is important when encountering impediments. Agency thinking is the motivational component in hope theory that reflects a person's cognitions about his or her ability to begin and sustain goal-directed behavior (Snyder et al. 2003). Therefore, agency thinking takes on special significance when people encounter challenges or obstacles (Snyder 2002). Pathways and agency thinking are positively related, additive and reciprocal, but neither component alone defines hope, nor are they synonymous. When a person has a robust level of hope they will convey messages such as: "I'll find a way to get this done!"; "I can do this.", and "I am not going to be stopped." Whereas other positive psychology constructs such as goal theory (Covington 2000; Dweck 1999), optimism (Scheier and Carver 1985), self-efficacy (Bandura 1982), and problem-solving (Heppner and Petersen 1982) give differentially weighted emphases to the goal itself or to the future-oriented agency- or pathways-related processes, hope theory equally emphasizes all of these goal-pursuit components (Snyder 1994).

The Development of Hope

In detailing the importance of hope to success in life, it is necessary to elucidate first the mechanisms through which hopeful thought develops. Snyder (1994, 2000a, b) established a developmental framework for how hopeful thought takes form. One of the first goals of a newborn is to predict and control its environment, a necessary ability for survival. In fact, many developmental theorists (e.g., Berlyne 1960; Kagan 1972) have held that feelings of disorientation and confusion motivate individuals to improve their causal understanding. These feelings reflect unfulfilled needs in infants that are ultimately sated by the development of hopeful thought (Snyder et al. 2002a, b). Pathways thinking is the first component of hope to develop in children. Upon birth, infants are inundated with a bewildering sensory input but with time each sensation is imbued with meaning and linked temporally with another sensation. These connections turn into anticipatory thoughts in the infant's mind. This anticipation is the mechanism by which children later are able to cognitively chain events together to form if-then thinking, the precursor to pathways thinking.

Agency thought also develops early in life. By the age of 12–21 months children establish a sense of self (Kaplan 1978) and further evincing self-awareness. This self-awareness is followed by the realization that one can act as a causal agent. This sense of self, combined with the recognition that one can initiate change in the environment, is the basis of agency thought (Snyder 1994, 2000a, b).

Hopeful thought becomes more refined as the child matures. This improvement in hopeful thinking sparks developmental gains in vocabulary, memory capacity, and abstraction, skills that, in turn, help children to use hope more productively and achieve personal goals. This maturation is parallel to school entrance and the connection between hope and school begins to assume particular importance. According to hope theory (Snyder 1994, 2002), high-hope students demonstrate superior academic performance compared to their low-hope counterparts. Performance in school, often related to one's ability to set concrete goals and then attain the goal, necessitates using adequate pathways and agency thoughts. Research has supported this link.

Research has also demonstrated that hope is built on a foundation of contingency thinking (Snyder 1994) and that it is socially primed (Snyder et al. 1997a, b). The way that key stakeholder (e.g., parents, teachers) communicate, set goals, view challenges, cope with problems influences the development of children's hope (Marques and Lopez 2011). Related to this point, Marques et al. (2007) identified a moderate relation between children's hope and their parents' in a sample of Portuguese students. Further research is needed to investigate these process mechanisms (see Hoy et al. 2013).

Hope System Beliefs and Measurement

Hope is not only a goal-directed cognitive process. It also is a hierarchically organized system of beliefs regarding one's ability to successfully engage in such a thought process. These beliefs are organized into four specific levels of abstraction: global or trait hope; domain-specific hope; goal-specific hope; and state hope. Peoples' overall evaluation of their capacity to construct sufficient pathways and generate the agency thoughts necessary to achieve goals is known as global or trait hope (Snyder et al. 2002b). Adult and child versions of the Hope Scale have been developed to measure such global hope (Snyder et al. 1997a, 1991). A second, more concrete level in the system of hope-related beliefs is domain-specific. Illustratively, people who are high in global hope have the tendency to manifest high hope in most life domains. However, a gap commonly is observed in students who, although quite hopeful about life in general, display low hope in the academic domain (Snyder et al. 2002a, b). To fill this need, the Domain-Specific Hope Scale (Sympson 1999) was developed to assess adolescents' and adults' hope in six life arenas: social relationships, romantic relationships, family life, academics, work, and leisure.

A more concrete level in the hope belief hierarchy is the goal-specific level, manifested regarding a specific goal. Even when an individual's global and domain-specific hope levels are quite high, it is still possible that he or she will evidence low hope regarding a specific goal. The goal-specific level of analysis, then, may be important in understanding perceived deficits in specific goal-pursuits. Additionally, Snyder et al. (1996) developed and validated the State Hope Scale for tapping a person's hope in a specific context. Without identifying the goals, this State Hope Scale measures a person's momentary hopeful thinking, providing a snapshot of a person's current goal-directed thinking. That is to say, in contrast to the more enduring type of motivational set, the State Hope Scale is related to the ongoing events in people's lives. Both trait and state are operative and useful depending on one's focus. People probably have dispositional hope that applies across situations and times, but they also have state hope that reflects particular times and more proximal events.

Theoretically, dispositional hope should relate to the intensity of state hope by setting a band or range within which state hope varies. As such, it is important to pay close attention not only to global hope, but also to domain- and goal-specific hope and state hope to understand the complex web of hope-related beliefs that individuals possess (Snyder et al. 2002a, b).

Hope Theory: 25 Years of Research

Over the last 25 years, researchers have gained a clearer understanding of the relationships between hope and areas that are most salient to people lives.

Hope and Social-Emotional Development

Accumulating evidence suggests that hope is positively related with life satisfaction, perceived competence, self-worth (Marques et al. 2009) and negatively associated with symptoms of depression (Snyder et al. 1991) and measures of internalizing and externalizing behavior problems (e.g., Gilman et al. 2006). Indeed, researchers have reported that children very high in hope (upper 10% of the distribution) differ from students with average (middle 25%) and very low hope (bottom 10%) on self-esteem and life satisfaction, with significant higher self-esteem and life satisfaction levels for the very high-hope group (Marques et al. 2015). As with self-worth, extremely high and average hope is associated with mental health benefits that are not found among adolescents reporting comparatively extremely low hope levels (Marques et al. 2015). Additional longitudinal evidence suggests that adolescents with lower levels of hope (and life satisfaction) who experienced several stressful events had a higher risk of developing low mental health 5 years later, while those with higher levels of hope (and life satisfaction) were not exposed to this vulnerability (Marques 2016).

Also, lower hope predicts more depressive symptoms (Kwon 2000), and it does so independently of appraisals and other coping strategies (Chang and DeSimone 2001). Results from a recent meta-analysis found that hope accounted for 23% of the strength of student assets, making its greatest contributions to self-worth, optimism, and life satisfaction (Marques et al. 2016). Those with high hope typically are more optimistic, more focused on success when pursuing goals, they develop many life goals, and they perceive themselves as being capable of solving problems that may arise (Snyder et al. 1991, 1997a). Likewise, higher hope is linked closely to having a greater perceived purpose in life (Feldman and Snyder 2005).

Hope, Spirituality and Religiosity

There remains a paucity of research on the relationships between hope and spirituality and religiosity. Preliminary findings suggest no significant differences between children's hope from families that practice and do not practice religion (Santos 2012). Longitudinal findings with adolescents (Marques et al. 2013) indicated that hope is moderately correlated with spirituality but shares weak relations with religious practice (as measured by attendance at a place of worship). These associations were stable 6 months and 1 year later. Nevertheless, further research from different countries and ages is clearly needed (including different indicators of religiosity).

Hope and Physical Health

Research suggests that hope may play a significant role in health. Berg et al. (2007) investigated the relation between hope and adherence to a daily inhaled steroid regimen among 48 asthma patients ages 8–12. A multivariate model with children's hope level entered in the second step predicted adherence (and no other demographic or psychosocial variables were significant predictors of adherence). These results support hope as a significant predictor of student adherence to prescribed medication. As a possible explanation for these findings is that low-hope individuals may not believe their medication will provide a pathway to their goals of improved health; or it may be that taking the medication is difficult or uncomfortable, thus affecting their agency beliefs (Snyder 2000a). These findings highlight the need to attend to psychosocial predictors of adherence, specifically hope, and might help practitioners target these factors in their efforts to increase adherence among pediatric asthma patients.

Similarly, research on adolescents with diabetes showed that those with higher hope were more likely to adhere to a medical regimen necessary for glycemic control (Lloyd et al. 2009). Past research (Lewis and Kliewer 1996) on children with sickle-cell disease found that those who had the disease but maintained high hope perceptions along with active coping strategies were less likely to experience the negative effects of anxiety. Hope can provide benefits for those struggling with their health, but it can also facilitate healthy behaviors. At the college level, students with high hope were less likely to binge drink and smoke, even when controlling for demographics (Berg et al. 2011). Further, these high-hope students were more likely to restrict fat in their diet and they engaged in more frequent exercise than low-hope students.

Hope and Academic Outcomes

As early as grade school, hope is significantly related to achievement test scores (Snyder et al. 1997b). This trend continues throughout the educational sequence.

For example, higher levels of hope are related to stronger academic performance, as measured by grade point average, in elementary school students (Marques et al. 2011b, Snyder et al. 1997b), in junior high school and high school (Ciarrochi et al. 2007; Lopez et al. 2000; Snyder et al. 1991; Worrell and Hale 2001), and college (Buckelew et al. 2008; Curry et al. 1999; Snyder et al. 1991, 2002a). Additionally, there is some evidence that high-hope students are less likely to experience anxiety or engage in self-deprecatory thinking in academic situations (Onwuegbuzie and Snyder 2000; Snyder 1999). This may be due in part to the tendency for high-hope students to engage in more problem solving and positive problem orientation than low-hope students (Chang 1998).

Hope is not merely a proxy for intelligence and personality variables often associated with academic performance. Findings suggest that the predictive power of hope remained significant even when controlling for intelligence (Day et al. 2010; Snyder et al. 1997a, b), prior grades (Gallagher and Lopez 2008; Snyder et al. 1991, 2002a), self-esteem (Snyder et al. 2002a; b), personality (Day et al. 2010), and college entrance examination scores (Gallagher and Lopez 2008; Snyder et al. 2002a), such as high school GPA and ACT/SAT. Furthermore, recent research suggested that very high hope Portuguese youths (top 10%) reported significantly higher academic achievement and school engagement (Marques et al. 2015) than youth in the average (middle 25%) and very low (bottom 10%) hope groups.

Based on the longitudinal findings (Marques 2016), students with high levels of hope at the mean age of 12 years were at a reduced risk of developing school difficulties (i.e., low levels of school engagement) at the mean age of 17. These associations remained significant after controlling for age, gender and preexisting difficulties on school engagement at the mean age of 12. Additionally, early adolescents with lower levels of hope who experienced several stressful events had a superior risk of developing difficulties of engagement at school during early adulthood, while those with higher levels of hope were not exposed to this vulnerability (Marques et al. 2016).

When analyzing the relationship between agency and pathways components of hope, some studies suggest a significant positive relation between both components of hope and academic achievement (Day et al. 2010), while other studies suggest differential relationships. For example, a study with a college sample of students (Buckelew et al. 2008) reported that scores on the Agency subscale correlated positively with semester GPA (even when intelligence and anxiety were controlled), but not those on the Pathways subscale and GPA. Further research is needed in this area.

Hope and Athletic Achievement

Researchers have found that higher hope is positively related to superior athletic (and academic) performances among student athletes (Curry et al. 1997, 1999), even after statistically controlling for variance related to their natural athletic abilities. For example, Curry et al. (1997) reported that high-hope student athletes performed significantly better in track and field events than their low-hope counterparts, with trait and state hope scale scores together accounting for 56% of the variance in subsequent track performances.

Curry et al. (1999) examined the efficacy of a semester-long academic class aimed to raise students' levels of hope. Results from this study revealed that students have increased confidence related to their athletic ability, academic achievement, and self-esteem, after taking the "hope" class. These gains were retained for at least a year after completion of the athlete class intervention. Also, high- as compared to low-hope children were less likely to consider quitting their sports (Brown et al. 1999).

Hope, Demographics and Social Contexts

Preliminary research has found that hope is unrelated to the type of family structure and living situation (Santos 2012), although it is positively correlated with parents' educational level (Marques et al. 2007; Santos 2012). Moreover, hope is significantly lower among students from families where both parents are unemployed compared to students with one or neither of the parents unemployed (Santos 2012).

Cross-sectional findings suggest that hope is unrelated to gender and age in the early ages (Marques et al. 2011a). However, when the results are analyzed across the life span, (using a large Portuguese ample), hope levels are average in childhood (ages 10–13) and drop during the adolescent years (ages 14–17), rise gradually throughout adulthood from ages 18–29 to ages 46–64, and then decline in old age (Marques 2016b). Further, the differences in the hope scores of children and adults across ethnic groups have been examined. Researchers have found that Caucasians tend to report fewer obstacles (e.g., oppression, prejudice) in their lives than their ethnic-minority counterparts, although there differences were not statistically significant, but that minority groups report higher average hope scores (see McDermott et al. 1997; Munoz-Dunbar 1993) and higher average levels of agency thinking (Chang and Banks 2007) than Caucasians.

To date, few studies have examined the relative levels of hope among other groups, such as gifted students, students with disabilities, and groups at risk (e.g., institutionalized youth), necessitating additional research among these populations. The limited research that has been conducted with students with disabilities suggests that students with disabilities report lower levels of hope than students without disabilities, but that environmental factors likely shape these differences (Shogren et al. 2006).

Hope: Potential for Programs and Interventions

Although hope is generally stable across the life span, with moderate test-retest correlations at 1, 2 year and 5-years (e.g., Marques 2016; Marques et al. 2016; Valle et al. 2004), research suggests that hope is malleable to change through intentional efforts in children, adolescents, adults and old adults (Cheavens et al. 2006; Curry et al. 1999; Feldman and Dreher 2012; Klausner et al. 2000; Lopez et al. 2000; MacLeod et al. 2007; Marques et al. 2011a).

One program, *Building Hope for the Future – A Program to Foster Strengths in School Students* (see Marques et al. 2011a for detailed description about the program) is designed for delivery using a group format over 5 weekly sessions, to help students to (1) conceptualize clear goals; (2) produce numerous range of pathways to attainment; (3) summon the mental energy to maintain the goal pursuit; and (4) reframe seemingly insurmountable obstacles as challenges to be overcome. This program is based on the theoretical and applied work of Snyder and colleagues (Lopez et al. 2000; Snyder et al. 2002a; McDermott and Snyder 1999) and uses a social-ecological perspective, integrating solution-focused, narrative and cognitive-behavioral techniques. It includes psycho-educational, skills training and group process components, as well as structured activities, roleplaying, and guided discussion. The five sessions focus on: (1) Learning about Hope, (2) Structuring Hope, (3) Creating Positive and Specific Goals, (4) Practice Makes Perfect, and (5) Review and Apply for the Future. The program can be delivered by key stakeholders such as parents, teachers and school peers. A variety of activities and hope-related information is included that parents and teachers can use to develop their own and their students hopeful thinking. The activities and resources are organized in three segments: (1) Learning about hope, (2) Instilling Hope (includes Hope Finding and Hope Bonding), and (3) Increasing Hope (includes Hope Enhancing and Hope Reminding). When implemented with middle-school students, their parents, teachers and peers, students showed increased hope, life satisfaction and self-worth for 1-year and 6-months after the program, in contrast to a matched comparison group.

References

Bandura, A. (1982). Self-efficacy mechanism in human agency. *American Psychologist, 37*, 122–147.

Berg, C. J., Rapoff, M. A., Snyder, C. R., & Belmont, J. M. (2007). The relationship of children's hope to pediatric asthma treatment adherence. *Journal of Positive Psychology, 2*, 176–184.

Berg, C. J., Ritschel, L. A., Swan, D. W., An, L. C., & Ahluwalia, J. S. (2011). The role of hope in engaging in healthy behaviors among college students. *American Journal of Health Behavior, 35*, 402–415.

Berlyne, D. E. (1960). *Conflict arousal and curiosity*. New York: McGrawHill.

Brown, M., Curry, L. A., Hagstrom, H., & Sandstedt, S. (1999, August). *Female teenage athletes, sport participation, self-esteem, and hope*. Paper presented at the Association for the Advancement of Applied Sport Psychology, Banff, Alberta, Canada.

Buckelew, S. P., Crittendon, R. S., Butkovic, J. D., Price, K. B., & Hurst, M. (2008). Hope as a predictor of academic performance. *Psychological Reports, 103*, 411–414.

Chang, E. C. (1998). Hope, problem-solving ability, and coping in a college student population: Some implications for theory and practice. *Journal of Clinical Psychology, 54*, 953–962.

Chang, E. C., & Banks, K. H. (2007). The color and texture of hope: Some preliminary findings and implications for hope theory and counseling among diverse racial/ethnic groups. *Cultural Diversity & Ethnic Minority Psychology, 13*, 94–103.

Chang, E. C., & DeSimone, S. L. (2001). The influence of hope on appraisals, coping, and dysphoria: A test of hope theory. *Journal of Social and Clinical Psychology, 20*, 117–129.

Cheavens, J. S., Feldman, D. B., Gum, A., Michael, S. T., & Snyder, C. R. (2006). Hope therapy in a community sample: A pilot investigation. *Social Indicators Research, 77*, 61–78.

Ciarrochi, J., Heaven, P. C., & Davies, F. (2007). The impact of hope, self-esteem, and attributional style on adolescents' school grades and emotional well-being: A longitudinal study. *Journal of Research in Personality, 41*, 1161–1178.

Covington, M. V. (2000). Goal theory, motivation, and school achievement: An integrative review. *Annual Review of Psychology, 51*, 171–200.

Curry, L. A., Snyder, C. R., Cook, D. L., Ruby, B. C., & Rehm, M. (1997). Role of hope in academic and sport achievement. *Journal of Personality and Social Psychology, 73*, 1257–1267.

Curry, L. A., Maniar, S. D., Sondag, K. A., & Sandstedt, S. (1999). *An optimal performance academic course for university students and student-athletes*. Unpublished manuscript. University of Montana, Missoula.

Day, L., Hanson, K., Maltby, J., Proctor, C., & Wood, A. (2010). Hope uniquely predicts objective academic achievement above intelligence, personality, and previous academic achievement. *Journal of Research in Personality, 44*, 550–553.

Dweck, C. S. (1999). *Self-theories: Their role in motivation, personality, and development*. Philadelphia: Taylor & Francis.

Feldman, D. B., & Snyder, C. R. (2005). Hope and the meaningful life: Theoretical and empirical associations between goal-directed thinking and life meaning. *Journal of Social & Clinical Psychology, 24*, 401–421. doi:10.1521/jscp.24.3.401.65616.

Feldman, D. B., & Dreher, D. E. (2012). Testing the efficacy of a single-session goal-pursuit intervention for college students. *Journal of Happiness Studies, 13*, 745–759.

Gallagher, M. W., & Lopez, S. J. (2008). *Hope, self-efficacy, and academic success in college students*. Poster presented at the annual convention of the American Psychological Association, Boston.

Gilman, R., Dooley, J., & Florell, D. (2006). Relative levels of hope and their relationship with academic and psychological indicators among adolescents. *Journal of Social and Clinical Psychology, 25*, 166–178.

Heppner, P. P., & Petersen, C. H. (1982). The development and implications of a personal problem solving inventory. *Journal of Counseling Psychology, 29*, 66–75.

Hoy, B., Suldo, S., & Mendez, L. (2013). Links between parents' and children's levels of gratitude, life satisfaction, and hope. *Journal of Happiness Studies, 14*, 1343–1361.

Kagan, J. (1972). Motives and development. *Journal of Personality and Social Psychology, 22*, 51–66.

Kaplan, L. (1978). *Oneness and separateness*. New York: Simon & Schuster.

Klausner, E., Snyder, C. R., & Cheavens, J. (2000). A hope-based group treatment for depressed older adult outpatients. In G. M. Williamson, P. A. Parmlee, & D. R. Shaffer (Eds.), *Physical illness and depression in older adults: A handbook of theory, research, and practice* (pp. 295–310). New York: Plenum.

Kwon, P. (2000). Hope and dysphoria: The moderating role of defense mechanisms. *Journal of Personality, 68*, 199–223.

Lewis, H. A., & Kliewer, W. (1996). Hope, coping, and adjustment among children with sickle cell anemia: Tests of mediator and moderator models. *Journal of Pediatric Psychology, 21*, 25–41.

Lloyd, S. M., Cantell, M., Pacaud, D., Crawford, S., & Dewey, D. (2009). Brief report: Hope, perceived maternal empathy, medical regime adherence, and glycemic control in adolescents with type 1 diabetes. *Journal of Pediatric Psychology, 34*, 1025–1029.

Lopez, S. J., Bouwkamp, J., Edwards, L. M., & Teramoto Pedrotti, J. (2000). *Making hope happen via brief interventions*. Paper presented at the second Positive Psychology Summit, Washington, DC.

Lopez, S. J., Snyder, C. R., & Pedrotti, J. T. (2003). Hope: Many definitions, many measures. In S. J. Lopez & C. R. Snyder (Eds.), *Positive psychological assessment: A handbook of models and measures* (pp. 91–107). Washington, DC: American Psychological Association.

MacLeod, A. K., Coates, E., & Hetherton, J. (2007). Increasing well-being through teaching goal-setting and planning skills: Results of a brief intervention. *Journal of Happiness Studies, 9*, 185–196.

Marques, S. C. (2016). Age Differences and short-term stability in hope: Results from a sample aged 15 to 80. *Submitted.*

Marques, S. C., Pais-Ribeiro, J. L., & Lopez, S. J. (2007). Validation of a Portuguese version of the students' life satisfaction scale. *Applied Research in Quality of Life, 2*, 83–94.

Marques, S. C., Pais-Ribeiro, J. L., & Lopez, S. J. (2009). Validation of a Portuguese version of the children hope scale. *School Psychology International, 30*, 538–551.

Marques, S. C., Lopez, S. J., & Pais-Ribeiro, J. L. (2011a). "Building hope for the future" – A program to foster strengths in middle-school students. *Journal of Happiness Studies, 12*, 139–152.

Marques, S. C., Pais-Ribeiro, J. L., & Lopez, S. J. (2011b). The role of positive psychology constructs in predicting mental health and academic achievement in children and adolescents: A two-year longitudinal study. *Journal of Happiness Studies, 12*, 1049–1062.

Marques, S. C., Lopez, S. J., & Mitchell, J. (2013). The role of hope, spirituality and religious practice in adolescents' life satisfaction: Longitudinal findings. *Journal of Happiness Studies, 14*, 251–261.

Marques, S. C., Lopez, S. J., Fontaine, A. M., Coimbra, S., & Mitchell, J. (2014). Validation of a Portuguese version of the Snyder Hope scale in a sample of high school students. *Journal of Psychoeducational Assessment, 32*, 781–786.

Marques, S. C., Lopez, S. J., Fontaine, A. M., Coimbra, S., & Mitchell, J. (2015). How much hope is enough? Levels of hope and students' psychological and school functioning. *Psychology in the Schools, 52*, 325–334.

Marques, S. C., Lopez, S. J., Reichard, R. J., & Dollwet, M. (2016). Relation of hope to academic outcomes: A meta-analysis. *Journal of Happiness Studies, 14*, 251–261.

McDermott, D., & Snyder, C. R. (1999). *Making hope happen*. Oakland: New Harbinger.

McDermott, D., Hastings, S. L., Gariglietti, K. P., Gingerich, K., Callahan, B., & Diamond, K. (1997). *A cross-cultural investigation of hope in children and adolescents*. Resources in Education, CG028078.

Munoz-Dunbar, R. (1993). *Hope: A cross-cultural assessment of American college students.* Unpublished master's thesis. University of Kansas, Lawrence, Kansas.

Onwuegbuzie, A. J., & Snyder, C. R. (2000). Relations between hope and graduate students' coping strategies for studying and examination-taking. *Psychological Reports, 86*, 803–806.

Santos, A. (2012). *Hope, family challenges and school context.* Unpublished master thesis, Escola Superior de Altos Estudos, Instituto Superior Miguel Torga, Portugal (in Portuguese).

Scheier, M. F., & Carver, C. S. (1985). Optimism, coping, and health: Assessment and implications of generalized outcome expectancies. *Health Psychology, 4*, 219–247.

Shogren, K. A., Lopez, S. J., Wehmeyer, M. L., Little, T. D., & Pressgrove, C. L. (2006). The role of positive psychology constructs in predicting life satisfaction in adolescents with and without cognitive disabilities: An exploratory study. *The Journal of Positive Psychology, 1*, 37–52.

Snyder, C. R. (1994). *The psychology of hope: You can get there from here.* New York: Free Press.

Snyder, C. R. (1999). Hope, goal blocking thoughts, and test-related anxieties. *Psychological Reports, 84*, 206–208.

Snyder, C. R. (2000a). Genesis: Birth and growth of hope. In C. R. Snyder (Ed.), *Handbook of hope: Theory, measures, and applications* (pp. 25–57). San Diego: Academic.

Snyder, C. R. (2000b). Hypothesis: There is hope. In C. R. Snyder (Ed.), *Handbook of hope: Theory, measures, and applications* (pp. 3–21). San Diego: Academic.

Snyder, C. R. (2002). Hope theory: Rainbows in the mind. *Psychological Inquiry, 13*, 249–275.

Snyder, C. R., Harris, C., Anderson, J. R., Holleran, S. H., Irving, L. M., Sigmon, S. T., Yoshinobu, L., Gibb, J., Langelle, C., & Harney, P. (1991). The will and the ways: Development and validation of an individual-differences measure of hope. *Journal of Personality and Social Psychology, 60*, 570–585.

Snyder, C. R., Sympson, S. C., Ybasco, F. C., Borders, T. F., Babyak, M. A., & Higgins, R. L. (1996). Development and validation of the state hope scale. *Journal of Personality and Social Psychology, 70*, 321–335.

Snyder, C. R., Hoza, B., Pelham, W. E., Rapoff, M., Ware, L., Danovsky, M., Highberger, L., Rubinstein, H., & Stahl, K. L. (1997a). The development and validation of the children's hope scale. *Journal of Pediatric Psychology, 22*, 399–421.

Snyder, C. R., Cheavens, J., & Sympson, S. C. (1997b). Hope: An individual motive for social commerce. *Group Dynamics: Theory, Research, and Practice, 1*, 107–118.

Snyder, C. R., Shorey, H. S., Cheavens, J., Pulvers, K. M., Adams III, V. H., & Wiklund, C. (2002a). Hope and academic success in college. *Journal of Educational Psychology, 94*, 820–826.

Snyder, C. R., Feldman, D. B., Shorey, H. S., & Rand, K. L. (2002b). Hopeful choices: A school counselor's guide to hope theory. *Professional School Counseling, 5*, 298–307.

Snyder, C. R., Lopez, S. J., Shorey, H. L., Rand, K. L., & Feldman, D. B. (2003). Hope theory, measurements, and applications to school psychology. *School Psychology Quarterly, 18*, 122–139.

Sympson, S. (1999). *Validation of the domain specific hope scale.* Unpublished doctoral dissertation, Department of Psychology, University of Kansas, Lawrence.

Valle, M. F., Huebner, E. S., & Suldo, S. M. (2004). Further evaluation of the children's hope scale. *Journal of Psychoeducational Assessment, 22*, 320–337.

Worrell, F. C., & Hale, R. L. (2001). The relationship of hope in the future and perceived school climate to school completion. *School Psychology Quarterly, 16*, 307–388.

Part VI
Action-Control Beliefs

Synthesis

Causal action involves engagement in skills related to volitional and agentic action that are motivated by efforts to satisfy basic psychological needs. In addition, however such actions are mitigated by beliefs that empower and enable individuals to act. The chapter in this part overviews action-control beliefs and Action-Control Theory. Action-control beliefs involve three general beliefs that reflect the relationship between the three components of an action sequence: control expectancy, which refers to the relation between agent and ends, meaning that individual's expectancy about their capability to achieve a given goal or end; means-ends beliefs, which represent the relation between means and ends; and agency beliefs, refer to an individual's beliefs of what means they are capable of utilizing when the self acts as an agent.

Chapter 22
Action-Control Beliefs and Agentic Actions

Rong Chang, Nicole Adams, and Todd D. Little

Abstract Throughout their lifespan, agentic individuals consistently update their understandings of situational and environmental contexts and frequently deconstruct and reconstruct their actions as well as the consequences of their actions that arose within these contexts. Highly agentic persons display high aspirations, are motivated to engage the environment, and persist through difficulty. Individuals who are not agentic have lower aspirations, believe that actions have little effect on their outcomes, and are lacking in basic problem-solving skills. These non-agentic individuals typically accept failures and do not reflect on the actions which led to the failure. This chapter overviews action-control beliefs and Action-Control Theory. Action-control beliefs involve three general beliefs that reflect the relationship between the three components of an action sequence: control expectancy, which refers to the relation between agent and ends, meaning that individual's expectancy about their capability to achieve a given goal or end; means-ends beliefs, which represent the relation between means and ends; and agency beliefs, refer to an individual's beliefs of what means they are capable of utilizing when the self acts as an agent.

As has been emphasized throughout this text, individuals with personal agency command a sense of empowerment by knowing both what it takes to achieve their goals and how they can reach them (i.e., what it takes and whether I've got it; Skinner et al. 1990; see also Little et al. 2002). Throughout their lifespan, agentic individuals consistently update their understandings of situational and environmental contexts and frequently deconstruct and reconstruct their actions as well as the consequences of their actions that arose within these contexts. Highly agentic persons display high aspirations, are motivated to engage the environment, and persist through difficulty. Individuals who are not agentic have lower aspirations, believe that actions have little effect on their outcomes, and are lacking in basic problem-solving skills. These non-agentic individuals typically accept failures and do not reflect on the actions which led to the failure.

R. Chang (✉) • N. Adams
Texas Tech University, Lubbock, TX, USA
e-mail: rong.chang@ttu.edu

T.D. Little
Educational Psychology and Leadership, Texas Tech University, Lubbock, TX, USA

M.L. Wehmeyer et al. (eds.), *Development of Self-Determination Through the Life-Course*, DOI 10.1007/978-94-024-1042-6_22

The personal agency perspective is a multilayered theory with reaching influences from Self-Determination Theory, Action-Control Theory, Resource-Control Theory, Symbolic-Action Theory and others (Boesch 1991; Little et al. 2002, 2006). Personal agency, as a core psychological construct, has its roots in the perspective of organismic assumptions about human behavior. Biological and psychological needs are inherent to human behavior and they motivate individuals to establish goals (both short-term and long-term) and master challenges that arise in their surrounding environment. People are intrinsically motivated to reach those goals that will ultimately satisfy their personal needs.

During their life-span development, individuals will seek out resources to accomplish their physical growth and development (Darwin 1859; Hawley 1999; Reckless 1979). Resources can be defined as supplements for personal growth such as food or partners (Little et al. 2002, 2006). Practically speaking, individuals alone are not able to access every resource. In order to have greater accessibility to diverse resources, individuals can integrate into a social group. Social groups, however, can potentially evolve to within-group competition for limited-access resources. Therefore, an individual who is part of a social group may experience either gains or loss. Winners are able to take advantage of certain resources, while losers are not extended this ready access to resources. People who have frequently experienced wins, learn that they are able to meet their needs and control their environment. Conversely, people who have experienced losses realize they are not able to achieve their goals without external support. Thus, both early and life-long win-loss experiences can influence a person's sense of agency (Baltes 1987; Heckhausen et al. 1989; Little et al. 2002, 2006).

As a complement to basic biological needs, Ryan and Deci (2002) proposed that there are three inherent psychological needs that influence people's behaviors. These inherent needs are competence, relatedness, and autonomy. The need for competence refers to the need to feel capable of mastering tasks and having successful interactions with others and the environment (Deci and Ryan 1985; Ryan and Deci 2000; Weiner 1986; White 1959). Relatedness is similar to belongingness, the need to feel belonging or connected to others (Deci and Ryan 1985; Ryan and Deci 2000). Autonomy is the need to feel a sense of control over one's actions, goals, and their interaction with their environment (Ryan and Deci 2000; Ryan 1993).

From this perspective, "humans have a need to be autonomous and engage in activities because they want to" (Schunk et al. 2008, p. 248). Undertaking an action autonomously is particularly important for individuals' intrinsic motivation behind their actions (Deci and Ryan 2000; Lindley 1986; Ryan 1993). Self-determined persons make choices based on their needs and decide how to attain these desired needs. In this regard, to ensure the goals and actions are determined by the self, a person's actions must be autonomously enacted. Therefore, autonomy functions as driving force behind actions, with the actions helping the individual to strive for self-realization and self-determination (Little et al. 2002, 2006).

These biological and psychological needs provide direction for individuals to know what they should strive for and the manner in which to act in order to achieve their self-prescribed goals (Schunk et al. 2008, p. 169). Throughout their lifespan, individuals have interactions with their environment and these interactions provide meaning to their actions. In other words, actions that are selected from the presented choices for mastering the challenges are a reflection of the self. From this organismic viewpoint, individuals are intentional, self-regulating, goal-oriented, with their behaviors being purposive, volitional and self-initiated (Boesch 1991; Brandtstädter 1998; Chapman 1984; Skinner et al. 1988; Little et al. 2002).

During the process of goal pursuit, actions are executed by each individual – that is, the self as agent, or the agentic self. To achieve a desired goal, agentic or self-determined persons must be aware of their strengths and weaknesses, be able to recognize their needs, and make choices that will satisfy those needs and ultimately take action (Malmberg et al. 2004; Nurmi 2001; Little et al. 2006). Accordingly, an individual's actions are "triggered, executed and evaluated" in the environment (Little et al. 2006). From an action-control perspective, an agentic action is represented in each choice that is made by individuals to satisfy their goals.

Individuals interpret their actions and the outcomes that the actions obtained. In conjunction with the self-evaluation of actions, individuals seek to discover who they are and what capabilities they possess in order to reach success in the designated context. Agentic individuals actively set up new goals in novel contexts. Such goals are an expression of each individual's understanding of the means needed to achieve the goal and the degree to which they possess or can implement the means that can obtain the desired end state. Stated differently, people are agents in their own development, acting for their own needs and goals, interpreting and evaluating their actions and outcomes. Developmentally, the actions of individuals are contextualized – actions are catalyzed by the challenges in the given context. By acting out to resolve the challenges, individuals also impart some degree of change in their environment. This perspective suggests that persons are "active contributors" to their actions and their own development (Little et al. 2006). A person with these inherent tendencies regarding their actions can be described as demonstrating personal agency or an agentic self.

Self-Determination Theory provides a strong theoretical foundation that helps guide the individual in reaching their potential of becoming an agentic self. An agentic person is intrinsically motivated to be competent in mastering life-course challenges and self-determined in their interaction with the environment (Deci 1980, p. 27; Zuckerman et al. 1978). Individuals want to feel autonomous; that they are able to take responsibility for their actions and free to make decisions based on their choices. For instance, individuals may want to be competent in math. Their autonomy will be satisfied if they are able to make decisions based on what they desire to learn. In this way, their actions are determined by their own choices. Self-determined people ensure their actions and behaviors are all "self-caused" (Ryan and Deci 2002). From this perspective, self-determination is a function of an agentic action. In order to achieve a goal, all actions are executed to ultimately maintain or enhance people's sense of agency (Little et al. 2006). As Bandura (1997) states "agency refers to acts done intentionally" (p. 3). Individuals' progress along their own self-determined path, while continually updating their own sense of self, and give meaning to their actions (Little et al. 2002, 2006).

The greatest difference that can be seen with people who have a greater sense of personal agency is in their behaviors when they are presented with an unexpected or novel challenge. Agentic individuals are willing and able to try various and creative means to overcome a challenge. Individuals with a high sense of personal agency persist and problem-solve through challenges or obstacles. If they do not succeed, agentic individuals learn from their failures and adopt new approaches the next time they are presented with similar challenges. Non-agentic individuals on the other hand, feel helpless, often unable to develop any alternative solutions to the presented challenge. In the face of an obstacle or challenge, individuals who do not have a sense of personal agency will not persevere to accomplish the task at hand.

An Action-Theoretical Perspective on Perceived Control

The notion of perceived control over one's actions and outcomes is a central thought of numerous motivation theories (Schunk et al. 2008, p. 24), including self-determination theory, which assumes that a person has the freedom to make choices on their own. The concept of control from this viewpoint refers to a person's awareness of their power in controlling both the means to achieve an outcome as well as the outcome itself. One of the early perspectives on control was Rotter's locus of control, which focused on the generalized beliefs about the reasons that bring about successful or failed outcomes. People who attribute their success or failure to external influences, such as luck, fate or other environmental factors, see their actions as having little effect on the outcomes. Such a belief system inhibits people from engaging in a task and expending more effort, potentially leading them to blaming outside sources for their failure. On the other hand, people with an internal locus of control believe that outcome attainment is under their influence and take ownership for their actions. Most theories of perceived control introduce the central role of intrinsic motivation in driving people's behaviors. Actions and choices, however, may not always be self-determined. In many situations, actions are extrinsically determined as a function of the environmental context.

In addition to looking at the impetus of actions, Skinner and colleagues developed three different types of beliefs that have helped to formulate the construct structure surrounding an agentic perspective on volitional behavior (Skinner 1995; Skinner et al. 1988, 1990). Specifically, every action sequence comprises three constituents or components: (1) an agent or actor, (2) the means that help the agent obtain selected outcome, and (3) the end or goal that the agent is trying to achieve. Stemming from this conceptualization of personal agency, the action-control beliefs framework posits that across the life span, people develop and refine their beliefs surrounding these components that direct their actions (Chapman 1984; Little 1998; Skinner 1995). Unlike the other perceived control theories, Action-Control Theory focuses more on the sequential components of actions (agent -> means -> ends) during goal pursuit (Little et al. 2002, 2006; Little and Wanner 1997; Skinner et al. 1988). Here, volitional behavior is seen as an action sequence.

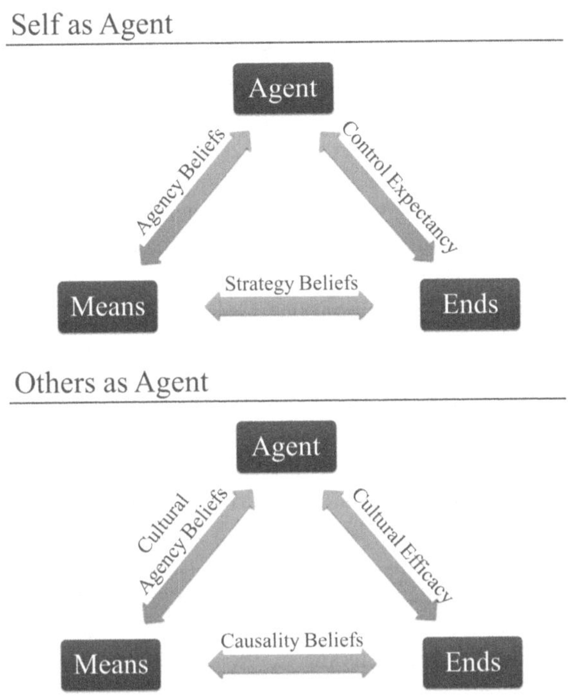

Fig. 22.1 The framework of action-control beliefs (From Little 1997)

The individual self which is termed as the "agent" functions as the central unit in the action-theory framework. A person's action-control beliefs are modulated and propelled by their sense of agency. By integrating a sense of personal agency and perceived control beliefs, the action-control beliefs can be seen as people's actions that are determined by their perceived global awareness on what the responsibilities are for certain outcomes, and their beliefs on whether they possess these means (Skinner et al. 1988). In other words, agentic actions reflect an individual's consciousness of their status in their environment, perceptions of the means to the end, and their beliefs about their ability to implement a self-chosen means in the actionable steps to pursue a goal (Champion and Skinner 1985; Cantor and Fleeson 1994). Agentic persons chose goals that are likely to satisfy perceived needs and define their actions in order to reach the goal. From this view, people's sense of agency provides the self-regulatory foundation for the actions (Little et al. 2002).

Action-control beliefs involve three general beliefs that reflect the relationship between the three components of an action sequence. Figure 22.1 portrays the three components and the belief types among these constituents of human actions, both for the self is agent and the others are the agent.

Control Expectancy Control expectancy refers to the relation between agent and ends, meaning that individual's expectancy about their capability to achieve a given goal or end. When the third-person as the agent (the generalized "other"), this control expectancy belief is a reflection of cultural efficacy, that refers to the tendency of others in one's cultural circle are capable of achieving the given goal. The difference in these two beliefs is the control expectancy of the self represents a personal judgment and expectation of the likelihood of goal attainment, whereas cultural efficacy represents a culturally generalized judgment about at typical group member's capacity to attain the goal. From this definition, control expectancy is similar as the concept of Bandura's outcome expectancy which is defined as "a person's estimate that a given behavior will lead to certain outcomes" (1997, p. 193). But control expectancy differs from outcome expectancy in two ways. First, instead of the expectation of success, control expectancy emphasizes the sense of agency and its perceived control (Skinner et al. 1988). From this view, the statements reflecting control expectancy should reflect people's expectancies on what outcomes they are able to produce; for example, a student's expectation on a math test can be "I can get 85 out of 100 in this math test". The second difference is that control expectancies of the outcome do not require the awareness of the means by which the goal can be achieved. For example, before a test, a student might have the expectancy to obtain the score of 85 without necessarily thinking about what they need to do in order to reach this outcome. In this sense, a student does not have to think about the specific means and whether he is able to access these means to achieve the goal.

Control expectancy reflects one's global desire about the expectancy of the outcome and is "a means-unspecified agency conception" of whether one can personally achieve the outcome (Little and Wanner 1997). Given this feature, control expectancy might is affected by personal desires and possibly wishful outcomes. For instance, young children tend to have higher expectancy due to their optimistic developmental stage; while the expectancy decreases as children get older (Heckhausen 1977, 1984; Little and Wanner 1997; Stipek 1984). The age differences in control expectancy may also reflect the effect of self-protective consciousness. Older children and adults tend to show lower expectancy in order to make the outcomes more desirable or avoid negative events (Abramson and Alloy 1980; Greenwald 1980; Harter 1982). The judgment of expectancy also appears to be influenced by the immediate environment (Little and Wanner 1997).

Means-Ends Beliefs Means-ends beliefs represent the relation between means and ends (see Fig. 22.1). As reflected in the action-control model, strategy beliefs of means-ends are defined as an individual's own global awareness of what resources or factors may produce the desired outcome. For the third-person in our model, means-ends beliefs are sometimes called causality beliefs which represent a person's general beliefs about causal factors for obtaining an outcome (Skinner et al. 1990; Skinner 1995). This type of belief reveal a general perception that if these strategies are accessible, then the goal can be reached. Means-ends beliefs reflect the global notion about the potentially effective strategies that allow individuals to reach their desired outcomes (Connell 1985; see also in Skinner et al. 1988; Oettingen et al. 1994). This type of general perception, however, is just personal naïve theories that are shaped through interactions in the sociocultural contexts (Little 1998; Little and Lopez 1997; Little and Wanner 1997; Skinner et al. 1988).

In school-age children, their perceptions about factors that may lead to success include effort, ability, luck, teachers' role and various other unidentified reasons. Students may hold a belief about their effort in the context of getting good grades; namely, it requires plenty of time to study such that "a good test score needs enough study time." The means-ends or strategy beliefs can be external forces that the student might think it is due to luck or some other unknown reasons, such as "there is no real reason that leads to the good test score." The various potential means can be further categorized into self-oriented (intra-self) and non-self-oriented (extra-self) causes (Little and Lopez 1997; Chapman and Skinner 1989). Effort and ability are the factors within the person that are a reflection of the self. Researchers (Graham 1991; Heckhausen 1984; Karoly 1993; Stetsenko et al. 1995) proposed that self-oriented awareness is derived from personal experiences and self-reflection on these experiences, combined with teachers' feedback and the learning environment created by adults. For example, teachers may underscore the importance of effort and ability in producing success. Meanwhile, luck, teachers and unknowns are outside the person which is non-self-oriented. Students' cognizance of these means emanates from the sociocultural influences such as how connected adults perceive outcomes and general notions reflected in a given sociocultural context.

Age difference can also be seen in children's means-ends beliefs. Skinner et al. (1988) found that all the middle-age children (i.e., 7–12 years old) perceived effort as the most effective factor leading to the desired outcomes. Children's perceived effectiveness of all the factors including both internal and external causes declined with increasing ages. These age change are culturally universal. Little and Lopez documented extensive cross-cultural similarities as well as some culture-specific differences in the age-related changes in children's means-ends beliefs.

Agency Beliefs Agency beliefs represent the link between agent and means (see Fig. 22.1), which refer to an individual's beliefs of what means they are capable of utilizing when the self acts as an agent. On the other hand, when others are fulfilling the agent role, the link between agent and means is termed cultural agency beliefs. Cultural agency beliefs appropriately refer to the common conception about agency for a defined sociocultural group.

Agency beliefs reflect the degree to which the individual believes that he or she possesses the means to an ends or can effectively manipulate the means toward achieved a desired ends. Individuals are not able to have agency beliefs of an unknown means because the not able to access to it. In other words, agency beliefs reflect an individual's awareness of his or her own capabilities to utilize a given means that is relevant for a given goal. For instance, a student's agency belief for effort is stated differently than the general means-ends beliefs: "When it comes this math test, I can put in enough effort to achieve a good grade." Thus, agency beliefs are very unique to learning and feedback history of the individual whereas means-ends beliefs are more a reflection of the sociocultural context. Because agency beliefs are the beliefs of personal beliefs about a specific means to achieve an outcome, they are very similar to self-efficacy beliefs, which refers to personal beliefs about one's capabilities to perform actions (Bandura 1977; Schunk 2012). Both of these beliefs focus on personal perceived sense of ability to access various means to reach the desired outcomes. Agency beliefs are specific to each potential means whereas self-efficacy is an unspecific amalgam across the various salient means for performing well and overlap, therefore, with control expectancy beliefs. Agency beliefs, on the other hand are clearly differentiated from control expectancy – agency beliefs are the perception of capability to perform certain behaviors that are the means to reach the desired outcome; whereas control expectancy are the judgments about the likelihood achieving an outcome without reference to personal ability or specific means.

Research has documented many ways that agency beliefs are different across the ages and gender. Findings in Skinner et al. (1988), for example, revealed that children in the middle school had high agency in their accessibility of internal causes, effort and ability. Interestingly, regarding the external causes, those children's agency beliefs on powerful others (the help from peers and teachers) increased with age, whereas beliefs about the influence of luck decreased. Stetsenko et al. (2000) identified a large gender bias in children's agency beliefs of ability across different sociocultural settings. Those school-age children from different countries held very similar views of what means generally produce the desired outcomes in schools (means-ends beliefs). Girls, however, reported lower beliefs in their ability in producing their school performance. Girls' agency beliefs about other means – effort, luck, and access to teachers were consistent with their school outcome and equal to boys. They found that girls from different sociocultural settings did assess themselves as being talented even though they achieved higher school grades than boys.

Conclusions

Action-Control Theory and the tripartite model of personal beliefs is a very effective model for dissecting and identifying deficiencies in how people perceive the causes of success and failure (means-ends beliefs) and whether or not the person believes they possess the means necessary to achieve an outcome. The profile of what it takes and whether one has it provides a precise and effective way to remedy maladaptive profiles of beliefs as well as structuring developmental contexts that enhance or promote adaptive action-control belief profiles. The precision in theoretical and operational definitions provided by the Action-Control Theory model offers researchers across many different contexts a high degree of comparability in the meaning and interpretation of similarities and differences. A less precise model mixes substantive differences with noisy operational differences that cannot be unconfounded. The Action-Control Theory model eliminates the imprecise operational and theoretical sources of mismeasurement that impact other similar models of perceived control.

References

Abramson, L. Y., & Alloy, L. B. (1980). Judgments of contingency: Errors and their implications. In A. Baum & J. Singer (Eds.), *Advances in environmental psychology* (Vol. 2, pp. 111–130). Hillsdale: Lawrence Erlbaum Associates Inc.

Baltes, P. B. (1987). Theoretical propositions of life-span developmental psychology: On the dynamics between growth and decline. *Developmental Psychology, 23*, 611–626.

Bandura, A. (1977). Self-efficacy: Toward a unifying theory of behavioral change. *Psychological Review, 84*, 191–215.

Bandura, A. (1997). *Self-efficacy: The exercise of control*. New York: Freeman.

Boesch, E. E. (1991). *Symbolic action theory and cultural psychology*. New York: Springer.

Brandtstädter, J. (1998). Action perspectives on human development. In W. Damon (Series Ed.) & R. M. Lerner (Vol. Ed.), *Theoretical models of human development: Vol. 1. Handbook of child psychology* (5th ed., pp. 807–863). New York: Wiley.

Cantor, N., & Fleeson, W. (1994). Social intelligence and intelligent goal pursuit: A cognitive slice of motivation. In W. Spaulding (Ed.), *Integrative views of motivation, cognition, and emotion* (pp. 125–179). Lincoln: University of Nebraska Press.

Champion, M., & Skinner, E. A. (1985). Action in development/development in action. In M. Frese & J. Sabini (Eds.), *The development of social cognition* (pp. 35–64). East Sussex: Psychology Press.

Chapman, M. (1984). International action as a paradigm for developmental psychology: A symposium. *Human Development, 27*(3–4), 113–144.

Chapman, M., & Skinner, E. A. (1989). Children's agency beliefs, cognitive performance and conceptions of effort and ability: Interaction of individual and developmental differences. *Child Development, 60*, 1229–1238.

Connell, J. P. (1985). A new multidimensional measure of children's perceptions of control. *Child Development, 56*, 1018–1041.

Darwin, C. (1859). *The origin of species*. London: John Murray.

Deci, E. L. (1980). *The psychology of self-determination*. Lexington: D. C. Heath (Lexington Books).

Deci, E. L., & Ryan, R. M. (1985). *Intrinsic motivation and self-determination in human behavior*. New York: Plenum.

Deci, E. L., & Ryan, R. M. (2000). The "what" and "why" of goal pursuit: Human needs and the self determination theory of behavior. *Psychology Inquiry, 11*, 227–268.

Graham, S. (1991). A review of attribution theory in achievement contexts. *Educational Psychology Review, 3*, 5–39.

Greenwald, A. G. (1980). The totalitarian ego: Fabrication and revision of personal history. *American Psychologist, 35*, 603–618.

Harter, S. (1982). The perceived competence scale for children. *Child Development, 53*, 87–97.

Hawley, P. H. (1999). The ontogenesis of social dominance: A strategy-based evolutionary perspective. *Developmental Review, 19*, 91–132.

Heckhausen, H. (1977). Achievement motivation and its constructs: A cognitive model. *Motivation and Emotion, 1*, 283–329.

Heckhausen, H. (1984). Emergent achievement behavior: Some early developments. In J. G. Nicholls (Ed.), *The development of achievement motivation* (pp. 1–32). Greenwich: JAI Press.

Heckhausen, J., Dixon, R. A., & Baltes, P. B. (1989). Gains and losses in development throughout adulthood as perceived by different adult age groups. *Developmental Psychology, 25*, 109–121.

Karoly, P. (1993). Mechanisms of self-regulation: A system view. *Annual Review of Psychology, 44*, 23–52.

Lindley, R. (1986). *Autonomy*. London: Macmillan.

Little, T. D. (1997). Mean and Covariance Structures (MACS) analyses of cross-cultural data: Practical and theoretical issues. *Multivariate Behavioral Research, 32*, 53–76.

Little, T. D. (1998). Sociocultural influences on the development of children's action-control beliefs. In J. Heckhausen & C. S. Dweck (Eds.), *Motivation and self-regulation across the life span* (pp. 281–315). New York: Cambridge University Press.

Little, T. D., & Lopez, D. F. (1997). Regularities in the development of children's causality beliefs about school performance across six sociocultural contexts. *Developmental Psychology, 33*, 165–175. doi:10.1037/0012-1649.33.1.165.

Little, T. D., & Wanner, B. (1997). *The Multi-CAM: A multidimensional instrument to assess children's action-control motives, beliefs, and behaviors* (Materialen aus der Bildungsforschung, Nr. 59, ISBN #3–87985-064-x). Berlin, Germany: Max-Planck Institute for Human Development and Education.

Little, T. D., Hawley, P. H., Henrich, C. C., & Marsland, K. W. (2002). Three views of the agentic self: A developmental synthesis. In E. L. Deci & R. M. Ryan (Eds.), *Handbook of self-determination research* (pp. 389–404). Rochester: University of Rochester Press.

Little, T. D., Snyder, C. R., & Wehmeyer, M. (2006). The agentic self: On the nature and origins of personal agency across the life span. In D. K. Mroczek & T. D. Little (Eds.), *Handbook of personality development* (pp. 61–79). Mahwah: LEA.

Malmberg, L.-E., Wanner, B., Nordmyr, A-M., & Little, T. D. (2004*). The teachers' control, agency, and means-ends (TCAM) questionnaire: Reliability and validity* (Monograph (No. 7) of the Faculty of Education, Abo Akademi University). Vasa: Multiprint Press.

Nurmi, J.-E. (2001). Adolescents' self-direction and self-definition in age-graded sociocultural and interpersonal contexts. In J.-E. Nurmi (Ed.), *Navigating through adolescence* (pp. 229–250). New York: Rutledge.

Oettingen, G., Little, T. D., Lindenberger, U., & Baltes, P. B. (1994). Causality, agency, and control beliefs in East versus West Berlin children: A natural experiment on the role of context. *Journal of Personality and Social Psychology, 66*, 579–595. doi:10.1037/0022-3514.66.3.579.

Reckless, R. E. (1979). *Ecology*. Portland: Chiron Press.

Ryan, R. M. (1993). Agency and organization: Intrinsic motivation, autonomy, and the self in psychological development. In J. E. Jacobs (Ed.), *Developmental perspectives on motivation, Nebraska Symposium on Motivation* (Vol. 40). Lincoln: University of Nebraska Press.

Ryan, R. M., & Deci, E. L. (2000). Self-determination theory and the facilitation of intrinsic motivation, social development and well-being. *American Psychologist, 55*, 68–78.

Ryan, R. M., & Deci, E. L. (2002). An overview of self-determination theory. In E. L. Deci & R. M. Ryan (Eds.), *Handbook of self-determination research* (pp. 3–33). Rochester: University of Rochester Press.

Schunk, D. H. (2012). *Learning theories: An educational perspective* (6th ed.). Boston: Pearson Education.

Schunk, D. H., Pintrich, P. R., & Meece, J. L. (2008). *Motivation in education* (3rd ed.). Upper Saddle River: Pearson Merrill Prentice Hall.

Skinner, E. A. (1995). *Perceived control, motivation, and coping*. Thousand Oaks: Sage.

Skinner, E. A., Chapman, M., & Baltes, P. B. (1988). Children's beliefs about control, means-ends and agency: Developmental differences during middle childhood. *International Journal of Behavioral Development, 11*, 368–388.

Skinner, E. A., Wellborn, J. G., & Connell, J. P. (1990). What it takes to do well in school and whether I've got it: The role of perceived control in children's engagement and school achievement. *Journal of Educational Psychology, 82*, 22–32.

Stetsenko, A., Little, T. D., Oettingen, G., & Baltes, P. B. (1995). Agency, control, and means€nds beliefs about school performance in Moscow children: How similar are they to beliefs of Western children? *Developmental Psychology, 31*, 285–299.

Stetsenko, A., Little, T. D., Gordeeva, T., Grasshof, M., & Oettingen, G. (2000). Gender effects in children's beliefs about school performance: A cross-cultural study. *Child Development, 71*, 517–527. doi:10.1111/1467-8624.00161.

Stipek, D. (1984). Young children's performance expectations: Logical analysis or wishful thinking? In J. Nicholls (Ed.), *The development of achievement motivation* (pp. 33–56). Greenwich: JAI Press.

Weiner, B. (1986). *An attributional theory of motivation and emotion*. New York: Springer.

White, R. W. (1959). Motivation reconsidered: The concept of competence. *Psychological Review, 66*, 297–333.

Zuckerman, M., Porac, J. F., Lathin, D., Smith, R., & Deci, E. L. (1978). On the importance of self-determination for intrinsically motivated behavior. *Personality and Social Psychology Bulletin, 4*, 443–446.

Conclusion

As noted in the Introduction to this text, the self-determination construct is one of the foundational constructs in the discipline of positive psychology. This text had two primary purposes: first, to provide a frame for understanding the development of self-determination and, second and relatedly, to align research in motivation on SDT with research on causal action derived from Causal Agency Theory. Self-determination in both theories has been situated within theories of human agency. Human agentic theories share meta-theoretical assumptions that organismic aspirations drive human behavior, where such aspirations can be understood as the drive to be active contributors to, or agents of, one's behavior. Human agentic theories assume that actions are volitional and that an agentic person uses self-regulated and goal-directed agentic actions to set an attain goals that are motivated by autonomous motivation and propelled by volitional and agentic action and action-control beliefs. Such actions enable one to be the causal agent in one's life. Repeated experiences of causal agency lead to enhanced self-determination. Self-determination, as a psychological construct, refers to self- (vs. other-) caused action—to people acting volitionally, based on their own will.

So, why detail a theoretical frame for the development of self-determination that aligns SDT and Causal Agency Theory? To date, SDT has contributed significantly to understandings of contexts and actions that support and animate intrinsic and autonomous motivation. Causal Agency Theory has contributed to understandings of autonomy-supportive interventions that enable individuals to engage in causal action and become causal agents in their lives. A description of the motivational and psychological elements that contribute to the fulfillment of basic psychological needs and the knowledge, skills, and beliefs that enable one to act as causal agents in one's life has both heuristic and practical value. Understanding the factors that result in enhanced self-determination and that mediate and moderate the development of self-determination will enable practitioners and others to create contexts that are autonomy-supportive; understanding the linkages between motivation and causal action will provide a means to maximize opportunities to enhance and promote self-determination; and understanding the sequence in causal action can lead

M.L. Wehmeyer et al. (eds.), *Development of Self-Determination Through the Life-Course*, DOI 10.1007/978-94-024-1042-6

to the development and evaluation of interventions that both enable causal agency and the fulfillment of basic psychological needs.

And, then, where to from here? Obviously, research is needed to examine and evaluate the proposed linkages between constructs associated with the development of self-determination as well as on development within individual constructs (e.g., problem solving, decision making, goal setting, self-initiation, etc.). Understanding the links between causal action and basic psychological need fulfillment and autonomous motivation is important as well. Broadly, the role of the development of self-determination in the context of adolescent psychological development is a critical area of research need. How does the development of self-determination contribute to identify formation, autonomous functioning, self-regulation processes, and emotional or cognitive development?

Finally, a developmental approach may enable researchers to better understand important contextual and cultural aspects of the development of self-determination and enable practitioners to implement and design practices that are culturally relevant and responsive.

Index

M.L. Wehmeyer et al. (eds.), *Development of Self-Determination Through the Life-Course*, DOI 10.1007/978-94-024-1042-6

The manufacturer's authorised representative in the EU is Springer Nature Customer Service Centre GmbH, Europaplatz 3, 69115 Heidelberg, Germany. If you have any concerns regarding our products, please contact ProductSafety@springernature.com

Printed and bound by CPI Group (UK) Ltd, Croydon, CR0 4YY
22/09/2026
02221058-0014